Evidence-Based Herbal Medicine

Michael Rotblatt, MD, PharmD

Assistant Clinical Professor
Department of Medicine
University of California School of Medicine
Los Angeles
    and
Primary Care Internist
Veterans' Administration
Greater Los Angeles Healthcare System
Sepulveda Ambulatory Care Center
North Hills, California

Irwin Ziment, MD, FRCP

Professor and Vice Chairman
Department of Medicine
University of California School of Medicine
Los Angeles
    and
Chief of Medicine and Chief of Division of Pulmonary
    and Critical Care Medicine
Olive View–UCLA Medical Center
Sylmar, California

Hanley & Belfus, Inc. / Philadelphia

Publisher: HANLEY & BELFUS, INC.
                    Medical Publishers
                    210 South 13th Street
                    Philadelphia, PA 19107
                    (215) 546-7293; 800-962-1892
                    FAX (215) 790-9330
                    Web site: http://www.hanleyandbelfus.com

Note to the reader: Although the information in this book has been carefully reviewed for correctness of dosage and indications, neither the authors nor the editors nor the publisher can accept any legal responsibility for any errors or omissions that may be made. Neither the publisher nor the editors make any warranty, expressed or implied, with respect to the material contained herein. Before prescribing any drug, the reader must review the manufacturer's current product information (package inserts) for accepted indications, absolute dosage recommendations, and other information pertinent to the safe and effective use of the product described.

Library of Congress Cataloging-in-Publication Data

Evidence-based herbal medicine / edited by Michael Rotblatt, Irwin Ziment.
    p. ; cm.
  Includes index.
  ISBN 1-56053-447-8 (alk. paper)
    1. Herbs—Therapeutic use—Handbooks, manuals, etc. 2. Evidence-based medicine—Handbooks, manuals, etc. I. Rotblatt, Michael, 1954–
II. Ziment, Irwin.
  [DNLM: 1. Medicine, Herbal. 2. Alternative Medicine. 3. Evidence-Based Medicine.
  WB 925 E935 2001]
  RM666.H33 E95 2002
  615'.321—dc21

                                                    2001039725

Evidence-Based Herbal Medicine   ISBN 1-56053-447-8

Last digit is the print number: 9   8   7   6   5   4   3   2   1

Table of Contents

Acknowledgments

We wish to thank our respective wives, Mia and Yda, for their help, encouragement, and patience, and for sharing with us their sensitive appreciation of the values of herbal and other alternative therapies. The office skills of Gus Chavez and Sylvia Anguiano were of tremendous help, as was the assistance of library technicians Suzanne Hill and Shirley Oles, which went far beyond the call of duty. We are thankful for our exceptional editor, Jacqueline Mahon, who from the beginning encouraged us and saw the value of a book of this kind for the medical establishment. We are grateful to our colleagues who prepared much of the basic work on many of the herbal summaries contained herein; this book could not have been as comprehensive without their contributions. Finally, this book is built on the foundation of many exceptional clinical investigators and authoritative writers who have contributed to the scientific literature on herbal therapeutics, whose work we reference throughout this book. We are grateful for all that they have done—this book would not exist without them.

~ M.R., I.Z.

Contributors

Claudine Armand, MD
Fellow, Women's Health, Department of Medicine, Veterans' Administration, Greater Los Angeles Healthcare System, Sepulveda Ambulatory Care Center, North Hills, California
Chapter contribution: papaya

Mitra Assemi, PharmD
Assistant Clinical Professor, Department of Clinical Pharmacy, University of California, San Francisco; Acting Director, UCSF-Fresno School of Pharmacy Programs, San Francisco, California
Chapter contribution: pygeum

Janet Au, MD, PharmD
Clinical Professor, Department of Internal Medicine, University of California School of Medicine, Los Angeles; Pulmonologist, Division of Pulmonary and Critical Care Medicine, Olive View-UCLA Medical Center, Sylmar, CA
Chapter contribution: astragalus

Cynthia D. Caffrey, MD
Associate Physician, Department of Internal Medicine, Kaiser Permanente, Lancaster, California
Chapter contribution: pokeroot

Mina Charon, MD
Physician, Department of Internal Medicine, Indian Health Service, Chinle Hospital, Chinle, Arizona
Chapter contribution: yucca

Michael D. Cirigliano, MD, FACP
Assistant Professor, Department of Medicine, University of Pennsylvania School of Medicine, Philadelphia, Pennsylvania
Chapter contribution: chamomile

Kevin A. Clauson, PharmD
Fellow, Natural Product Research, and Adjunct Faculty Member, Division of Pharmacy Practice, University of Missouri, Kansas City, Missouri
Chapter contributions: gotu kola, PC-SPES

Cathi Dennehy, PharmD
Assistant Clinical Professor, Department of Clinical Pharmacy, University of California School of Pharmacy, San Francisco, California
Chapter contribution: hawthorn, milk thistle

Daniel Garcia, MD
Associate Clinical Professor, Department of Medicine, University of California School of Medicine, Los Angeles; Primary Care Internist, Veterans' Administration, Greater Los Angeles Healthcare System, Sepulveda Ambulatory Care Center, North Hills, California
Chapter contribution: aloe vera

Arthur Gomez, MD
Associate Clinical Professor, Department of Medicine, University of California School of Medicine, Los Angeles; Associate Program Director, UCLA-San Fernando Valley Internal Medicine Residency Program; Primary Care Internist, Veterans' Administration, Sepulveda Ambulatory Care Center, North Hills, CA
Chapter contribution: cat's claw

Juan Jaime Guzman, MD
Internist, Private Practice, Dana Point, California
Chapter contribution: horse chestnut seed

John Han, PharmD
Clinical Pharmacist, Department of Pharmacy, Harbor-UCLA Medical Center, Torrance, California
Chapter contribution: American ginseng

Mary L. Hardy, MD
Medical Director, Integrative Medicine Program, Division of General Internal Medicine, Cedars-Sinai Medical Center, Los Angeles; Assistant Clinical Professor, Department of Medicine, University of Southern California, Los Angeles, California
Chapter contribution: Herb-Drug Interactions (Reports in Humans)

Helen Mingfen Hsiao, MD
Rheumatologist, Department of Rheumatology, Kaiser-Permanente, Woodland Hills, California
Chapter contribution: Siberian ginseng

Maga Jackson-Triche, MD, MSHS
Associate Clinical Professor, Department of Psychiatry, University of California School of Medicine, Los Angeles; Director, Consultation Liaison Service, UCLA-San Fernando Valley Psychiatry Training Program; Veterans' Administration, Sepulveda Ambulatory Care Center, North Hills, California
Chapter contribution: St. John's wort

Charles I. Hong Lu, MD
Fellow, Nephrology, UCLA-San Fernando Valley Nephrology Training Program, Olive View-UCLA Medical Center, Sylmar, California
Chapter contribution: Asian ginseng

Glenn E. Mathisen, MD
Clinical Professor, Department of Medicine, University of California School of Medicine, Los Angeles; Chief, Division of Infectious Diseases, Olive View-UCLA Medical Center, Sylmar, California
Chapter contribution: wormwood

Cydney E. McQueen, PharmD
Assistant Clinical Professor, School of Pharmacy, and Assistant Director, Drug Information Center, University of Missouri, Kansas City, Missouri
Chapter contributions: glucosamine, chondroitin, PC-SPES, tea tree oil

Giulia Michelini, MD
Associate Clinical Professor, Department of Medicine, University of California School of Medicine, Los Angeles; Primary Care Internist, Veterans' Administration, Greater Los Angeles Healthcare System, Sepulveda Ambulatory Care Center, North Hills, California
Chapter contribution: ginkgo

Elsa J. Brochmann Murray, PhD
Associate Research Professor, Department of Medicine, University of California School of Medicine, Los Angeles; Research Chemist, Geriatric Research, Education and Clinical Center, Veterans' Administration, Greater Los Angeles Healthcare System, Sepulveda Ambulatory Care Center, North Hills, California
Chapter contribution: bilberry

Samuel S. Murray, MD
Associate Professor, Department of Medicine, University of California School of Medicine, Los Angeles; Staff Physician, Geriatric Research, Education and Clinical Center, Veterans'

Administration, Greater Los Angeles Healthcare System, Sepulveda Ambulatory Care Center, North Hills, California
Chapter contribution: bilberry

Phuong-Chi T. Pham, MD
Assistant Clinical Professor, Department of Medicine, Division of Nephrology, University of California School of Medicine, Los Angeles; Nephrologist, Olive View-UCLA Medical Center, Sylmar, California
Chapter contribution: nettle

Phuong-Thu T. Pham, MD
Clinical Instructor, Department of Medicine, Division of Nephrology, University of California School of Medicine, Los Angeles, California
Chapter contribution: nettle

Sheree R. Poítier, MD
Associate Clinical Professor, Department of Medicine, Division of Infectious Diseases, University of California School of Medicine, Los Angeles; Clinical Consultant, Olive View-UCLA Medical Center, Sylmar, California
Chapter contribution: feverfew

Victoria Rand, MD
Assistant Clinical Professor, Department of Medicine, Division of General Internal Medicine, University of California, San Francisco; Urgent Care Internist and Primary Care Teacher, Moffitt Hospital Ambulatory Care Center, San Francisco, California
Chapter contribution: evening primrose

Mark J. Rosenthal, MD
Associate Professor, Department of Medicine, University of California School of Medicine, Los Angeles; Internist and Geriatrician, Geriatric Research, Education and Clinical Center, Veterans' Administration, Greater Los Angeles Health Care System, Sepulveda Ambulatory Care Center, North Hills, California
Chapter contributions: yarrow, yohimbe

Michael Rotblatt, MD, PharmD
Assistant Clinical Professor, Department of Medicine, University of California School of Medicine, Los Angeles; Primary Care Internist, Veterans' Administration, Greater Los Angeles Healthcare System, Sepulveda Ambulatory Care Center, North Hills, California

Mina L. Ryu, MD
Staff Internist, Cedars-Sinai Medical Group, Beverly Hills, California
Chapter contribution: devil's claw

Candy Tsourounis, PharmD
Assistant Clinical Professor, Department of Clinical Pharmacy, University of California School of Pharmacy, San Francisco; Acting Director, Drug Information Analysis Service, San Francisco, California
Chapter contributions: Co-enzyme Q10, melatonin, MSM, SAMe

Swamy Venuturupalli, MD
Fellow, Health Services Research and Clinical Rheumatology, Department of Medicine, Division of Rheumatology, University of California School of Medicine, Los Angeles; Veterans' Administration, Sepulveda Ambulatory Care Center, North Hills, California
Chapter contribution: fenugreek

Irwin Ziment, MD, FRCP
Professor and Vice Chairman, Department of Medicine, University of California School of Medicine, Los Angeles; Chief of Medicine and Chief of Division of Pulmonary and Critical Care Medicine, Olive View-UCLA Medical Center, Sylmar, California

Foreword

A New Era in Herbal Medicine

I have written and said it so often that I hesitate to state it again: evidence-based herbal medicine must not, and will not, remain a contradiction in terms. Why do I believe this to be true?

The facts show the impressive degree of acceptance of herbal medicinal products (HMPs), and this reality renders rigorous research into the safety and efficacy of HMPs an ethical, legal, and scientific imperative. The public is often misled into believing that anything natural must also be safe. Clearly this is an illusion that is naive at best and dangerous at worse. The public is also often misled into believing that herbs that have been used medicinally for millennia must be efficacious. This too is an illusion. This does not, however, amount to saying that traditional use and experience is of no value at all. On the contrary, they are essential for generating hypotheses. If we want to test these hypotheses, we require tools of evidence-based medicine, such as randomized clinical trials and systematic reviews.

This book by Drs. Rotblatt and Ziment has adopted such an evidence-based approach. Thus, it is far ahead of most books on this topic, since even respected texts are not evidence-based and therefore mislead their readers. This is a laudable, well-researched text that has the potential to fill the information gap that currently exists. I believe that we are at the beginning of a new era of herbal medicine, with an evidence-based approach at last taking hold of this area of health care. The most important question must be whether a given remedy does more good than harm to suffering patients, and only the evidence-based approach will find conclusive answers.

This book makes an important contribution to modern medical herbalism. It adopts the clinician's perspective, authoritatively guides the reader through the complex and, at times, contradictory lines of evidence, and attempts to provide sound recommendations for clinical practice. In other words, it is excellently suited for the new era of evidence-based herbalism, and it complements the efforts that myself and others have made to bring rationality to this important component of current health care.

EDZARD ERNST, MD, PHD, FRCP
DEPARTMENT OF COMPLEMENTARY MEDICINE
SCHOOL OF SPORT AND HEALTH SCIENCES
UNIVERSITY OF EXETER, ENGLAND

Preface

Physicians and other healthcare practitioners are feeling the pressure to inform themselves about herbal medicines. They are barraged with data about herbal medicines from their patients, the media, and the internet, but this information is often confusing because it is based on incomplete or biased knowledge. Many clinicians are therefore uncertain whether to encourage, discourage, or simply accept their patients' use of these traditional remedies, which are mostly unproven and controversial. Although new studies on herbs and their uses are increasingly being conducted and published, there are few high-quality resources that objectively review the burgeoning information.

Most of the herbal therapies in use around the world were not developed based on the findings of controlled clinical studies or modern scientific investigations. The persistence of herbs in phytomedicinal practice results from an amalgam of long-held traditional beliefs and the wide-ranging knowledge of dedicated empirical practitioners. We acknowledge the potential value of the plants used in many traditional systems of herbal medicine; however, we feel that it is now essential to address the information on the therapeutic effects of herbs with a more critical, scientific, and evidence-based approach.

In this book, we have taken care to analyze the large and often controversial primary literature on controlled clinical trials and toxicities, and to provide reliable and practical clinical information on the uses, pharmacology, efficacy, and adverse effects of a selection of the most popular medicinal herbs. This book is written to enable health practitioners to offer more confident answers to their patients' questions about self-selected herbal remedies. It also should help clinicians select a rational herbal formulary that could confidently be incorporated into their medical practice.

We have approached this book with several concepts in mind. The evaluations encompass about 65 herbal medicines (including a few non-herbal dietary supplements), most of which are well known. We chose to include a few herbs of historical interest that have become less acceptable because of their toxicity or lack of effectiveness, although they are still available in today's herbal marketplace. For each herb, an extensive literature search was conducted (including Medline, the Cochrane Collaboration, and evaluations of bibliographies of major herbal texts and relevant published articles), and the available evidence was analyzed and assessed using our judgment as practicing physicians. When a prior high-quality analysis or systematic review was available in the medical literature, we quoted those findings that we found to be appropriate.

We wish to acknowledge that we have derived valuable insights from the work of Professor Edzard Ernst of the University of Exeter in England. The many careful analyses of herbs that have been published by his group are outstanding contributions, and they constitute a standard for systematically evaluating the evidence in many fields of complementary health care. In evaluating each herb for this book we have given it a benefit and safety rating that is strictly based on the quality of published evidence that we obtained from the accessible clinical literature. We recognize that our analyses of some of the less-studied herbs may therefore give an inappropriately unfavorable impression of their effectiveness. At times we are in conflict with the favorable recommendations published by authorities on herbalism, as well as the less critical information provided in the lay press.

Our evaluations have dealt primarily with Western herbs, but we have also reviewed the evidence and provided monographs on a limited number of other commonly used herbs. Several chapters summarize the use of traditional Chinese, Indian (Ayurvedic), and Mexican herbal medications. The evidence for most of these agents is frustratingly inadequate, but such herbs are widely advertised and sold directly to consumers, and we recognize the need to familiarize health professionals with their use. Thousands of herbal remedies continue to be employed by peoples from every culture; the vast numbers of herbs and their wide variety of traditional uses have precluded our attempt at a comprehensive listing.

In separate chapters, we discuss herbal quality assurance, herbal dosage forms, herb-drug interactions, and the chemistry of herbal medicines. These discussions are designed to give clinicians a basic understanding of many of the important issues and some of the controversies that are characteristic of herbal medicine. In the appendices, recommended herbal medicine information resources are listed. Other selected herbs that are available in North America are also tabulated, although the majority of these agents have not been subjected to adequate clinical studies.

A major concern about herbs is that some are proving to be less harmless than formerly believed. A growing literature, often of single case reports, provides evidence of harmful properties and raises the possibility that many effective herbal medicines can be toxic to certain individuals or can interact unexpectedly with pharmaceutical drugs. Many published lists of side effects and interactions are of dubious or unknown significance. Therefore, we chose to focus on those adverse or toxic effects for which there is reasonable clinical evidence. Many active pharmaceutical drugs are also plant-based medicines, and we strongly caution all prescribers and users of herbs to recognize that any effective remedy that has pharmacologic effects (whether it is called an "herb" or a "drug"), may also be capable of causing an adverse outcome.

Many leading writers and practitioners of Complementary and Alternative Medicine, as well as some practitioners of integrative medicine, consider herbal therapies to be qualitatively unlike orthodox medicines. The two may have different types of pharmacologic effects—for example, herbs are considered to be effective adaptogens, tonics, or immune modulators, or are used for detoxification and purification, thereby helping the body heal itself. The implication is that the art and science of herbal therapeutics should be viewed from a different platform than that which is the basis for understanding Western allopathic medicine. We have not reviewed or discussed the many nonscientific herbalist properties or philosophies in this book. However, we acknowledge and are in sympathy with the concept that individualized healing can be accomplished through a personal relationship with a sensitive practitioner offering a harmless token of healing, and we discuss the significance, benefits, and legitimacy of the therapeutic power of the placebo effect in several chapters in the latter section of this book.

After careful analysis of the literature, the authors are satisfied that a limited number of herbs have effective and beneficial medical properties, while most others must be considered to be of uncertain or dubious value. Nevertheless, we understand that experienced and sensitive clinicians acknowledge the usefulness of numerous herbs for many patients either as a potential therapy that has not been adequately proven, or simply as a valued placebo. We accept that it can be appropriate to advocate or at least to condone the use of herbal medicines that are apparently harmless, even if their value is not established.

A current book on herbal medicine would be deficient if certain ethical issues in today's marketplace were not addressed. The tendency for claims of efficacy to be based on inadequate data creates an additional responsibility for physicians and other professionals to protect the public. Consumers and patients are confronted with numerous herbal preparations that are promoted with exaggerated or inaccurate claims by ill-informed or exploitative merchandisers. We share the concerns of those ethical herbalists who condemn marketers that employ pseudo-science to create misleading advertising, and this concern is particularly directed at potentially harmful products.

This misuse of herbs is extremely disturbing when it is targeted at desperate patients with serious illnesses who may be led to the incorrect belief that herbs should replace effective orthodox medical care. The deficit of high-quality science and the relative absence of governmental regulations in herbal medicine are accompanied by an excess of commercial exploitation. It is therefore important for the herbal industry to police itself and to try and eliminate fraudulent or unacceptable marketing. Fortunately, most marketing keeps to the middle ground, in which a large number of relatively harmless and potentially beneficial herbs are promoted for appropriate indications. It is evident that there is an urgent need for organized, controlled studies to be carried out on the more promising herbs, and physicians should participate in such investigations using the same careful criteria for examining phytomedicines as are used in evaluating orthodox medications.

In the preparation of this book, many judgments have been required, and our own experiences and biases have determined selections and exclusions. Readers may dispute our decisions and arbitrary choices, or disagree with our assessments; careful reviewers will undoubtedly find factual or technical errors in our data. In assembling this book, we called upon our colleagues who have interest in specific herbs and supplements, but we, in the dual role of author/editor, worked jointly to review, discuss, and extensively edit every contribution, and therefore we take full responsibility for the final printed version. We welcome criticisms and corrections, since these will enable us to provide more accurate and better-informed education in the future.

The scientific field of herbal medicine is rapidly evolving as new information is revealed and clinical trials are conducted. We hope that this book will effectively meet the needs of interested health practitioners who are searching for a source of reputable herbal information. Evidence-based herbal medicine should constitute a basis for encouraging orthodox medical professionals, herbalists, and marketers to work together to raise the standards of herbal therapeutics, and thereby enable selected herbs to become part of standard medical practice.

MICHAEL ROTBLATT, MD, PHARMD
IRWIN ZIMENT, MD, FRCP

I: Introduction to Herbal Medicine

Evidence-Based Herbal Medicine

Much of the medical and popular literature on herbal medicines is difficult to interpret. Quasi-scientific studies, folklore, exaggerations, and imaginative claims continue to be promoted in preference to (or in the absence of) high-quality clinical trials in support of claims about the efficacy or safety of a variety of herbal medicines. In general, conclusions that a particular herbal medicine is useful or useless, safe or toxic, are based on suboptimal evaluations of the available data. Many herbal medicines have little or no reliable clinical data to back up their claims, and indications are based on traditional uses.

Scientific professionals should keep an open mind and accept that although a substance may lack evidence of efficacy, this does not mean that it is ineffective, or that it cannot be useful in any clinician-patient interaction. There are a variety of reasons why many potentially beneficial herbal therapies have not been adequately evaluated, including lack of funding, inability to obtain patent protection (true for all crude herbs), or lack of research interest. Lack of *evidence* of effect is not the same as lack of effect. As discussed in several chapters in this book, an unproven herb or drug can nevertheless be beneficial for many patients and for many disorders. However, tradition, experience, enthusiasm, and anecdotes can be misleading when accepted and applied without sufficient critical examination.

An evidence-based approach to the herbal literature is needed to enable professional health providers to place therapeutic claims in an appropriate clinical perspective. Health advisors must incorporate reliable information from clinical research into their medical decision-making, rather than rely solely on the nonscientific findings of poorly controlled clinical experience, inadequate animal or *in vitro* studies, anecdotal unsubstantiated reports, and advertising by marketers. Although the overall evidence for many herbal medicines is often markedly deficient or of unacceptably poor quality, the efficacy and safety of an increasing number of potentially useful herbal products have been evaluated in well-designed clinical studies, including randomized controlled trials (RCTs).

Problems With the Herbal Literature

Qualified investigators in many Western countries outside the U.S., primarily in Europe, have been scientifically evaluating herbal preparations for decades. From 1980 to 1988, over 300 clinical trials were carried out with standardized phytopharmaceuticals in Germany alone (where the traditional art of herbal medicine has evolved into a modern science).[1] Because most of these studies have been published in foreign journals, and some articles are not in English, it has been difficult for American practitioners to access and evaluate them. In addition, much of the literature on herbal and other "complementary" therapies can be criticized for being based on suboptimal study methodology and questionable reliability of outcome measures. Moreover, many herbal studies are published in nonclinical or nonpeer-reviewed journals and are characterized by a lack of scientific standards, which is a common problem with the material in many of these potentially biased publications. These criticisms are particularly applicable to earlier investigations (especially prior to the early 1990s) and to studies from Asian or Eastern European countries.[2–4]

The organization and size of herbal clinical trials have rarely been given adequate statistical attention, leaving doubt as to the power of a study for reliable detection of important differences in clinical outcomes. Only in the last few years has this analytical approach been considered, and it is now evident in increasing numbers of studies of herbal medicines.

Clinical studies of herbs have a unique set of problems, particularly when evaluating heterogeneous or nonstandardized preparations. There are few herbal "generic equivalents"; each product or formulation is unique and may differ considerably from apparently equivalent products. Additionally, a given manufacturer's product may not maintain uniformity over time (see chapter "Quality Assurance and Choosing a Brand or Product"). Furthermore, suggested herbal doses are often based on original empirical observations that may date back several centuries; relatively few dose-response studies of herbs have been carried out. There is also major difficulty in double-blinding studies using crude substances with particular odors or tastes.[4] Other more subtle or unknown biases may also affect outcomes. For example, many European studies are not only sponsored by, but appear to be conducted by, the manufacturer of the herbal product without any external monitoring. It is difficult to rely on even the most scientific-appearing trial or study that is conducted under such circumstances.

Searching and Evaluating the Herbal Literature

High-quality, critical, systematic reviews and meta-analyses of the available herbal literature are now being conducted, to evaluate foreign articles that are difficult to locate, as well as to judge the appropriateness of the clinical trials. Such reviews reduce the effect of biased investigations as much as possible, and are published by well-established, peer-reviewed medical journals that employ high standards to assure quality.

The Department of Complementary Medicine at the University of Exeter in England, under the leadership of Professor Edzard Ernst, has published a pioneering series of systematic reviews and meta-analyses in a range of different journals. The reviewers carefully analyze controlled clinical trials on herbal and other complementary therapies. They search multiple databases of the worldwide literature; invite experts and manufacturers to contribute unpublished material; and translate studies from other languages into English. The Exeter group uses standard objective criteria to assess methodologic quality and potential biases of each study. Their herbal systematic reviews include evaluations of popular agents such as aloe vera, feverfew, garlic, ginger, ginkgo biloba, ginseng, kava, St. John's wort, valerian, and yohimbine, and they have written reviews categorizing information on adverse effects and interactions with drugs.

American researchers and international medical organizations, such as the U.S. Agency for Healthcare Research and Quality and the Cochrane Collaboration,[5] have also published a number of rigorous, systematic reviews of the clinical herbal literature, which emphasize the results of high-quality clinical trials. These reviews, as well as the primary literature, can generally be found using Medline, the Cochrane Library, or other key resources.[6,7] Many articles on herbal therapy published in foreign journals are not indexed in Medline, however, and must be searched for in other, less familiar, bibliographic databases (e.g., EMBASE, AMED). They can also be located in increasingly available tertiary herbal information sources, some of which offer summaries or critiques of articles originally written in other languages (see appendix "Resources for Herbal Medicine Information"). All of these sources, including the published systematic reviews, were examined to produce this book.

Current U.S. Research

While few large herbal medicine studies have been conducted in the United States due to a lack of financial incentives, this trend is beginning to change. At the National Institutes of Health (NIH), the budget for the National Center for Complementary and Alternative Medicine (NCCAM) has increased dramatically over the last several years ($89.1 million for FY 2001). The NCCAM is funding large multi-institutional RCTs of herbal medicines, including St. John's wort, ginkgo, echinacea, and saw palmetto, as well as other alternative therapies.[8] The NIH's Office of Dietary Supplements is also helping to fund botanical research centers at academic institutions throughout the U.S.[9] Some of the herbs to be evaluated include soy, red clover, black cohosh, ginger, turmeric, boswellia, grape polyphenols, and green tea. In addition, herbal medicine manufacturers are starting to fund well-designed RCTs by experienced American clinical investigators. High-quality, controlled clinical trials are now being published at an increasing rate, and these studies will add considerably to the growing database of evidence-based herbal information.

Conclusion

Although there may be numerous shortcomings in the existing herbal database, evidence-based medicine takes the best available evidence to make clinical decisions. The evidence obtained from high-quality RCTs (as emphasized in the herbal summaries in this book) should remain the gold standard for herbal medicines;

this is certainly the case for conventional drug therapies. Systematic reviews, meta-analyses, and high-quality clinical research are currently helping to bring this information and appropriate conclusions to the attention of health professionals.

references

1. Wagner H. Phytomedicine research in Germany. Environ Health Perspect 107:779–781, 1999.
2. Vickers A, Goyal N, Harland R, Rees R. Do certain countries produce only positive results? A systematic review of controlled trials. Control Clin Trials 19:159–166, 1998.
3. Tang J-L, Zhan S-Y, Ernst E. Review of randomised controlled trials of traditional Chinese medicine. BMJ 319:160–161, 1999.
4. Mahady GB. Botanicals: the complexities associated with assessing the clinical literature on efficacy. P&T 25:127–132, 2000.
5. Ezzo J, Berman BM, Vickers AJ, Linde K. Complementary medicine and the Cochrane collaboration. JAMA 280:1628–1630, 1998.
6. Glanville J, Lefebvre C. Identifying systematic reviews: Key resources. ACP J Club 132(May/June):A11–12, 2000.
7. Haynes B, Glasziou P, Straus S. Advances in evidence-based information resources for clinical practice. ACP J Club 132(1):A11–14, 2000.
8. National Center for Complementary and Alternative Medicine. Accessed March 9, 2001 at http://nccam.nih.gov/nccam/research/grants/rfb/index/html
9. Office of Dietary Supplements. Accessed March 9, 2001 at http://ods.nih.gov/grants/grants/html

Herbal Practices in the U.S.

Herbal products are increasingly available in most industrialized countries of the world, as part of a resurging belief in natural and traditional remedies. This unexpected phenomenon has occurred, in part, as a reaction to the expense and personal frustration that patients sometimes encounter during interactions with orthodox medical services, and also as a result of the explosion of information and products made available on the internet and by creative marketers. Additionally, many people find ancient, traditional herbal remedies to be appealing and comforting. Others, who recognize that nonscientific philosophies and magical thinking are inherent components of historical herbal traditions, prefer the emerging scientifically-oriented, modern herbal pharmacotherapy, which was unknown to our ancestors.

A variety of herbs is increasingly available at health food stores, in supermarkets and pharmacies, at farmers' markets, and from religious, ethnic and other special outlets, mail-order houses, and internet advertisers. There is a wide choice of herbal medicine practices available to anyone who wishes to explore the range of ancient and modern options (see table).

European Origins of Herbal Medicine

Conventional U.S. and European herbal practices are based on ancient Greek-Roman experiences, particularly the writings of the herbalist Pedanius Dioscorides (dating back to about 60 A.D.) and the physician Claudius Galen (138–201 A.D.), who used complex mixtures subsequently known as galenicals.

Following the Roman Empire's decline, herbal medicine stagnated, although some additions and refinements were added by Arab physicians in the Middle Ages. The Renaissance gave rise to the influential iconoclastic thinker, Paracelsus (1493–1541), who, despite his brilliance, continued to honor the romantic, nonscientific concept of the Doctrine of Signatures, whereby the shape or color of a plant was thought to signify its possible use. This thinking led to fallacious naming of plants, such as "eyebright,"

Varieties of Herbal Medicine Practices in the U.S.*

Systems	Sources/Characteristics
Greek/Roman—based on Dioscorides/Galen, others; use of single herbs	
European	Modified by Gerard, Culpeper, others
German	Modern scientific studies; very popular, including unique commercial combinations
North American/U.S.	European, Native American, Mexican, etc.
Mexican	Spanish, Mayan, Aztec, etc.
Chinese Traditional—based on formulas using multiple herbs	
Kampo (Japanese)	Closely related to Chinese herbal practices
Jamu (Indonesian)	Chinese, with regional modifications and additions
Filipino, Thai, etc.	Local traditional herbs
Indian—based on use of herbs and spices	
Ayurveda	Based on ancient experience
Unani-Tibb	Ayurveda modified by Persian/Greek herbalism
Siddha	Herbs and spiritual practices
Indosyunic (Pakistani)	Similar to Ayurveda
Tibetan	Combines Indian and Chinese practices
Psychospiritual—use of herbs for psychic stimulation	
Incenses, oils, candles	Used in churches, in prayers, or witchcraft
Aromatherapy	Aromatic oils, mainly for inhalation or massage
Homeopathy	Uses extraordinarily diluted herbal extracts
Flower remedies	Combine aromatherapy and homeopathy
Nutraceuticals—use of foods, food extracts, and natural supplements	
Established foods	Vitamins, minerals, amino-acids, certain vegetables
Functional foods	Chemical extracts and variants, e.g., lycopene from tomatoes
Dietary extenders	Grasses, leaves, seeds, etc. used for health
Dietary extracts	Juices, essences, and other liquid products
Diet control agents	Anorexiant or stimulant herbs, bulk herbs

(Table continued on next page.)

Systems	Sources/Characteristics
Naturopathy—holistic therapy based on prevention and healthy lifestyle	
Classical	Elimination of dietary "poisons"
Current	Eclectic use of diet, health practices and alternative therapies

* In addition, herbal products such as tobacco, cocaine, marijuana, opium, and other psychoactive and addictive phytochemicals have powerful pharmacologic properties, and were formerly regarded as medicines.

"lungwort," and "mandrake," implying beneficial effects on the eyes, lung, or total body.[1] Famous herbalists in the 16th and 17th centuries, such as Brunfels, Turner, and Gerard, relied on their own observations to supplement the traditional teachings of their ancient predecessors. Culpeper (1616–1654) created an imaginative herbal compendium that was written for popular reading; he liberally employed astrology and witchcraft concepts to make the herb-book more acceptable to the typically educated patients of the pre-scientific era,[1] and thus emphasized the "magical" quality of herbs.

American Herbal Medicine

In the U.S., Samuel Thomson (1769–1843) gained enormous recognition with a practical and simple approach that avoided excessive use of dangerous herbs. His followers, the Thomsonians, who accepted his 70 or so herbs, believed in the healing power of nature (the *vis mediatrix naturae*); they emphasized his use of cayenne pepper (to restore body heat, as a "life promoter") and strongly favored lobelia, myrrh, and bayberry.[2] Thomsonian medicine was based on sensible, basic principles coupled with semi-scientific faith in concepts that lacked any validity other than all-too fallible dogmatic misinterpretation of personal experience. Thus, natural healing that occurred spontaneously was incorrectly assumed to be caused by the coincidental administration of herbal therapy by practitioners who lacked training in science and logic.

In contrast to the unsophisticated teaching of country herbalists such as Thomson, American doctors with training, such as John King, Wooster Beach, and John Scudder, developed Eclectic Medicine in the mid-19th century. Their practices were based on the extraction of chemicals such as resinoids from a number of

North American plants that had a tradition of healing value primarily for Native Americans.[3] A pharmacist, John Uri Lloyd, helped these physicians develop and market high-quality botanical products. In 1897, Lloyd and Harvey Fetter published a revised edition of "King's American Dispensatory," emphasizing the values of herbal medicines.[3] However, this era of refined herbalism was evolving at a time when the formal drug industry was able to introduce increasing numbers of synthetic medications that showed greater effectiveness in treating specific disease.

At the beginning of the 20th century, herbal medicine gradually became outdated, and the scene was set for the dominance of allopathic medical remedies. These increasingly seemed to have the potential to cure all diseases, as drug discoveries accelerated in the middle half of the 20th century. In addition, the 1938 U.S. Federal Food, Drug, and Cosmetic Act stipulated that all new drugs must be proved safe, and the 1962 Kefauver-Harris Amendment ensured that all new drugs, and those marketed after 1938, must be proved effective as well. Many common herbal preparations, sold as over-the-counter (OTC) products, were removed over the next several decades from the U.S. market due to lack of proven efficacy, or because of lack of willingness of marketers to submit claims to the National Academy of Science panels that were charged with examining this evidence.[4] Many herbal manufacturers in the U.S. simply removed therapeutic claims from their labels, and began to market their herbal products "underground," as simple nutritional supplements or food additives that could be purchased along with other natural dietary and cosmetic products. These found a growing acceptance in outlets such as health food stores.

Herbal Regulation. In 1993, these "second-class" medicines again became the focus of attention when the U.S. Food and Drug Administration (FDA) proposed that herbal medicines and other nutritional supplements not already regulated as drugs should undergo stringent marketing regulations. Intense opposition by consumer groups and the supplement industry led to a compromise decision, passed by Congress in 1994, called the Dietary Supplement Health and Education Act (DSHEA). DSHEA, which classified herbal medicines as "dietary supplements" (along with many vitamins, minerals, amino acids, enzymes, and just about any other substance used for improving health that was not already marketed as a drug), has radically changed the marketplace and created a multi-billion dollar industry in the U.S. Under DSHEA, herbs can be labeled with suggested doses and advertised as having certain healthful or nutritional properties, as long as no definite therapeutic claims implying prevention or treatment of specific diseases are made. Instead, manufacturers can describe how the supplement is *intended to affect* the "structure and function" of the human body, or they can emphasize its recognized physiological effect.

The subtle distinction between medical claims and suggestions for improving health has resulted in a parallel health industry that is less restricted than the orthodox pharmaceutical industry. As an example, the popularity of saw palmetto is attributed to the numerous European controlled clinical trials that have demonstrated its value in the treatment of the symptoms of benign prostatic hypertrophy (BPH). In the U.S., saw palmetto cannot be advertised as treatment for BPH (a therapeutic claim), but it can be advertised more generally "to support healthy prostate function" or "to maintain normal urine flow." Cat's claw, an herbal medicine that has no defined indications established by published clinical trials, is even more vaguely advertised as "helping to support the body's natural defenses" or "as a daily immune system protectant." Thus, manufacturers are permitted to allude to a therapeutic use of an herb, whether it is effective or not. The current lack of oversight that permits such provocative claims in labeling statements results in the seduction of health-seeking consumers and promotes skepticism and confusion among healthcare professionals.

Herbal medicines and other dietary supplements in the U.S. are not subject to evaluation and approval of their claimed effects by the FDA prior to marketing. Theoretically, manufacturers are expected to be able to substantiate their "structure and function" claims, but they do not need to share this information with the FDA or make it publicly available. The FDA only reviews the wording of the product labels, and the manufacturers are not required to notify the FDA of label claims until 30 days after their products are first marketed.

The recent rise of herbal medicine use in the U.S. is a consequence of both DSHEA and the increasing complexities of modern medical practice. The final decades of the 1900s contributed to the general disillusionment with pharmaceuticals because of their side effects, high costs, and monitoring requirements (which are expensive), and because of the restricted availability of potent prescription drugs. In contrast, the simplicity of readily accessible herbal remedies has made them an increasingly attractive option. The success of old and new herbs has been fostered by their national availability in the form of modern, scientific-appearing versions of the successful simple herbal medicines of the prior century. Moreover, they are now marketed by major producers with large advertising budgets.

Influences on U.S. Herbal Medicine. In Germany, the tradition of herbal medicine has prospered over the centuries and is well accepted by physicians and regulatory authorities.[5] Many, if not most, of the scientific and clinical studies on Western herbs come from investigators in Germany, where official acceptance of herbal products occurs with the favorable findings of the Commission E of the German Regulatory Authority, the Federal Institute for Drugs and Medical Devices. However, the scientific standards for accepting the value of an herb or its chemical extract as a "phytomedicine" fall far below the existing requirements of the U.S. FDA for establishing the value of pharmaceutical drugs. The basic indications and recommendations that are given by the Commission E for "approved" herbs in Germany emphasize long-established conventional practices, supplemented by extrapolations from pharmacologic principles and preliminary clinical evaluations.

More effort is now being directed at establishing greater validity for herbal research in Germany (and the U.S.). Current studies are more often based on rigorous, randomized, double-blind, and placebo-controlled trials with adequate statistical power. The increasing popularity and interest in alternative therapies is leading modern researchers to focus investigations on herbs with the intent of deriving reliable efficacy and safety data. In the U.S., the National Center for Complementary and Alternative Medicine and the Office of Dietary Supplements are funding large, randomized, controlled trials, by academic research institutions and others, to scientifically study herbal medicines and other dietary supplements.

In North America, most popular herbs of European background have been readily incorporated into herbal practice, while significant indigenous ones have been discovered or reintroduced in recent years. Several of the U.S. herbs that were first used by Native Americans, and were strongly promoted by the Eclectic practitioners in the late 19th and early 20th centuries, have become established as major therapies throughout the industrialized world. The most important examples are echinacea and saw palmetto.

In the southwest U.S., many of the local herbs have been used by people of Mexican descent for centuries, but these agents remain largely unknown in the world market. Nevertheless, there is reason to expect that some Mexican herbs may also offer significant benefits in managing certain diseases, such as diabetes.[6]

New American herbs as well as foreign herbs are frequently added to the marketplace. It is expected that many of the more promising herbs will be studied in a standardized, scientific fashion, and thus clearer indications for their use will gradually emerge.

Asiatic Herbalism

The cultural melting-pot that characterizes the population of the U.S. is now being reflected elsewhere in the industrialized world, with migrant groups and the internet introducing ethnic medical systems into cities throughout the Americas, Europe, and Australasia. In the U.S., the most important ancient herbal system that is becoming increasingly available is Traditional Chinese Medicine (TCM). This empiric and philosophic system was never based on science during its several millennia of development, and historic and cultural barriers hinder our ability to evaluate the claims of benefit of many Chinese herbs and formulations. Unlike other herbal medicine systems, TCM usually employs numerous plants (as well as minerals and animal parts) in complex mixtures with many variants.[7,8] It is difficult to study the effects of the individual herbs that are used in traditional mixtures, and the true benefits of combinations of herbs cannot be investigated comprehensively due to the complexity of the formulations (see chapter "Chinese Herbs").

Other traditional ethnic systems from Asia—such as Indian Ayurveda, Japanese Kampo (Kanpo), and Indonesian Jamu—do not enjoy the same level of acceptance in the U.S. that is accorded to TCM. The explanation is that Chinese herbal medicine was imported along with the large Chinese immigrations of the late 19th and early 20th centuries, whereas much of the immigration from Asiatic countries occurred in the late 20th century, after most FDA regulatory policies had become established. Nevertheless, Ayurvedic medicine from India, the second most important Asiatic herbal system, is making inroads in America and throughout the industrialized world (see chapter "Ayurvedic Herbs").

The importance of many ethnic traditional systems, such as Ayurveda, is that they incorporate holistic practices that emphasize disease prevention through dietary and lifestyle adjustments, appropriately adapted to individual patient requirements. The increasing popularity of Tibetan Medicine can be attributed to its combination of the important elements of traditional Chinese and Indian health systems along with mysticism, spirituality, and philosophy, and the use of foods and herbs in synergy as medicines.[9]

Aromatherapy

Herbs are, of course, not just sources of active constituents for botanical remedies. When herbs are used as foods and condiments, the psychological satisfaction provided by their flavor is as important as their nutritive, preventative, and curative properties. Herbs offer oral and olfactory stimulation, and these benefits are essential to our esthetic appreciation of the natural world, whether manifested in herb gardens, perfumes, pomanders, or appetizing meals.[10] Incenses and aromas were of importance in the past to counteract bad odors, but their use today is primarily for pleasure.

The extraordinary growth in the popularity of aromatherapy cannot be denied. This ancient medical practice credits aromatic herbs, and extracts containing their essential oils, with healing properties that combine poetic imagination with sensual awareness. Since patients who indulge in aromatherapy experience relief of both psychological and physical symptoms, this therapy is indeed of clinical relevance. An uplifting experience can be as important as a measurable clinical outcome resulting from orthodox drug therapy. Such experiences emphasize the deep significance of token healing, whereby a body-mind benefit is attained by an immaterial dose of a potential medicine. This effect may be similar to the placebo effect, which has a major role in all therapeutic practices. The placebo effect is a validated, useful property that can be employed advantageously by medical practitioners, and it serves as a crucial component in the healing arts of alternative and complementary practices (see chapter "The Placebo Effect and Herbs").

Nutraceuticals

In recent years, a new industry has arisen which blurs the distinction between "nutritional" and "medicinal" products by recognizing that inexpensive foods can be converted into expensive medicines. The basic effects of antioxidants, vitamins, minerals, and other chemicals that the body requires for maintaining healthy function and for fighting disease can be obtained from an optimal diet that incorporates a variety of fruits, vegetables, and spices. The nutraceutical (or nutriceutical) industry applies specific food components or chemicals, individually and in mixtures, in the form of proprietary products to promote or maintain health, prevent degeneration, and treat diseases such as arthritis, menopausal symptoms, fatigue, and even cancer. Such herbal products provide attractive and convenient sources of chemicals for people who cannot or prefer not to rely on a balanced diet of wholesome natural foods.

More persuasive forms of nutraceuticals are the "functional food" products that are based on extracts or derivatives of herbs or natural substances for specific health-related purposes, such as lycopene, quercetin, and linoleic acid. However, the benefit and the cost-effectiveness of such products need to be further determined; more effort will have to be exerted by the health professions to guide consumers in selecting from this growing market of alternative therapies. At present, there is no regulation of the production of these supplements, and little reliable advice is available regarding their use. Many of the promoters' claims for health benefits are imaginative; based on indirect or preliminary scientific evidence; and, all too often, misguided if not frankly fraudulent. Concern is repeatedly expressed by responsible health professionals who point out that much more scientific study is required to justify those claims.

Dietary supplement manufacturers and food suppliers are enthusiastically introducing the public to innovative health-providing natural products, such as phytomedicinal juices or "functional beverages." Interesting products range from grasses (e.g., wheatgrass juice) to seeds (e.g., flaxseed, chia) and grains (e.g., amaranth) to fruits (e.g., noni). In addition, commercial juice and other drink manufacturers are marketing beverages that contain token amounts of herbal or other additives (usually in amounts much smaller than those thought to be therapeutically active), thus exploiting the popularity of herbs and nutraceuticals such as ginseng, ginkgo, kava, echinacea, and glucosamine. Despite the increased numbers of health-seeking users of fruit and vegetable juices and seed extracts, who are attracted by these nutraceutical products, there is no reliable evidence that these fashionable refreshments, especially when imbibed sporadically, improve health or prevent disease. Nevertheless, many are more healthful (or at least nutritional) than mainstream commercial soft drinks that primarily consist of simple sugars, chemical additives, and water.

Perhaps the most successful functional foods that have entered the marketplace are soy or tofu and similar products derived from soybeans. These are alleged to be of benefit for postmenopausal symptoms and in the prevention of osteoporosis, atherosclerosis, and breast and prostate cancers, but their exact value is less certain than is commonly claimed. Similarly, the medical justification for exotic mushrooms, seaweeds, algae, and other unusual supplementary food-herb products has not been established. It is an interesting social phenomenon that the grape—the ancient source of the good and evil of alcohol—has now gained a new status in the dietary supplement market in the form of grape skin and grape seed antioxidants, such as reservatol and the pycnogenols.

Naturopathy

The emerging clinical practice of naturopathy combines many of the best concepts of treatment, prevention, and holistic health care by emphasizing good diet and the selective use of foods, herbs, exercise, relaxation, and massage as the means of improving or preserving health or treating illness.[3] Many of these principles are now being incorporated into modern conventional health practices, and early naturopathic therapies and other holistic systems of healing should be given full credit for their emphasis on an optimal approach to health based on sensible combinations of appropriate diets and lifestyles. The challenge for naturopaths and other advocates of natural or traditional healing is to avoid being overly responsive to the public's fascination with herbs, since it is all too easy to succumb to the opportunity to exploit humankind's desire to be medicated "naturally."

Conclusion

A wide variety of herbal practices are available and are used by today's U.S. consumers. Market forces are helping to promote legitimate herbal medicines with beneficial properties, but are also creating a climate in which questionable or misguided therapies are marketed just as easily. A careful examination of the evidence regarding the safety and efficacy of individual herbal medicines should be regarded as being preferable to an automatic, uncritical acceptance of natural products as natural healers. Over-reliance on nature's herbs may be as inappropriate as was the unquestioning tolerance of the use of leeches, phlebotomy, and purges as dominant forces in medical practices not so many generations ago.

references

1. Porter R (ed). Medicine: A History of Healing. Ancient Traditions to Modern Practices. New York, Marlowe & Company, 1997.
2. Griggs B. Green Pharmacy: A History of Herbal Medicine. New York, The Viking Press, 1981.
3. Brinker F. The role of botanical medicine in 100 years of American naturopathy. HerbalGram 42:49–54, 1998.
4. Foster S, Tyler VE. Tyler's Honest Herbal: A Sensible Guide to the use of Herbs and Related Remedies, 4th ed. New York, Haworth Herbal Press, 1999.
5. Blumenthal M (ed). The Complete German Commission E Monographs. Therapeutic Guide to Herbal Medicines. Boston, MA, Integrative Medicine Communication, 1998.
6. Yarnell E. Southwestern and Asian botanical agents for diabetes mellitus. Altern Complement Therap 6:7–11, 2000.
7. Reid D. A Handbook of Chinese Healing Herbs. Boston, Shambhala, 1995.
8. Ziment I. Five thousand years of attacking asthma. Respir Care 31:117–136, 1986.
9. Bradmaev V. Tibetan medicine. In Jonas WB, Levin JS (eds): Essentials of Complementary and Alternative Medicine. Philadelphia, Lippincott Williams & Wilkins, 1999, pp 252–274.
10. Ziment I. The messianic relationship between inspiration and expectoration. In Baum G, Priel Z, Roth Y, et al (eds): Cilia, Mucus, and Mucociliary Interactions. New York, Marcel Dekker, 1998, pp 383–389.

Quality Assurance and Choosing a Brand or Product

Prior to the current availability of mass-marketed herbal medicines and dietary supplements, herbalists and patients made their own phytomedicinal preparations. Often the herb was grown and obtained locally, and compounded by hand into a particular formula or concocted into a simple infusion (tea) or decoction (see chapter "Understanding Herbal Dosage Forms"). Doses and effects were acceptable even if variable and inconsistent, and there was little thought of standardization or quality control.

However, the art and science of herbal medicine has become more sophisticated, and is adapting to the "big-business" side of mass-market appeal; numerous herbal products are now grown worldwide and are distributed internationally. In addition, as herbs are increasingly packaged and advertised to compete with pharmaceutical drugs, consumers and healthcare providers increasingly expect botanical products to meet comparable quality standards.[1]

Problems With Herbal Quality Assurance

Currently, there are no government regulations that assure manufacturing standards and quality control, other than the Good Manufacturing Practice regulations required for foods. Numerous factors affect the ultimate ingredients and quality of an herbal product, including the growing conditions, method of drying and grinding, different processing methods and solvents used for extraction, and storage conditions. Thus, each manufacturer produces a unique product or formulation. Different marketed brands may vary substantially in quality and in the quantity of active phytomedicines, as well as in the absolute or relative concentrations of the chemical constituents in the different products. An analogy can be made with the wine industry, which also manufactures a botanical product. Wines from the same species of grape vary substantially from different wineries, and even year to year from the same vineyard.

Standardization of specific active constituents within herbal medicines, unlike that of drug products with a single chemical entity, is complex and unreliable. Standardization often implies that the preparation contains a designated amount or percentage of a certain chemical component thought to be therapeutically active. Botanicals may contain hundreds of bioactive chemicals, however, and the individual contributions of compounds responsible for therapeutic activity are usually not known. Moreover, additive or synergistic activity of several constituents may be required for effectiveness. In the case of herbal preparations, although standardization of chemical components may be used to assist with batch-to-batch replicability, the process fails to provide reliable controls for pharmacologic activity.

Standardization practices, if they are in place at all, can vary considerably between manufacturers. It is not uncommon for laboratory analyses of different brands of herbal medicines to find that important constituents vary by 5-, 10-, or even 40-fold[2–5]; some contain no labeled product at all.[6–7] In addition, substitution or contamination of the declared ingredients with toxic herbs that may be dangerous[8,9] or environmental pollutants (e.g., micro-organisms, pesticides, toxic metals),[10,11] and adulteration with drug products (reported particularly in Asian patent medicines)[12–15] have all been well described. These disturbing problems are probably vastly underreported, since only serious adverse outcomes are likely to be investigated. It is also recognized that currently there is a worldwide problem with counterfeit or substandard pharmaceutical drugs, and it is reasonable to assume that misrepresentation in herbal preparation marketing may similarly increase in the coming years unless vigorous efforts are directed against such practices.

Choosing a Brand or Product

Since there is little regulatory oversight of quality assurance among herbal preparations, there is a risk of unsafe contaminants. Moreover, since there are no herbal "generic equivalents," selecting from the multitude of different brands and products on today's market is a daunting task. Although many ethical herbal medicine manufacturers are producing high-quality products that are based on careful identification procedures, batch-to-batch standardization, and assays for impurities, it is difficult to determine which brands and products meet even basic quality standards. In the absence of any clear-cut evaluation criteria, the following recommendations may help consumers select more reliable herbal products.

1. Use products tested in positive, controlled clinical trials. If controlled clinical trials have been conducted and have demonstrated an herb's effectiveness, favor choosing the product used in those trials if it is available. Many of these products are tested and formulated in Europe and may be more expensive, but they are also considered to be manufactured to high quality standards; thus they are presumably the most reliably effective, and have been safety-tested as well (see table). For example, EGb 761 and LI 1370, the standardized ginkgo GBE extracts used in most of the European clinical trials, are imported to the U.S. and sold by several different companies. Other herbal products, manufactured in North America or elsewhere, are also increasingly being tested, and those that are found to be effective in controlled clinical trials should be favored. Note that the clinically tested brands available in the U.S. are included in the "Preparations & Doses" section of each herbal evaluation in this book

Clinically Tested European Products Marketed in the U.S.*

Herb	U.S. Product (Importer)	Equivalent European Product (Manufacturer)
Bilberry	Bilberry Extract (Enzymatic Therapy/PhytoPharmica)	Tegens (Synthelaso/Sanofi)
	Bilberry Extract (Solaray)	Tegens (Synthelabo/Sanofi)
Black Cohosh	Remifemin (GlaxoSmithKline)	Remifemin (Schaper & Brümmer)
Cat's Claw	Saventaro (PhytoPharmica/ Enzymatic Therapy)	Krallendorn (Immodal Pharmaka)
Chamomile	Camo Care (Abkit) [Topical]	Kamillosan (Asta Medica)
Echinacea	Echinaguard (Nature's Way) **Esberitox (Enzymatic Therapy/PhytoPharmica)	Echinacin (Madaus AG) **Esberitox N (Schaper & Brümmer)
Elderberry	Sambucol (Nature's Way)	Sambucol (Razei Bar)
Garlic	Kwai (Lichtwer Pharma)	Kwai (Lichtwer Pharma)
Ginkgo	Ginkgold (Nature's Way)	Tebonin [EGb761] (Schwabe)
	Ginkoba (Pharmaton)	Tebonin-Forte [EGb761] (Schwabe)
	Ginkai (Lichtwer)	Kaveri [LI-1370] (Lichtwer)

(Table continued on next page.)

Clinically Tested European Products Marketed
in the U.S. (*Cont.*)*

Herb	U.S. Product (Importer)	Equivalent European Product (Manufacturer)
Ginseng, Asian	Ginsana (Pharmaton)	Ginsana [G115] (Pharmaton-Switzerland)
Hawthorn	HeartCare (Nature's Way)	Crataegutt-forte [WS 1442] (Schwabe)
Horse chestnut	Venastat (Pharmaton)	Venostasin-retard (Klinge Pharma)
Lemon balm (Melissa)	Herpalieve (PhytoPharmica) Herpilyn (Enzymatic Therapy)	Lomaherpan (Lomapharm) Lomaherpan (Lomapharm)
Milk thistle	Thisylin (Nature's Way)	Legalon (Madaus)
Pygeum	Pygeum Extract (Solaray) **Saw Palmetto Complex (Enzymatic/PhytoPharm) **Nettle-Pygeum Complex (Enzymatic/PhytoPharm)	Pygenil (Synthelabo/Sanofi) Prunuselect [extract] (Indena) Prunuselect [extract] (Indena)
Saw palmetto	Prost Active (Nature's Way) Propalmex (Chattem)	Prostagutt (Schwabe) Talso/Uno (Synthelabo/ Sanofi Winthrop)
St. John's wort	Kira (Lichtwer Pharma) Movana (Pharmaton) Perika (Nature's Way)	Jarsin 300 [LI-160] (Lichtwer Pharma) Neuroplant (Schwabe) Neuroplant (Schwabe)
Valerian	**Valerian Nighttime (Nature's Way) Sedonium (Lichtwer Pharma)	**Euvegal forte (Spitzner Arznel-mitel) Sedonium (Lichtwer Pharma)
Vitex (Chaste-berry)	Femaprin (Nature's Way)	Agnolyt (Madaus)

* This table includes frequently prescribed herbal products that are: (1) clinically tested in controlled trials, and (2) manufactured in Europe and also marketed in the U.S. These products are generally manufactured to highly regulated European standards, and can thus be considered to be high-quality preparations. Inclusion in this table does not guarantee efficacy, however, and the herb evaluations (see page 63) should be referred to for overall efficacy recommendations. Products manufactured in the U.S. and other countries are also being clinically tested and are available on the U.S. market (see herb evaluations).

**Combination herbal product

References consulted in constructing this table:
1. Blumenthal M, Goldberg A, Brinckmann J (eds). Herbal Medicine: Expanded Commission E Monographs. Newton, MA, Integrative Medicine Communications, 2000 [Appendix, Table 5, pp. 479–480].
2. Tyler VE. A guide to clinically tested herbal products in the U.S. market. Healthnotes Rev Complement Integr Med 2000;7:279–287.

2. Rely on independent laboratories to evaluate product quality. In the absence of clinical trials, consider using products that meet quality assurance standards (correct plant identity, minimum concentrations of major constituents, and absence of toxic impurities) by an independent testing laboratory. Currently, the most useful source is ConsumerLab.com, which provides independent quality-control laboratory testing of different brands of herbs, supplements, and related health and nutrition products. Herbal products that have been tested include St. John's wort, Asian and American ginsengs, Ginkgo biloba, saw palmetto, and echinacea. Dietary supplements include CoQ10, SAMe, glucosamine, and chondroitin. A few brand names that meet their quality criteria are posted on their website (www.ConsumerLab.com), but details on all the brand names are available for a yearly subscription fee (about 20–30 different brands for each herb or supplement), and are updated regularly. Products that pass their laboratory tests may carry a "ConsumerLab.com" seal of approval on their label.

Consumer Reports has also tested different brands of St. John's wort, kava, saw palmetto, and SAMe, to date, and is expected to publish more laboratory analyses on a continuing basis.[16,17] The American Botanical Council's authoritative Ginseng Evaluation Program is publishing the analyses of many commercially available ginseng products.[19]

3. Consider other quality assurance standards. The United States Pharmacopeia (USP), the official organization that sets drug and other health-product standards, has established analytical standards for many botanical products.[18] Manufacturers who meet these standards can place an official "NF" (for National Formulary) on their labels, although the use of these standards are voluntary and do not appear to be popular among herbal manufacturers at this time. Choosing a product that carries an "NF" designation does provide some guarantee of quality assurance, however. In addition, other scientific organizations, the herbal medicine industry, and some trade groups are also developing their own standardized analytical methods and quality standards.[1] Adhering to any of these quality assurance standards is voluntary for U.S. manufacturers, unlike their European counterparts who are more rigorously controlled by government agencies.

4. Consider products manufactured by pharmaceutical firms. Consider products manufactured or distributed by large, ethical pharmaceutical companies, for example, Boehringer

Ingelheim's Pharmaton division or Centrum Herbals by American Home Products/Whitehall-Robbins.[1] These large companies have experience with and can presumably ensure a high level of quality control. Pharmaton also markets products that have demonstrated beneficial effects when evaluated in clinical trials. Warner-Lambert's Quanterra division previously manufactured or marketed herbal medicines that were demonstrated effective in clinical trials, but has not actively marketed herbal products since September 2000.

5. Research individual herbal manufacturers. There are many herbal manufacturers who care deeply about product quality and produce high-quality products. However, there are no good criteria to logically assess the excellence of a producer other than by relying on general reputation and researching individual companies. It is appropriate to question manufacturers about their individual quality assurance and standardization procedures. Marketed products should provide detailed information on the label, including batch number, expiration date, and manufacturer contact information.

Conclusion

Many users of herbal medicines may be tempted to purchase inexpensive or "bargain" products, but there is a higher risk that such herbal medications are lacking in potency, contaminated with impurities, and/or produced without the benefit of some essential quality-assurance process. Consumers should recognize that no government agency currently regulates the production and quality of herbs, and should exercise discretion in selecting any phytomedicinal product. The introduction of voluntary standards and oversight criteria by the organized herbal industry is beginning to have a positive impact on herbal product quality, but it is expected that improvements in standards will not significantly occur without independent or government controls in place.

references
1. Rotblatt MD. Herbal medicines: a practical guide to safety and quality assurance. West J Med 1999;171:172–175.
2. Monmaney T. Labels' potency claims often inaccurate, analysis finds. Los Angeles Times 1998 August 31, p A10.
3. Herbal roulette. Consumer Reports 1995;60(Nov):698–705.
4. Gurley BJ, Gardner SF, Hubbard MA. Content versus label claims in ephedra-containing dietary supplements. Am J Health-Syst Pharm 2000;57:963–969.

5. Schardt D, Schmidt S. Garlic: Clove at first sight? Nutrition Action Healthletter 1995; 22(July/Aug):3–5.
6. Cui J, Garle M, Eneroth P, Bjorkhem I. What do commercial ginseng preparations contain? Lancet 1994;344:134.
7. Ross SA, ElSohly MA, Wilkins SP. Quantitative analysis of *Aloe vera* mucilaginous polysaccharide in commercial *Aloe vera* products. J AOAC Internat 1997;80:455–457.
8. Slifman NR, Obermeyer WR, Aloi BK, et al. Contamination of botanical dietary supplements by *Digitalis lanata*. NEJM 1998; 339:806–811.
9. Nortier JL, Martinez M-CM, Schmeiser HH, et al. Urothelial carcinoma associated with the use of a chinese herb (*Aristolochia fangchi*). N Engl J Med 2000;342:1686–1692.
10. De Smet PAGM. Toxicological outlook on the quality assurance of herbal remedies. In De Smet PAGM (ed): Adverse Effects of Herbal Drugs, Vol. 1. Berlin, Springer, 1992, pp 1–72.
11. Beigel Y, Ostfeld I, Schoenfeld N. A leading question. N Engl J Med 1998;339:827–830.
12. Ko RJ. Adulterants in Asian patent medicines. N Engl J Med 1998;339:847.
13. Keane FM, Munn SE, duVivier AWP, Higgins EM. Analysis of Chinese herbal creams prescribed for dermatological conditions. West J Med 1999;170:257–260.
14. Dreskin SC. A prescription drug packaged in China and sold as an ethnic remedy. JAMA 2000;283:2393.
15. Tomlinson B, Chan TYK, Chan JCN, et al. Toxicity of complementary therapies: An Eastern perspective. J Clin Pharmacol 2000;40:451–456.
16. Herbal Rx for prostate problems. Consumer Reports 2000;65(9):60–62.
17. Emotional "aspirin'"?: We tested what's in the alternative "mood" pills. Consumer Reports 2000;65(12):60-62.
18. United States Pharmacopeia at www.usp.org.
19. Hall T, Lu Z-Z, Yat PN, et al. Ginseng evaluation program. Part one: Standardization phase. HerbalGram 2001;52:27–47.

Understanding Herbal Dosage Forms

Most physicians and healthcare providers have little formal background in botanical medicine and herbal dosage forms. The amount of herb or chemical constituents contained in a specific extract, tincture, or other herbal formulation is often difficult to calculate, or is confusing to the nonherbalist. How many health professionals know what a 1:10 liquid extract really means?

Moreover, common herbal dosage forms have been affected by market forces in the last decade. Previously, crude dried herbs (whole or powdered) were used to make teas or decoctions, or products were prepared and sold as liquid tinctures and extracts. Currently, with the recent marketing explosion of dietary supplements in North America, the majority of commercial herbal products (especially those sold in conventional pharmacies and mass-market outlets) are now available in solid dosage forms such as tablets or capsules. This is also true for a variety of popular products in Western Europe, where many of the best known herbal medicines (e.g., *Ginkgo biloba*, St. John's wort, valerian, saw palmetto) were originally researched and then standardized in solid forms for marketing.

American consumers and health professionals are often more comfortable purchasing or recommending solid dosages, because they are familiar with this form in the arena of pharmaceutical drugs. Additionally, there is a feeling that such products are more reliable. Nevertheless, traditional liquid forms such as teas, decoctions, tinctures, and extracts are readily available and are used by many patients.

Because solid dosage forms are widely available, generally preferred by U.S. consumers, and often evaluated in clinical trials, their use is more likely to be supported by evidence-based recommendations. For these reasons, liquid forms such as fluid extracts and tinctures are not emphasized in this book. The following pages will help healthcare professionals understand the most common, traditional herbal dosage forms (both liquid and solid) that can be purchased from retail outlets, or that are recommended in many herbal books.

Interpreting Herb-to-Extract Ratios

Although some herbal medicines are dosed as the crude or minimally processed herb (e.g., 2 g of dried root, or 500 mg of dehydrated or freeze-dried leaves), an increasing proportion of herbal medicines purchased by U.S. consumers are extracts (e.g., 900 mg of a 5:1 extract product). The amount of crude herb that a particular extract contains (or is equivalent to) is not always obvious, as many labels on herbal products do not provide details of their proprietary extract. However, if the herb-to-extract ratio is known, the amount can be roughly calculated. This ratio expresses the weight of dried herb in the original starting material, to the volume or weight of finished product, in that order.

For example, in a 1:5 tincture, 1 g of dried herb would be used to make 5 ml of the final tincture. A more potent formulation would be a 1:1 fluid extract, in which 1 g of dried herb is used to make 1 ml of the final extract. In a solid formulation, a 10:1 product represents 10 g of dried herb concentrated into 1 g of finished solids. The equivalent of 1 g of dried herb parts (leaf, root, flower, etc.) is thus used to make (or is contained in) each of the following:

- 5 ml of a 1:5 liquid
- 1 ml of a 1:1 liquid
- 250 mg of a 4:1 solid extract
- 200 mg of a 5:1 powder

Note that while herb-to-extract ratios can be used to calculate the amount of starting material used in an herbal preparation, they allow only rough estimates of the product's ultimate chemical constituents. Herbal preparations from different manufacturers with identical herb-to-extract ratios should not be considered to have identical potencies and/or effects. There are numerous factors that affect the ultimate ingredients of an herbal product, including quality of the starting material, method of drying and grinding, different processing methods and solvents used for extraction, and storage conditions. There may even be significant batch-to-batch variability, and each manufacturer has different quality assurance processes to help minimize variability and standardize their products (see chapter "Quality Assurance").

Traditional Liquid Dosage Forms

Liquid dosage forms (infusions, decoctions, tinctures, and extracts) are widely used in traditional herbal medicine. They are readily absorbed; dosing is flexible; and they are easy to take. Disadvantages include a disagreeable or bitter taste, and a small amount of alcohol in most tinctures and extracts (ethanol typically is used as a solvent). There is also some confusion about dosing and potency. For example, as mentioned above, a 1:1 liquid extract should be 5 times more potent than a 1:5 tincture. However, the actual potencies and doses recommended in the herbal literature do not always correspond with these ratios. This discrepancy is due to widely variable manufacturing techniques and standardizations among different products. Broad dosing ranges and dosing inconsistencies in different herbal pharmacopoeias result in lack of standardized prescribing.

Water Extractions. These time-honored, simple preparations are often prepared by herb users, and are employed both orally and topically. Infusions and decoctions are obtained by the extraction of water-soluble or polar constituents such as tannins and glycosides, although water is not a good solvent for many other active chemicals. They are the safest type of extract, however, as toxic alkaloids are usually water insoluble. Water extracts have a short shelf-life (unless they contain antimicrobial additives) due to bacterial contamination, and thus should be refrigerated and discarded after a few days. They are also difficult to standardize, and are often bitter or unpleasant tasting unless flavor additives are incorporated.

An **infusion** is another name for a strong tea, and is the preferred extraction method for delicate plant parts such as leaves, flowers, soft stems, and fruit. Infusions are commonly prepared by pouring boiling water over an herb and allowing it to steep or "brew." Typically, 8 ounces of water is poured over 2–3 teaspoons of herb and allowed to steep for 10–15 minutes. The solids are strained out, and the resultant liquid is available for use.

A **decoction** is similar to boiled coffee or soup: the herb and water are boiled together. Decoctions are generally more concentrated than infusions, and the method is useful for fibrous plant material such as roots, stems, and bark. Typically, 2–3 teaspoons of herb are placed in 12 ounces of cold water, which is then brought to a boil and simmered under cover for 5–15 minutes or longer. Again, the solids are strained out.

Solvent or Hydroalcoholic Extractions. Tinctures and fluid extracts can be commercially prepared for retail sale because they have a long shelf-life. Tinctures were traditionally made by placing the herb in an organic solvent and leaving it to soak for days to weeks. An alternative and faster method is for the solvent to be percolated through the herb. Percolation has been used mainly for fluid extracts, but is also used for tinctures. The liquid that is obtained from the herbal material is the medicine, and the remainder of the herb is discarded. The solvent is usually a 30–70% ethanol and water mixture. Glycerol can be substituted for ethanol for certain herbs in which an alcoholic solution is undesirable.

Alcohol-based solvent extracts generally have a shelf-life of 2–3 years. They are usually stronger than infusions or decoctions, as alcohol can extract additional constituents that are lipophilic or water-insoluble. Tinctures and fluid extracts are typically mixed in water or a beverage and administered 2–4 times daily. Although often used interchangeably, technically there is a difference between a tincture and a fluid extract.

A **tincture** is generally defined as a solvent (e.g., alcohol) extract in a 1:5 or weaker ratio (e.g., 1:10). For many herbs, a typical tincture dose is several ml (perhaps a teaspoonful), which is equivalent to about 1 g of the crude or dried herb.

A **fluid extract** is similar to a tincture, but by definition it is a 1:1 or 1:2 ratio (i.e., 1 g of herb is contained in 1 or 2 ml of liquid) or stronger. It is supposed to be about 5–10 times more potent than a tincture, and smaller doses are used (often dosed in drops). Currently, fluid extracts are also made by reconstituting solid concentrates.

Solid Dosage Forms

Tablets and capsules are currently preferred by many patients because they are convenient and familiar dosage forms that do not present problems with taste or alcohol content. Crude herbs can be air-dried, freeze-dried, or ground and used to fill gelatin capsules or compressed into tablets. However, because limited amounts of whole herb can be incorporated into these solids forms, more concentrated extracts are often required.

To prepare a solid extract, the herb is first combined with a solvent, as in preparing a liquid extract. However, the resultant liquid (which would otherwise be used as a liquid extract) is then evaporated by various methods, and a concentrated solid is left.

Therefore, the product is usually at least 4–5 times as potent as a typical 1:1 fluid extract (e.g., 5:1 ratio, or 5 g of dried herb is concentrated to 1 g of finished extract).

Many highly concentrated solid extracts are also produced (10:1, 50:1, etc.). For example, EGb 761, a standardized proprietary extract of *Ginkgo biloba* leaves, is a 50:1 solid extract. This means that 50 g of dried leaves was used to make 1 g of the final solid extract preparation.

Summary

Herbal medicines are available in a wide range of solid and liquid forms. The herb-to-extract ratio allows you to calculate how much of the dried herb is used to prepare a particular extract, although multiple factors in the manufacturing process affect the ultimate concentration of chemical ingredients. Traditional water extracts (infusions and decoctions) are generally safe and are easy to make at home, but they are difficult to standardize and have a short shelf-life. Solvent extracts (tinctures and fluid extracts) are typically made with ethanol-water solvents, are more potent, and are generally commercially available. Many popular herbal medicines in the U.S. are sold as solid extract products, and are readily available in pharmacies and other conventional outlets.

references

1. Mills S, Bone K. Principles and Practice of Phytotherapy: Modern Herbal Medicine, Edinburgh, UK, Churchill Livingstone, 2000.
2. Schulz V, Hänsel R, Tyler VE. Rational Phytotherapy: A Physicians' Guide to Herbal Medicine, 3rd ed. New York, Springer, 1998.
3. McCaleb R, Leigh E, Morien K. The Encyclopedia of Popular Herbs. Roseville, CA, Prima Health, 2000.
4. Low Dog T. Key to understanding herbal preparations. Botanical Medicine in Modern Clinical Practice, 3rd Annual Course, Columbia University, New York, May 1998.

Chemistry of Herbal Medicines

There are numerous complex chemicals in plants, and rigid classification is impossible. In this summary, the classes of "secondary" metabolites that often serve as therapeutic chemicals will be discussed (Table 1). These agents are found in specific groups of plants, and they exert a protective influence by being toxic to various predators. These products are also biologically active in humans, and are often used as phytomedicines.

Major Components

Alkaloids

Alkaloids have some of the most potent effects on animals and humans, and they demonstrate both therapeutic and toxic properties. They are basic amines; they are not volatile and lack odor; and they have a bitter taste and are insoluble in water, although their salts are soluble. Included in this class of over 12,000 known agents are purines, pyrrolidines, piperidines, pyridines, and quinolines. Some of the best known herbal drugs are alkaloids, including atropine, emetine, capsaicin, cocaine, morphine, quinine, methylxanthines (such as caffeine and theophylline), strychnine, and nicotine. Ephedrine is related; it is sometimes classified as a protoalkaloid.

There are 13 or more subclasses of alkaloids (Table 2). Alkaloids have multiple therapeutic effects. Many are too dangerous to be used in herbal practice, and they are therefore usually regarded as allopathic drugs. They cross the blood-brain barrier and act on neurotransmitter receptors.

Bioflavonoids

Several thousand bioflavonoid (or flavonoid) compounds are known, occurring freely or as glycosides. They lack nitrogen, and usually contain two 6-carbon rings joined by three carbon atoms,

Table 1. Important Categories of Phytomedicinal Chemicals

Class	Definition	Properties
Alkaloids	Basic amines (names end in "-ine").	Includes potent drugs and narcotics. Over 12,000 known; over 13 classes.
Bioflavonoids	Plant pigments; vitamin-like.	Most medical effects are questionable. Over 4000 known; over 14 classes.
Essential Oils	Isoprene derivatives: oxidized terpenes and phenylpropanoids.	Used in perfumes and in aromatherapy. Over 9 classes. Also known as volatile oils, ethereal oils, essences.
Glycosides	Sugar derivatives attached to aglycones.	Over 10 classes. Over 3000 known.
Resins	Oxidation products of terpenes; resins are insoluble in water.	Includes oleoresins, gum resins and balsams.
Saponins	Soap-like glycosides; cause hemolysis if directly introduced into the blood stream.	Various groups of chemicals. Some are involved in steroid metabolism.
Sterols	Steroid and vitamin D precursors.	Found in soy and other plants; also produced by microorganisms (e.g., sitosterol, stigmasterol).
Tannins	Polyphenolics, mostly based on gallic acid.	Astringent compounds, bind to protein (tanning); reduce diarrhea, act as hemostatics.
Terpenes (Terpenoids)	Derived from 5-carbon isoprene units (10, 15, 20, 30, 40, >40).	Over 20,000 known; 6 classes. Most structurally varied phytochemicals.

but 5-membered rings (aurone) and open-chain (chalcone) compounds are included in this group (Table 3). There are about 8000 plant phenolic compounds, half of which are flavonoids; these polyphenols are based on phenylpropanoid units. The flavonoids are often pigmented, appearing as yellow or other colors of

Table 2. Alkaloids

Classes	Examples	Common Sources	Major Uses
Imidazoles	colchicine	autumn crocus	gout
	ephedrine	ma huang	asthma
Indoles	ergotamine	ergot	migraine
	reserpine	snakeroot	hypertension
	vincristine	periwinkle	leukemias
	yohimbine	yohimbe	aphrodisiac
Isoquinolines	berberine	goldenseal	diarrhea, colds
	emetine	ipecacuanha	emetic, amebiasis
	hydrastine	goldenseal	diarrhea, colds
	morphine, codeine, papaverine	poppy	narcotics
Piperidine Amides	piperidine	black pepper	stimulant
Piperidines	lobeline	lobelia	asthma
Purines	caffeine, theophylline	coffee, tea	stimulants, asthma
Pyridines	nicotine	tobacco	stimulant
Pyrrolidines	cocaine	coca plant	anaesthetic, stimulant
	tropanes (e.g., atropine)	nightshade	anticholinergics
Pyrrolizidines	senkirkine	coltsfoot	expectorant
	symphytine	comfrey	dermatologic
Quinolines	quinine	cinchona	malaria
Quinolizidines	lupanine	broom	oxytocic
Steroidals	veratrine	veratrum	hypertension
Terpenoids	aconitine	monkshood	cardiac failure

petals, fruits, and berries in higher plants. They are found in high concentrations in many flowers, and in foods such as citrus fruits, tomatoes, red wine, onions, and tea. Flavonoids commonly are antioxidants with free-radical scavenging properties. They are believed to be anti-inflammatory and protective against various cancers. They are usually water soluble, and are made available in many fruit and vegetable juices.

Table 3. Major Bioflavonoids*

Classes	Examples	Common Sources	Claimed Effects
Flavonoids			
Flavone glycosides	apigenin luteolin	chamomile thyme	anti-inflammatory anti-inflammatory
Flavonol glycosides	rutin quercetin kaempferol	rose onion elder	antioxidant antiallergy anti-inflammatory
Flavanones and Dihydro-flavonols	hesperetin eriodictyol liquiritin naringenin	yerba santa artemesia licorice grapefruit	antifungal antimalarial antitussive antimicrobial
Flavans (Catechins)	epigallocatechin-3-gallate	tea	antioxidant
Isoflavonoids			
Isoflavones	daidzein genistein	soy red clover	estrogenic estrogenic
Isoflavonones	cyclokievitone	bean	antifungal
Isoflavans	licoricidin	licorice	antifungal
Proantho-cyanidins (condensed tannins)	pycnogenol	pine	antioxidant
Anthocyanidins (Anthocya-nosides)	cyanidin delphinidin	elderberry bilberry	food colorant food colorant
Rotenoids	rotenone puerarin	derris kudzu	insecticide for alcoholism
Chalcones	isoliquiritigenin	licorice	MAO-inhibition
Aurones	hispidol	coreopsis	colorant
Coumestans	coumestiol	alfalfa	estrogenic
Flavonolignans	silymarin	milk thistle	hepatoprotective

* Flavonoids may also be combined with tannins and catechins.

The main flavonoids are the very common and structurally variable flavones (which are oxidation products of flavanones), flavonols (which are often glycosides), and the often bitter flavanones (including related dihydroflavonols). The other major constituents in this group are the ubiquitous colorful plant pigments, anthocyanins, and their glycosides, the anthocyanidins. Chalcones and aurones are isoflavonoids and are sometimes included as separate groups or are classified with other neoflavonoids. The isoflavonoids are fewer in number (around 700) and are mainly found in plants belonging to the *Leguminosae* family. Rotenoids are present in the kudzu vine (*Pueraria lobata*) which is used by herbalists to treat alcoholism. Additional classes that are sometimes recognized include isoflavenes, flavenes, and similar variants.

The best known flavonoids are those in green tea (epigallocatchin-3-gallate, catechin, etc.) and citrus fruits (kaemferol, quercetin and its derivatives, rutin and hesperidin). These latter, along with anthocyanins, are known sometimes as vitamin P, because they were thought to decrease capillary permeability in peripheral vascular disease. However, there is little evidence for such activity, and the concept of vitamin P has generally been discarded. Soy bioflavonoids (especially genistein and daidzein) are well known food supplements that are being promoted as phytoestrogens. Of particular interest is the product pycnogenol, composed of oligomeric proanthocyanidins (OPCs). These chemicals are obtained from the bark of maritime pine trees, and are promoted as powerful antioxidants with a myriad of preventive and therapeutic effects. Grape seed has a similar content of OPCs, while red wine offers the grape skin antioxidant, resveratrol, a polyphenol that is promoted as a preventive of atherosclerosis and cancer.

Essential Oils

These volatile compounds constitute the attractant odors of flowers, and the attractant or defensive components of the other parts of the plant. They are sometimes referred to as volatile oils or essences. They are common in many herbs that are favored for use in treating skin and respiratory disease. Odiferous or pungent essential oils can evoke responses varying from mucus secretion in the airways to rubefaction, manifested by reddening and tingling of the skin. Essential oils are of particular interest to the perfume and fragrance industry, and are used both therapeutically and hedonistically in aromatherapy.

The important essential oils are found in ten classes (Table 4). The more pleasurable oils are mainly derived from terpenes and

Table 4. Essential Oils

Classes*	Examples	Common Sources
Alcohols (often based on monoterpenes)	camphor oil citronellol menthol thujone zingiberol	camphor rose mints wormwood ginger
Aldehydes (partially oxidized primary alcohols)	benzaldehyde cinnamaldehyde citronellal	almonds cinnamon cintronella
Esters (terpene alcohol combined with an organic acid)	acetates allyl esters methyl esters	lavender mustard wintergreen
Ethers (include oxides and peroxides)	anethole cineole (eucalyptol) myristicin	anise eucalyptus nutmeg
Furans	menthofuran	mints
Hydrocarbons (often are terpenes)	limonene phellandrene pinene turpentine	citrus fruits parsley conifers pine
Ketones (from oxidation of secondary alcohols)	carvone menthone pulegone	caraway peppermint pennyroyal
Phenols (benzene ring structure)	capsaicin eugenol thymol	capsicum clove thyme
Sesquiterpinoids (includes lactones)	caryophylline 4-hydroxycoumarin	clove sweet clover
Sulfur Compounds (Thiosulfinates)	methyl disulfide diallyl disulfide	onion garlic

* Sometimes, the essential oils are further subclassified as monoterpenes, sesquiterpenes and phenylpropanoids (including allylphenols and pro-penylphenols).

alcohols, while the pungent ones that are used also to flavor food include sulfides and their derivatives. Essential oils have a less important role in herbal therapeutics, although several specific agents, such as the essential oils of the mint family, are extensively used as flavors and drugs. Some essential oils are in popular use.

For example, essential oils of thyme are believed to serve as weak antibacterials in products such as mouthwashes.

Glycosides

Numerous plant chemicals contain a carbohydrate residue, or glycone, attached to a noncarbohydrate residue, or aglycone, to form a glycoside. If hydrolysis yields glucose, the originating glycoside is termed a glucoside, in contrast to non-glucosides that yield other sugars. The glycosides are difficult to classify as their aglycone components are variable, but a common therapeutic classification is shown here (Table 5). Glycosides are usually bitter-tasting, but some are sweet.

The cardiac glycosides, such as digoxin, are major drugs in allopathic medicine. Anthraquinones are glycosides that are in common use as laxatives, whereas isothiocyanates are valued as flavors, being characteristic of pungent herbs and vegetables. The

Table 5. Glycosides*

Glycoside	Agylycone Component	Examples of Major Drugs	Plant Sources	Claimed Effects
Cardiac Glycosides	steroids	digitoxin hellebrin	foxglove hellebore	cardiotonic cardiotonic
Saponins	sapogenins: neutral (steroids) acid (triterpenoids)	glycyrrhizin ginsenosides	licorice ginseng	peptic ulcer adaptogen
Anthraquinones	anthracene	cascarocides barbaloin sennosides	cascara aloes senna	laxative laxative laxative
Cyanogenic glycosides (Cyanophores)	hydrocyanic acid	amygdalin prunasin sambunigrin	apricots prunes elderberry	anti-cancer anti-cancer anti-cancer
Isothiocyanates	glucosinolates	alliin sinigrin	garlic mustard	cholesterol reduction expectorant
Aldehydes	aldehydic	vanillin	vanilla	flavor
Phenolics	phenols	hydroquinone	uva ursi	urinary disinfectant
Alcohols	salicyl alcohol	salicin	willow	analgesic
Lactones	hydroxycinnamic acid	aesculin	horse chestnut	venous insufficiency
Coumarins	coumarin	dicumarol	sweet clover (+fungus)	anticoagulant

* Many flavonoids exist as glycosides.

isothiocyanates are the pungent chemicals that are liberated by enzyme activity in members of the mustard, radish, and cabbage family. Alliaceous plants, such as garlic, onions, and chives, also have sulfur-based pungent chemicals that are produced when enzymes are released by crushing the cells of the bulbs; however, these organosulfur agents are not glycosides. The cyanogenic glycosides are sometimes used as unorthodox medicines; laetrile, derived from apricot pits, was a notorious, ineffective agent promoted for use in cancer. Saponins are soaplike; some are considered to be poisons ("sapotoxins," which are mainly irritants of the gastrointestinal tract), but most are harmless.

Many glycosides exist as the cyclic esters known as lactones. Coumarins are the lactones of 2-hydroxycinnamic acid; phytomedicines such as aesculin of horse chestnut, and less common agents in folk medicine such as scopoletin, khellin, and visnagin, are related. Other glycosides include phenolic compounds, such as hydroxyquinone, which is derived from arbutin by hydrolysis. Many of the glycosidic β-lactones are considered to be carcinogenic.

Phenylpropanoids

This is a large group of compounds. Phenylpropanoids are usually based on the aromatic amino acids, phenylalanine and tyrosine. They do not contain nitrogen, and are often classifed as plant phenolics. Their major precursors are cinnamic acid and 2-hydroxycinnamic acid, which are derived from amino acid precursors by the shikimic acid pathway.

Phenylpropanoids include phenylpropenes, which contribute odor to plants and are associated with terpenes. So-called "abridged" phenylpropanoids include capsaicin and salicin. Derivatives of 2-hydroxycinnamic acid (also called coumaric acid) can be classified as glycosides; the corresponding lactone is coumarin, from which the anticoagulant dicumarol and related furanocoumarins can be obtained. Chromones are related to coumarins; the best-known example is khellin, the compound that led to the discovery of the anti-asthma drug, cromolyn. Other phenylpropanoid derivatives include lignans and neolignans; these have antitumor and antiviral properties. Flavonoids and tannins also arise from phenylpropanoids.

Table 6. Resins

Category	Composition	Examples
Pure Resins	solid complexes	guaiac (guaifenesin) hashish
Oleoresins	resins mixed with volatile oils	turpentine (terpene hydrate)
Oleo-Gum Resins	complex oleoresins	frankincense (olibanum)
Balsams	incorporate cinnamic or benzoic acids or their esters	benzoin storax tolu balsam
Resin Acids	contain dipteroid oxyacids	myrrh
Resinotannols	complex alcohols with a tannin reaction	benzoin

Resins

When a plant is injured it may exude a hard-setting material to cover the wound. Such resins (Table 6) are composed of resin alcohols, resenes, esters, and other compounds. The main components are oxidation products of terpenes. They may be mixed with volatile oils to form oleoresins, and these may be present as oleo-gum-resins. If cinnamic acid or benzoic acid or their esters are in the mixture, the product is a balsam.

Saponins

These are glycosides with terpenoid aglycone components. They possess two major characteristics: they have soaplike surfactant effects, and they cause hemolysis when directly introduced into the blood stream. They are usually poorly absorbed, and do not cause hemolysis when taken orally. There are three classes of saponins, and a number of them have potential medicinal effects, including anti-inflammatory, anti-venous permeability, and expectorant properties (Table 7). Their surfactant qualities have made them popular for use as mucolytics and expectorants, but there is little evidence to suggest that they have significant surfactant action on mucus. They probably are capable of inducing an emetic-expectorant reflex originating in the stomach and causing vagal stimulation of mucous secretion in the airways.

Table 7. Saponins

Classes	Examples	Common Sources	Claimed Effects
Steroidal (Sapogenins)	digitoxin diosgenin hederosaponins sarsasapogenin	foxglove yam ivy yucca	cardiotonic steroid precursor expectorant anti-inflammatory
Terpenoid (Triterpenes)	aescin astragalosides cycloartanes ginsenosides glycyrrhizin quillaja saikosaponins	horse chestnut astragalus black cohosh ginseng licorice soapbark bupleurum	venous insufficiency immunostimulant estrogenic adaptogen peptic ulcer, cough expectorant anti-inflammatory
Glycoalkaloids (Alkaloid Glycosides)	solasodine	Solanum species	steroid precursor

Ivy is an example of an herb that is employed for its saponin effects. Sapogenins are used in steroid hormone synthesis, but the native herbal compounds lack endocrine effects. Licorice contains important saponin-like agents, such as glycyrrhizin, while ginseng contains a group of saponins called ginsenosides.

Sterols

These compounds are precursors of steroids, including ergosterol, dihydrotachysterol, and ergocalciferol, which are part of the vitamin D complex. The important phytosterols are ß-sitosterol, stigmasterol, and campesterol; they are found in popular sources such as olive oil and soy. They may reduce low-density lipoproteins and lower serum cholesterol. Similar sterol combinations in ginseng are credited with adaptogenic properties. Other phytosterol benefits that are claimed include anti-inflammatory properties, immune enhancement, anti-cancer activity, antioxidant effects, and reduction of prostatism symptoms.

Tannins

These polyphenolic compounds have an astringent effect, and can precipitate proteins in the tanning process that produces leather. Many tannins can be classified as glycosides, while others are classified as complex tannins or as pseudotannins. Hydrolyzable tannins release gallic acid, while nonhydrolysable or condensed tannins are proanthocyanidins and anthocyanins. These products have been strongly promoted as potent antioxidants that have a wide range of properties, although adequate evidence for clinical benefits is lacking. Galls (wasp-induced pathologic growths) from a variety of plants contain tannic acid (gallotanic acid or tannin), which is used as a dermal astringent. Tannins are also found in oak (quebracho), hawthorn, rhatany, witch hazel, and tea.

Terpenes

Terpenoid compounds are made up of 5-carbon isoprene units, which are synthesized from acetyl-CoA. They are among the most common phytochemicals, comprising over 20,000 structures, and they are the most varied in structure. They occur commonly in green vegetables, soy, and grains, and many have antioxidant properties. The prototype of this class is pinene, which characterizes the turpentine of pine oil. The low-molecular-weight monoterpenes and sesquiterpenes are volatile, and many are found in the odorous essential oils of plants (Table 8). The most important of the terpenes are 40-carbon atom tetraterpenes that encompass the large group of over 600 carotenoid pigments, which are antioxidants and vitamins.

Other Phytochemicals

Numerous other classes of compounds are recognized in plants, and many may have a role in phytomedicines (Table 9). Many are toxic and could be considered as poisons. Some of these are used in aromatherapy, but they should not be ingested; if they are ingested, due care must be exercised to avoid excessive dosing (e.g. thujone, pulegone).

Antioxidants

Many foods and most popular spices possess antioxidant properties. Antioxidants are also present in many herbal remedies and nutraceuticals, including ashwagandha, astragalus, bilberry, cat's claw, chapparal, co-enzyme Q10, cordyceps, ginkgo, ginsengs, grapeseed, green tea, guava, gymnema, horehound, huperzine A,

Table 8. Terpenoids

Classes	Examples	Sources	Properties
Monoterpenes (including iridoids, which are lactones; many are essential oils)	cineole pinenes terpinenes	spices pine coriander	essential oil voltaile essences carminatives
Sequiterpenes (including lactones; many are essential oils)	artemesin caryophyllene zingiberene	wormwood clove ginger	antimalarial essential oil essential oil
Diterpenes (non-volatile, very variable structures)	balsams capsianosides forskolin ginkgolides taxol marrubin	conifers capsicum coleus ginkgo yew horehound	resins counterirritants bronchospasmolytic anti-inflammatories anticancer bitter
Triterpenes (including steroids, saponins, and phytosterols)	digitoxin (glycoside) ergosterol (saponin)	foxglove yeast	heart failure provitamin D
Tetraterpenes (including carotenoids and xanthophylls)	carotene lycopene	carrot tomato	antioxidant anticancer
Polyterpenes (complex molecules)	rubber	rubber tree	non-drug
Meroterpenes (partial terpenes)	vincristine tetrahydro-cannabinol	periwinkle marijuana	anticancer anti-nauseant

kelp, kudzu, milk thistle, mullein, oats, Oregon grape, pycnogenol, red yeast rice, reishi mushroom, schisandra, and scullcap. The extreme popularity of these herbal agents justifies special consideration of their chemical classifications and properties. The body relies on its own antioxidant defenses to inactivate excessive oxidants that are produced during metabolic processes, inflammatory disorders, and responses to infections. The highly "reactive oxygen species" include several important free radicals: superoxide anions, hydroxyl radicals, and hydrogen peroxide. These agents, and other oxidants entering the body in the diet and through smoking, can damage cell membranes, release proteolytic enzymes, alter protein linkages, and damage DNA. Such processes, when

Table 9. Some Common Phytochemical Classes

Classes	Chemical Structure	Occurrence/Properties
Acids	May be saturated or unsaturated	Widespread (e.g., citric, malic, oxalic, tartaric acids)
Alcohols	May be free or combined as esters with one or more hydroxyl groups	Found widely: volatile oils (e.g., geraniol), balsams (e.g., cinnamyl alcohol, glycerol)
Amino Acids	Free molecules; basic units of peptides and proteins	Nitrogen reserve of plants; important in nutrition
Bitters	Members of bioflavonoid, glycosides, and terpene classes	Distinguished by taste (e.g., gentian, wormwood)
Enzymes	Proteins which act as catalysts	Important in garlic (alliinase), mustard (myrosinase), etc.
Esters	Combination of alcohols and acids	Widely dispersed in volatile oils, balsams, etc. (e.g., linalyl acetate, benzyl benzoate)
Fats/Lipids	Glycerides of fatty acids (i.e., carboxylic acids)	Various oils (e.g., olive, palm, castor, soy)
Fatty Acids	Esters of glycerol; may be saturated or unsaturated	Found in oils, resins and waxes (e.g., myristic, linoleic, palmitic)
Furanocoumarins	Derivatives of coumarin; furanochromones are related	Widely distributed (e.g., psoralens, khellin, vasaka)
Glucosilonates (Thioclycosides)	Glycosides containing nitrogen and sulfur, such as isothiocyanates	Pungent agents of vegetables and some flowers (e.g., mustard, garlic, radish, nasturtium)
Iridoids	Monoterpenes	Bitter agents (e.g., chicory, quassia)
Lignans	Derived from condensation of two units of phenylpropane	Active principles of mayapple, milk thistle, schizandra, etc.
Mucilages/Gums	Acidic polysaccharides derived from uronic acid	Hygroscopic agents, used as demulcents and bulk laxatives (e.g., marshmallow, psyllium, flax, slippery elm)

(Table continued on next page.)

Table 9. Some Common Phytochemical Classes *(Cont.)*

Classes	Chemical Structure	Occurrence/Properties
Peptides	Derived from amino acids; subunits of proteins	Include agents that are antibiotics, hormones, and antioxidants
Phenols	Simple hydroxy substitutions of benzene ring	Caustics, antiseptics (e.g., phenol, salicylic acid, thymol)
Phytoestrogens	Members of bioflavonoid (especially isoflavones) and lignan classes	Mainly estrogenic activity (e.g., genistein)
Polysaccharides	Polymers of sugar and uronic acid	Present in mushrooms, aloe, etc. (e.g., acemannan)
Vitamins	Essential agents in human nutrition	Include antioxidants (A, C, E); some are "medicinal" (e.g., vitamin C has antihistaminic activity)

acting for prolonged periods, can hasten aging processes, tissue damage, heart disease, and cancers.

Although herbal antioxidants (Table 10) are vigorously promoted in a variety of forms to neutralize the potentially harmful reactive oxidant species, their value as supplements has not been adequately established. Many of the deduced health benefits of antioxidants are based on demographic correlations between diet and disease; however, such studies do not prove a cause-and-effect relationship. There is a concern that many antioxidant products have never had their clinical value determined by careful scientific studies; many claims are based on inappropriate extrapolation of *in vitro* evidence or overreaction to preliminary human investigations. Some studies have even suggested that antioxidants could be harmful: beta-carotene supplementation has been associated with increased lung cancer risk in smokers; vitamin E supplements have been associated with a higher incidence of bladder cancer; and large amounts of vitamin C may also increase the risk of cancers.

Supplemental antioxidants may be no more beneficial than a correctly balanced, normal diet that includes natural antioxidants in fruits and vegetables. Indeed, the uncertain state of the role of antioxidants suggests that the recommended nutritious diet of health-conscious people is not only at least as effective as commercial antioxidant supplements, but may prove to be safer.

Table 10. Major Herbal Antioxidants*

Classes	Examples of Antioxidants	Typical Herbal Sources
Vitamins	A (carotenoids)	tomato (lycopene), carrot, (carotenes)
	C (ascorbic acid)	capsicums, citrus fruits
	E (tocophenols)	spinach, brocolli, nuts
	B group (B_2, B_3, B_6)	yeasts, cereals, green vegetables
Bioflavonoids	isoflavonoids (phytoestrogens)	soy (daidzein, genistein), beans
	proanthocyanidins	pine (pycnogenol), grape (resveratrol)
	quercetin	colored fruits
Organosulfurs	allicin	garlic, onions, leeks, chives
Metals	selenium	cereals, garlic
Ubiquinol	reduced co-enzyme Q10	leafy vegetables
Coumarins	lactones of 2-hydroxy-cinnamic acid	carrots, celery, beets, citrus fruits
Lignans	phenylpropanoids	milk thistle (silymarin)
Polyphenols	catechins	green tea, red wine, nuts spices
Phenolics	flavonols	wine, grapefruit, carrots, nuts, grains
Saponins	glycosides	beans, legumes, licorice (glycyrrhizin)
Terpenoids	ginkgolides	ginkgo
Curcuminoids	curcumin	turmeric

* The most potent antioxidant foods include, in descending order, tea, prune, raisin, blueberry, blackberry, strawberry, raspberry, garlic, kale, spinach, brussel sprout, plum, alfalfa sprout, brocolli floret, beet, orange, red grape, red pepper, cherry, kiwi, grapefruit, white grape, bell pepper, onion. (Data from Cao G, Sofic E, Prior RL: Antioxidant capacity of tea and common vegetables. J Agric Food Chem 1996;44: 3426–3431.)

references

1. Bruneton J. Pharmacognosy, Phytochemistry, Medicinal Plants. Secaucus, NY, Lavoisier Publishing Inc., 1995.
2. Chevallier A. The Encyclopedia of Medicinal Plants. London, Dorling Kindersley, 1996.
3. Crouteau R, Kutchan TM, Lewis HG. Natural products (Secondary metabolites). In Buchanan BB, Grusheim W, Jones RL (eds): Biochemistry and Molecular Biology of Plants. Rockville, MD, American Society of Plants Physiologists, 2000.
4. Dewick PM. Medicinal Natural Products. A Biosynthetic Approach. Chichester, England, John Wiley & Sons, 1997.

5. Evans WC. Trease and Evans' Parmacognosy, 14th ed. London, WB Saunders Company Ltd, 1996.
6. Fetrow CW, Avila JR. Professional's Handbook of Complementary and Alternative Medicines. Springhouse, PA, Springhouse Corporation, 1999.
7. Harborne JB, Baxter H, Moss GP. Phytochemical Dictionary. A Handbook of Bioactive Compounds from Plants. London, Taylor & Francis, 1999.
8. Lawless J. The Illustrated Encyclopedia of Essential Oils. New York, Barnes & Noble, 1995.
9. Leung AY, Foster S. Encyclopedia of Common Natural Ingredients Used in Food, Drugs and Cosmetics, 2nd ed. New York, John Wiley & Sons, Inc., 1996.
10. Mills SY. The Essential Book of Herbal Medicine. London, Penguin Books, 1991.
11. Mills S, Bone K. Principles and Practice of Phytotherapy: Modern Herbal Medicine. Edinburgh, Churchill Livingstone, 2000.
12. Robbers JE, Speedie MK, Tyler VE. Pharmacognosy, 8th ed. Philadelphia, Lea & Febiger, 1981.
13. Scott TA, Mercer EL. Concise Encyclopedia. Biochemistry and Molecular Biology, 3rd ed. Berlin, Walter DeGruyter, 1997.
14. Tisserand R, Balacs T. Essential Oil Safety. A Guide for Health Care Professionals. Edinburgh, Churchill Livingstone, 1995.

Websites (Accessed May/June 2001)

http://friedli.com (Flavonoids)

http://www.looneyware.com (Phytochemicals)

http://www.realtime.net/anr (Austin Nutritional Research. Marcia Zimmerman: Nutraceuticals Phytochemicals Phytonutrients—Nutritional Value)

http://www.aspp.org (Biochemistry and Molecular Biology of Plants

Herb-Drug Interactions: Reported Vs. Potential Effects

Herb-drug interactions appear to be much less frequent and less serious than drug-drug interactions. This primarily reflects a weaker pharmacologic profile for herbs compared to their potent pharmaceutical counterparts, but most likely also reflects under-recognition, under-reporting, and less research.[1] Many important plant chemicals are known to interact with drugs, but only a few clinical interactions are proven or well studied. Examples of well-documented and clinically important interactions include vitamin K–rich plants antagonizing warfarin[2,3]; grapefruit juice inhibiting intestinal cytochrome P450 3A4 enzymes to enhance bioavailability of many drugs[4]; and St. John's wort *inducing* the same cytochrome enzyme system to *reduce* bioavailability of drugs.[1] Other herbs with extensively researched pharmacologic constituents or activity include yohimbe, which contains yohimbine, an alpha$_2$-antagonist[5]; ephedra, which contains ephedrine and other alkaloids with alpha- and beta-agonist properties[6]; and licorice, which can inhibit 11-beta-dehydrogenase, thereby causing pseudo-hyperaldosteronism.[7]

All of these pharmacologically active herbs, when given in large-enough doses, are known to interact, or can be predicted to interact, with specific drugs or drug classes. Nevertheless, these well-studied interactions and pharmacologic properties are rarities; in general, there is a dearth of well-documented data in this area, and there are few studies that have specifically evaluated herb-drug interactions in humans.

Problems With the Herb-Drug Interaction Literature

Much of the known information on herb-drug interactions is based on case reports of varying quality. These limited and sometimes anecdotal associations often fail to establish a firm cause-effect relationship. Inconsistencies of product formulations, combinations of herbs, and poor quality control (leading to adulteration or contamination) also limit the conclusions and generalizations that can be derived. Nevertheless, case reports can warn of possible interactions (especially when multiple reports are published that help to confirm an association) that merit further study.

Many authors in the herbal and medical literature have extrapolated conclusions from *in vitro*, animal, or other experimental studies. Such indirect data of toxic reactions should be considered preliminary or speculative "potential interactions," because most of these effects are never proven, and many are controversial. Many potential toxicities or interactions that have become established in the popular herbal or medical literature are difficult to disprove.

For example, St. John's wort was initially declared to interact with monoamine oxidase inhibitor (MAOI) drugs based on weak *in vitro* data[8]; however, as yet there have been no reported cases. In Germany, echinacea has been considered a potent immunostimulant based on *in vitro* studies, but it has never been reported to adversely interact with any medical therapy or disease.[9] Other herbs inhibit platelet aggregation in *in vitro* experiments (e.g., feverfew, ginger, turmeric, clove), but there are no reports of hemorrhagic effects or interactions with anticoagulant or antiplatelet drugs.

Many potential adverse outcomes or toxicities listed in herbal texts, having been extrapolated from *in vitro* or animal studies, are not described in the appropriate context. An extensive review on herb-drug interactions that was published in a peer-reviewed journal contained many such overgeneralizations, inappropriate extrapolations, and even inaccuracies (e.g., suggestions about hormonal effects of saw palmetto or hepatotoxic properties of echinacea).[10] Without clearly distinguishing the theoretical from the well-documented, the media reported on this information without placing the preliminary data in a proper context.[11,12] In contrast to case reports, which are clinically applicable but cannot prove causality, *in vitro* and animal experiments can demonstrate causality—but may not be clinical applicable.

Pharmacologic Effects and Interactions of Herbs

Numerous herbal medicines have potential pharmacologic activity, and therefore may also interact with pharmaceutical drugs, although there is very little clinical evidence of such interactions. Many common plants used as foods or spices are included in published lists. Alleged pharmacologic properties are often based on traditional experience with the plant, or are indirectly extrapolated from *in vitro* or animal experiments (which are not necessarily transferable to humans), or are based on unsubstantiated reports and observations.

Although many plants contain alkaloids and other active constituents, the pharmacologically significant effects of common food plants or herbal medicines are usually weak or nonexistent, and are unlikely to cause harmful drug or disease interactions. Nevertheless, interactions or effects can be significant in susceptible patients or specific situations, especially with toxic or pharmacologically potent plants. Adverse interactions with potent medicinal herbal products (especially with a large dose or in a susceptible patient) are occasionally observed.

The clinical result of a specific interaction may be harmful, neutral, or beneficial. An herb used to lower blood sugar may interact with anti-diabetes drugs, adding to the hypoglycemic effect. This would usually be considered beneficial for most diabetics (to help improve blood glucose levels), but could potentially be harmful in labile or tightly controlled patients, as it could cause hypoglycemia. Most herbs classified in herbal texts as hypoglycemic or hyperglycemic, hypotensive or hypertensive, sedating or stimulating, immunostimulating or immunosuppressive, anticoagulant or coagulant, etc. lack adequate clinical evidence to support these potential effects. The actual clinical effects of the vast majority of such "active" herbs may be very weak or have no effect at all in usual oral doses, and they are unlikely to cause clinically significant interactions. In many texts, opposing actions (such as sedating and stimulating) are ascribed to individual herbs without explanation, presumably because neither of the contrasting effects has been authenticated.

Mechanisms of Herb-Drug Interactions

Herbs and drugs usually interact in two general ways: pharmacokinetically and pharmacodynamically. **Pharmacokinetic interactions** result in alterations of an agent's absorption, distribution, metabolism, or elimination—quantitatively increasing or decreasing the amount that becomes effective in the body. **Pharmacodynamic interactions** alter the way the herb or drug affects a target tissue, organ system, receptor, etc. These latter interactions can affect drug actions qualitatively, usually enhancing or antagonizing the drug's properties, but they may also have indirect effects (e.g., an herb that increases potassium excretion can increase the risk of digoxin toxicity). Outcomes will also vary considerably based on the herb's route of administration, the portion of the herb used (e.g., root, leaf, or flower), the dose or concentration, and the patient's individual tolerance.

Reports in Humans

Not all detrimental or unexpected interactions reported in humans are generalizable, as causality (especially from case reports) is difficult to prove. In the following table of reported clinical interactions, they are rated as likely (√√√), possible (√√), or doubtful (√), based on the cited literature. For further details and discussion of these interactions, good reviews are available.[13–20] "Potential" interactions based on preliminary *in vitro* and animal studies, traditional usage or anecdotes, and hypotheses are excluded. (Many of these preliminary or potential interactions are addressed in the following section. Note that we include primarily Western herbs; objective data for most Asiatic or other ethnic herbal traditions is less well documented.)

Herb-Drug Interactions Reported in Humans*

Herb and Drug	Effect on Drug or Patient	Type of Evidence and Rating; Comments
Betel nut (*Areca catechu*)		
Asthma drugs	Decreases asthma control	Case report and small clinical study[1] [√√]
Phenothiazines	Extrapyramidal effects	Case report[2]; betel nut contains arecoline, a cholinergic alkaloid [√√]
Capsicum (cayenne) pepper† (*Capsicum annuum*)		
ACE inhibitors	Increased cough	Case report (topical capsaicin)[3] [√√]
Theophylline (sustained release)	Increased absorption	Controlled clinical study (highly spiced meal with cayenne)[4] [√√√]
Danshen (*Salvia miltiorrhiza*)		
Warfarin	Increased INR	Case reports, and decreased warfarin metabolism in animal study[5] [√√√]
Devil's Claw† (*Harpagophytum procumbens*)		
Warfarin	Purpura/enhanced effect	Case report (no details)[6] [√]
Dong quai† (*Angelica sinensis*)		
Warfarin	Increased INR, bruising	Case reports[7,8] [√√]
Ephedra† (*Ephedra sinica*)		*Sympathomimetic stimulant*
Phenelzine (MAOI)	Severe MAOI toxicity	Case reports (with ephedrine)[9]; expected pharmacologic effect [√√√]

(Table continued on next page.)

Herb-Drug Interactions Reported in Humans* *(Continued)*

Herb and Drug	Effect on Drug or Patient	Type of Evidence and Rating; Comments
Fenugreek† *(Trigonella foenum-graecum)* and boldo *(Peumus boldus)*		
Warfarin	Increased INR	Case report (herbs used together)[10] [√√]
Fiber *(supplements and dietary)*		
Digoxin *(w/guar gum, others)*	Slight decrease/delay in absorption	Controlled clinical studies (depends on fiber type)[11–14] [√√]
Glyburide *(w/gluco-mannan)*	Decreased/delayed absorption	Controlled clinical study[15] [√√]
Lithium *(w/psyllium)*	Decreased serum level	Case report[17] [√]
Lovastatin *(w/pectin, oat bran)*	Decreased effect	Case series[18] [√√]
Metformin *(w/guar gum)*	Decreased absorption	Controlled clinical study[19] [√√]
Penicillin V *(w/guar gum)*	Decreased absorption	Controlled clinical study[20] [√√]
Tricyclic antidepressants *(w/bran, oats, other dietary fibers)*	Decreased absorption	Case series[21] [√√]
Iron (w/bran, psyllium)	Decreased absorption	Controlled clinical study[16] [√√]
Garlic† *(Allium sativum)*		*May have antiplatelet effects*
Warfarin	Increased INR	Case report (no details)[22] [√]
Ginkgo† *(Ginkgo biloba)*		*May have antiplatelet effects*
Aspirin, warfarin	Bleeding	Case reports[23,24] [√√]
Thiazide diuretic	Antihypertensive effect counteracted	Case report[6] [√]
Trazodone	Enhanced sedation	Case report[25] [√√]
Ginseng, Asian† *(Panax ginseng)*		
Phenelzine (MAOI)	Headache, tremor, mania	Case reports[26,27] [√√]
Warfarin	Decreased INR	Case report[28]; no effect in animal model[29] [√√]
Ginseng, Siberian† *(Eleutherococcus senticosus)*		
Digoxin	Increased digoxin level in assay (no toxicity)	Case report[30]; probably due to contamination with another herb[31] [√]
Grapefruit juice	Increases drug bio-availability (inhibits intestinal CYP3A4)	Clinical studies[32] [√√√]; *may enhance absorption of many drugs‡*
Amiodarone[33]		
Artemether (antimalarial)[32]		
Benzodiazepine (esp. diazepam, midazolam, triazolam)[32]		
Calcium antagonists (esp. dihydropoyridines such as felodipine)[32]		
Carbamazepine[32]		
Cisapride[32]		
Cyclosporin[32]		
Ethinyl estradiol[32]		
Psychiatric drugs (esp. buspirone, clomipramine, sertraline)[32]		
Saquinivir[32]		
Statins (esp. atorvastatin, lovastatin, simvastatin)[32]		

(Table continued on next page.)

Herb and Drug	Effect on Drug or Patient	Type of Evidence and Rating; Comments
Kava[†] *(Piper methysticum)*		
Alprazolam/cimetidine/ terazosin	Severe disorientation	Case report (pt taking all 3 drugs)[34] [√√]
Levodopa	Extrapyramidal-like effects	Case reports[35] [√√]
Licorice[†] *(Glycyrrhiza glabra)*		
Antihypertensive drugs	Decreased effect	Chronic high doses can cause pseudohyperaldosteronism[36–38] [√√√]
Diuretics	Exacerbate K+ loss, myopathy	Case reports (high doses)[39] [√√√]
Prednisolone	Increased drug level (decreases metabolism)	Clinical study with glycyrrhizin[40] [√√√]
Papaya extract[†] *(Carica papaya)*		
Warfarin	Increased INR	Case report (few details)[6] [√]
Shankhapusphi (Ayurvedic herbal combination)		
Phenytoin	Decreased serum level; loss of seizure control	Case report and animal study[41] [√√√]
St. John's wort[†] *(Hypercium perforatum)*		*May enhance CYP3A4 metabolism of many drugs*
Amitriptyline	Decreased serum level	Clinical study[42] [√√]
Anaesthetic, general	Hypotension	Case report[43] [√√]
Cyclosporin	Decreased serum level; transplant rejections	Case series and reports[44,45] [√√√]
Digoxin	Decreased serum level	Controlled clinical study[46] [√√√]
Indinavir	Decreased serum level	Clinical study[47] [√√√]
Oral contraceptives	Decreased effect	Case reports (no details)[48,49] [√√]
SSRI antidepressants	Mild serotonin syndrome	Case reports[50–52] [√√]
Theophylline	Decreased serum level	Case report[53] [√√]
Warfarin	Decreased effect	Case reports (no details)[49,50] [√√]
Tamarind *(Tamarindus indica)*		
Aspirin	Increased absorption	Controlled clinical study (highly spiced meal with tamarind)[54] [√√√]
Yohimbe[†] *(Pausinystalia yohimbe)*		*Sympathomimetic stimulant*
Clonidine	Antagonizes effects	Case reports,[55] expected pharmacologic effect[56] [√√√]
Tricyclic anti- depressants	Enhanced autonomic and central effects of yohimbine	Case series and clinical studies[55] [√√√]

Level of evidence rating: √√√ = likely interaction; convincing reports or well studied

√√ = possible interaction; reports or studies need validation

√ = doubtful interaction; poorly evaluated or documented

* Apart from dietary fiber and grapefruit juice, reports of drug interactions with other plant products that are generally not used as herbal medicines (e.g., coffee, tobacco, alcohol), are not included here.

† For further details, see the individual evaluations in this book.

‡ See reference 32 for important potential drug interactions with grapefruit juice

MAOI = Monoamine Oxidase Inhibitor; INR = International Normalized Ratio; CPY3A4 = 3A4 isozyme of cytochrome P450.

"Potential" Effects & Interactions

The following compilation of potential pharmacologic effects and interactions is culled from general herbal texts and resources. It is not an evidenced-based summary, and annotations are designed to place these potential effects in perspective. Herbs, irrespective of their botanical parts, are listed by their common name.

Herbs That May Affect Absorption of Other Drugs

Tannin-containing herbs[1,2,4,9]:

Tannins are broadly distributed throughout the plant kingdom. They can complex with proteins, resulting in an astringent effect on skin or mucous membranes. Herbs with high tannin content can precipitate neuroleptic or alkaloid drugs and metal ions *in vitro*. Although herbs with high tannin content may decrease absorption or effects of these agents *in vivo*, clinical interactions have not been documented. Tannic acid, a specific extract found in certain tannin-containing herbs, can be a gastrointestinal irritant when taken in large amounts, and this may limit the intake of such herbs.

Examples: Agrimony, bayberry, betel nut, bilberry, black walnut, blackberry, eucalyptus, guarana, horse chestnut, oak, pomegranate, raspberry, rhubarb, sorrel, Spanish chestnut, St. John's wort, tea (black, green, oolong), uva ursi, witch hazel, white willow, yellow dock, yerba maté

High fiber (mucilage) herbs[1,4,9]:

Herbs that contain water-soluble hydrocolloidal fiber (forming a mucilage or gel) can theoretically impair absorption of many different drugs. A few interactions have been documented in humans (see table). These herbs are often utilized as bulk-forming laxatives.

Examples: Acacia (gum arabic), algae products (agar, alginate, carageenan), aloe vera gel, fenugreek, flax, guar gum, karaya, marshmallow, oats (and other cereals), okra, pectin, psyllium (ispaghula), quince, slippery elm, tragacanth

Cathartic herbs[1–4]:

Most stimulant laxative herbs contain anthranoids, particularly anthraquinone glycosides, which stimulate colonic peristalsis, and thus may reduce absorption of other drugs by reducing gut transit time. Laxative abuse can lead to hypokalemia and other electrolyte disturbances that can result in interactions with drugs such as digoxin.

Examples: Aloe vera juice/latex, buckthorn, cascara, castor seed oil, frangula, mayapple, rhubarb, senna, yellow dock.

Herbs That May Interfere With Coagulation

Antiplatelet herbs[1–3,10–12]:

Many herbs have been reported to inhibit platelet aggregation *in vitro*; several common spices (e.g., allspice, basil, marjoram, tarragon, thyme, turmeric) have this property. However, other than case reports for garlic and ginkgo, there are no reports of significant bleeding properties when these herbs are orally administered. Health professionals may wish to check bleeding times for patients at high risk of bleeding (e.g., taking warfarin, preop for surgery).

Examples: Asian ginseng, bromelain, cayenne, Chinese skullcap, cinchona, clove, danshen, feverfew, garlic, ginger, ginkgo, licorice, onion, salicylate- or salicin-containing herbs (black cohosh, European aspen, meadowsweet, poplar, sweet birch, willow, wintergreen), papaya/papain, reishi mushroom, turmeric

Coumarin-containing herbs[1,3,10,11,13,14]:

Coumarin-containing plants are often considered to enhance the effects of anticoagulant or antiplatelet drugs. However, coumarin (1, 2-benzopyrone, which is not an anticoagulant) and many coumarin derivatives (a large class of over 1300 natural chemicals) have been confused by herbalists and orthodox health professionals with the semi-synthetic drug Coumadin or warfarin. One particular mold converts a specific coumarin compound in alfalfa (4-hydroxycoumarin) to the anticoagulant bishydroxycoumarin (dicoumarol); this is the cause of bleeding in cattle grazing on moldy alfalfa hay (sweet clover). Anticoagulant effects occurring with the numerous other coumarin-containing plants are unlikely. Dong quai has been reported to interact with warfarin (see table page 48 and the individual herb evaluation), but it is not known if the mechanism is based on the potential coumarin constituents. Health professionals may wish to monitor the PT/INR more closely in patients taking warfarin who start or discontinue these herbs, but interactions are not expected.

Examples: Alfalfa, anise, arnica, buchu, celery, chamomile, dong quai, fenugreek, horse chestnut bark, horseradish, licorice, lovage, meadowsweet, nettle, passion flower, parsley, prickley ash, quassia, red clover, reishi mushroom, rue, sweet clover, tonka bean, vanilla, wild lettuce

Vitamin K-rich plants[1]:

These plants, mostly green leafy vegetables, may diminish the anticoagulant effects of warfarin, especially when consumed habitually.

Examples: Alfalfa, beet, cruciferous vegetables (broccoli, brussel sprout, cabbage, collard, kale, turnip), green tea, lettuce, nettle, parsley, plantain, shepherd's purse, spinach, sunflower, watercress

Herbs With Other Purported Effects

Diuretic herbs[3,7,15–17]:

This property is primarily based on traditional usage or animal experiments. Diuretic herbs may potentially deplete potassium, while "aquaretic" herbs are said to enhance water elimination without depleting electrolytes. However, with the possible exception of caffeine-containing plants, there is little evidence that any of these herbs have significant diuretic-type effects in humans.

Examples: Agrimony, artichoke, asparagus, birch, blackcurrant, borage, buchu, burdock, caffeine-containing herbs (cocoa bean, coffee seed, cola seed, guarana, maté, tea - black, green, oolong), celery, corn silk, couch grass, dandelion, elderberry, ephedra/ma huang, goldenrod, gravel root, horsetail, juniper berry, kidney bean, licorice, lovage, nettle, parsley, pokeroot, sassafras, Scotch broom, squill, uva ursi, yarrow

Hypertensive herbs[3,18]:

Herbs known to contain sympathomimetics (ephedra, yohimbe) or caffeine, especially in large doses, may increase blood pressure and counteract antihypertensive drugs. All the other herbs in this list are primarily supported on the basis of animal experiments, often with large parenteral doses.

Examples: Asian ginseng, bayberry, blue cohosh, caffeine-containing herbs (cocoa bean, coffee seed, cola seed, guarana, maté, black and green tea), capsicum, coltsfoot, ephedra/ma huang, ginger, goldenseal, licorice, Scotch broom (contains tyramine), vervain, yohimbe

Hypotensive herbs[3,4,18,19]:

Apart from Indian snakeroot (containing rauwolfia alkaloids) and garlic, these herbs are classified as having hypotensive effects based on traditional usage or animal experiments.

Examples: Asian ginseng, agrimony, black cohosh, calamus, celery, cornsilk, devil's claw, fenugreek, garlic, ginger, goldenseal, green helebore, hawthorn, horseradish, Indian snakeroot, mistletoe, nettle, olive leaf, parsley, plantain, poke root, prickly ash, reishi mushroom, sage, Siberian ginseng, squill, St. John's wort, vervain, wild carrot, yarrrow.

Hypoglycemic herbs[3,20–22]:

Several herbs have shown hypoglycemic potential in clinical trials; American ginseng, bitter melon, fenugreek, gurmar (gymnema), prickly pear and stevia have been best studied, although clinical effects are not conclusively established. More than 400 plants with possible glucose-lowering effects are known. Some are traditionally used for diabetes, while other extracts or chemical constituents have hypoglycemic effects only in animal or *in vitro* studies. Some high-fiber/mucilage herbs (see above) may impair carbohydrate absorption and reduce hyperglycemia in diabetics.

Examples: Agrimony, alfalfa, aloe vera, American ginseng, Asian ginseng, barley sprouts, bilberry, bitter melon, burdock, celery, cinnamon, corn silk, cucumber, cumin, damiana, dandelion, devil's club, elecampine, eucalyptus, fenugreek, fig leaf, garlic, ginger, goat's rue, gurmar (gymnema), hamula, holy basil, horse chestnut seed, jambul, juniper berry, lotus, lupin, Madagascar periwinkle, matarique, mullberry, myrrh, nettle, olive leaf, onion, prickly pear, reishi mushroom, sage, spinach, stevia, sweet broom, tansy

Immunostimulant herbs[3,4]:

These herbs have a reputation of having tonic or immune benefits, or have been reported to cause nonspecific immune stimulation in laboratory tests. Stimulation could theoretically activate autoimmune processes or interfere with immunosupressive drug treatment. However, there are no documented clinical reports of adverse interactions.

Examples: Ashwagandha, astragalus, alfalfa sprouts, boneset, calendula, echinacea, elderberry, ginsengs, licorice, mistletoe, wild indigo

Phytoestrogen herbs[3,4,23,24]:

A number of plants are rich in phytoestrogenic compounds, primarily the isoflavones (e.g., soybeans, red clover) and lignans (e.g., flaxseed), but most have very weak affinity for the estrogen receptor. Anti-estrogen effects are also possible due to competition for estrogen receptors. Clinical effects are difficult to demonstrate. The phytoestrogen effects of most herbs in this list are deduced from traditional usage, *in vitro* or animal experiments, or from case reports.

Examples: Alfalfa, anise, Asian ginseng, black cohosh, bloodroot, chasteberry (Vitex), dong quai, flaxseed, hops, licorice, mandrake, motherwort, pleurisy root, red clover, sheep sorrel, soy, thyme, turmeric, yellow dock, yucca, wild carrot

Sedative herbs[1,3,4]:

Many herbs are traditionally used as mild sedatives, hypnotics, and anxiolytics. Some have effects in animal studies, or bind to the benzodiazepine-GABA receptor complex *in vitro*. With the exception of kava and valerian, few have been documented to have effects in humans at usual oral doses.

Examples: Ashwagandha, black cohosh, bupleureum, catnip, celery, chamomile, couchgrass, elecampine, goldenseal, hops, kava, lavender, lemon balm, marigold, nettle, passion flower, sage, sassafrass, sheperd's purse, Siberian ginseng, skullcap, St. John's wort, valerian, wild carrot, wild lettuce, yerba mansa.

Stimulant herbs[1,2,4]:

Herbs containing sympathomimetics (e.g., ephedra, yohimbe), caffeine, or other constituents can stimulate the cardiovascular and nervous systems, and can potentiate drugs that have similar properties. They may also reduce the effectiveness of antihypertensive, sedative, and anxiolytic drugs. Sympathomimetic herbs can interact with monoamine oxidase inhibitors to cause a hypertensive crisis. In low doses, these herbs are commonly used beverages and stimulants; in large enough doses all of these herbs can cause serious toxicity.

Examples: Caffeine-containing herbs (cocoa bean, coffee seed, cola seed, guarana, maté, black and green tea), ephedra/ma huang, yohimbe, other "hypertensive herbs"

Toxic/poisonous herbs[2,8,25–27]:

Pharmacologically active plants with narrow therapeutic windows (potentially toxic effects at lower doses) are appropriately regarded as poisons rather than medicines. Certain toxic herbs can be used with relative safety in low doses or for short periods, but most herbs that contain the following substances are too toxic to justify being used in herbal therapies.

Examples: Aristolochic acid which causes nephrotoxicity (most Aristolochia plants); atropine and related anticholinergic alkaloids (e.g., nightshades, henbane, mandrake, jimson weed); cardiac glycosides (e.g., false hellebore, foxglove, lily of the valley, oleander, squill) and other cardioactive herbs; cyanogenic glycosides (e.g., apricot, bitter almond, and peach pits); emetic herbs (e.g., lobelia, pokeroot); pyrrolidizine alkaloids with hepatotoxic unsaturated necine bases (e.g., borage leaf, coltsfoot, comfrey, life root) and other hepatotoxic herbs (e.g., chaparral, germander, pennyroyal oil); thujone which causes neurotoxicity (e.g., wormwood oil).

references for pages 45–48

1. Ernst E. Herb-drug interactions: potentially important but woefully under-researched. Eur J Clin Pharmacol 2000;56:523–524.

2. Walker FB. Myocardial infarction after diet-induced warfarin resistance. Arch Intern Med 1984;144:2089–2090.

3. Pedersen FM, Hamberg O, Hess K, Ovesen L. The effect of dietary vitamin K on warfarin-induced anticoagulation. J Intern Med 1991;229:517–520.

4. Kane GC, Lipsky JJ. Drug-grapefruit juice interactions. Mayo Clin Proc 2000:75:933–942.

5. Hoffman BB, Lefkowitz RJ. Catecholamines, sympathomimetic drugs, and adrenergic receptor antagonists. In Hardman JG, Limbird LE (eds): Goodman & Gilman's The Pharmacological Basis of Therapeutics, 9th ed. NY, McGraw-Hill, 1996, Chapter 10, pp. 199–248.

6. Ziment I. Respiratory Pharmacology and Therapeutics. Philadelphia, WB Saunders Company, 1978.

7. Walker BR, Edwards CRW. Licorice-induced hypertension and syndromes of apparent mineralocorticoid excess. Endocrinol Metab Clin N Am 1994;23: 359–377.

8. Nathan PJ. The experimental and clinical pharmacology of St John's wort (*Hypericum perforatum* L.). Molec Psych 1999;4:333–338.

9. Blumenthal M, Goldberg A, Brinckmann J (eds). Herbal Medicine: Expanded Commission E Monographs. Newton, MA, Integrative Medicine Communications, 2000.

10. Miller L. Herbal medicinals: selected clinical considerations focusing on known or potential drug-herb interactions. Arch Intern Med 1998;158:2200–2211.
11. Fugh-Berman A. Herbal medicinals: selected clinical considerations, focusing on known or potential drug-herb interactions. Arch Intern Med 1999;159: 1957–1958 (letter).
12. Awang D, Fugh-Berman A. Myths and mistakes about herb-drug interactions. Alternative Therapies in Women's Health, May 1999.
13. Fugh-Berman A. Herb-drug interactions. Lancet 2000;355:134–138.
14. Griffin JP, D'Arcy PF. A Manual of Adverse Drug Interactions. Amsterdam, Elsevier, 1997.
15. DeSmet PAGM, D'Arcy PF. Drug interactions with herbal and other non-orthodox remedies. In D'Arcy PF, McElnay JC, Welling PG (eds). Mechanisms of Drug Interactions (Handbook of Experimental Pharmacology, Vol. 122). Berlin, Springer, 1996, pp. 327–352.
16. Pennachio DL, Cott J, Fugh-Berman AJ, Rakel D. Drug-herb interactions: how vigilant should you be? Patient Care 2000(Oct. 15):41–69.
17. Lambrecht JE, Hamilton W, Rabinovich A. A review of herb-drug interactions: documented and theoretical. US Pharmacist 2000;(August):42–53.
18. Brinker F. Herb Contraindications and Drug Interactions, 2nd ed. Sandy, Oregon, Eclectic Medical Publications, 1998.
19. Vaes LPJ, Chyka PA. Interactions of warfarin with garlic, ginger, ginkgo, or ginseng: nature of the evidence. Ann Pharmacother 2000;34:1478–1482.
20. Heck AM, Dewitt, BA, Lukes AL. Potential interactions between alternative therapies and warfarin. Am J Health-Syst Pharm 2000;57:1221–1230.

references for table (pp 48–50)

1. Taylor RFH, Al-Jarad N, John LME, et al. Betel-nut chewing and asthma. Lancet 1992;339:11341136.
2. Deahl M. Betel nut-induced extrapyramidal syndrome: An unusual drug interaction. Movement Disord 1989;4:330–333.
3. Hakas JF Jr. Topical capsaicin induces cough in patient receiving ACE inhibitor. Ann Allergy 1990;65:322–323.
4. Bouraoui A, Toumi A, Bouchacha S, et al. Influence de l'alimentation épicée et piquante sur l'absorption de la théophylline [Influence of spiced and pungent food on the absorption and bioavailablility of theophylline]. Therapie 1986;41:467–471.
5. Chan TYK. Interaction between warfarin and danshen (Salvia miltiorrhiza). Ann Pharmacother 2001;35:501–504.
6. Shaw D, Leon C, Kolev S, Murray V. Traditional remedies and food supplements: a 5-year toxicological study (1991–1995). Drug Safety 1997;17: 342–356.
7. Page RL, Lawrence JD. Potentiation of warfarin by dong quai. Pharmacother 1999;19:870–876.
8. Ellis GR, Stephens MR. Untitled (photograph and brief case report). BMJ 1999;319:650.
9. Dawson JK, Earnshaw SM, Graham CS. Dangerous monoamine oxidase inhibitor interactions are still occurring in the 1990s. J Accident Emerg Med 1995;12:49-51.
10. Lambert JP, Cormier J. Potential interaction between warfarin and boldo-fenugreek. Pharmacother 2001;21:509–512.

11. Brown DD, Juhl RP, Warner SL. Decreased bioavailability of digoxin produced by dietary fiber and cholestyramine. Am J Cardiol 1977;39:297 (Abstract).

12. Kasper H, Zilly W, Fassl H, Fehle F. The effect of dietary fiber on postprandial serum digoxin concentration in man. Am J Clin Nutr 1979;32:2436–2438.

13. Lembecke B, Häsler K, Kramer P, et al. Plasma digoxin concentrations during administration of dietary fibre (guar gum) in man. Z Gastroenterol 1982; 20:164–167.

14. Reissell P, Manninen V. Effect of administration of activated charcoal and fibre on absorption, excretion and steady state blood levels of digoxin and digitoxin. Evidence for intestinal secretion of the glycosides. Acta Med Scand 1982;668(Suppl):88–90.

15. Rossander L. Effect of dietary fiber on iron absorption in man. Scand J Gastroenterol 1987;22(Suppl.129):68–72.

16. Shima K, Tanaka A, Ikegami H, et al. Effect of dietary fiber, glucomannan, on absorption of sulfonylurea in man. Horm Metabol Res 1983;15:1–3.

17. Perlman BB. Interaction between lithium salts and ispaghula husk. Lancet 1990;335:416.

18. Richter WO, Jacob BG, Schwandt P. Interaction between fibre and lovastatin. Lancet 1991;338:706.

19. Gin H, Orgerie MB, Aubertin J. The influence of guar gum on absorption of metformin from the gut in healthy volunteers. Horm Metabol Res 1989;21: 81–83.

20. Huupponen R, Seppälä P, Iisalo E. Effect of guar gum, a fibre preparation, on digoxin and penicillin absorption in man. Eur J Clin Pharmacol 1984;26: 279–281.

21. Stewart DE. High-fiber diet and serum tricyclic antidepressant levels. J Clin Psychopharmacol 1992;12:438–440.

22. Sunter W. Warfarin and garlic. Pharmaceut J 1991;246:722.

23. Rosenblatt M, Mindel J. Spontaneous hyphema associated with ingestion of Ginkgo biloba extract. N Engl J Med 1997; 336:1108.

24. Matthews MK. Association of Ginkgo biloba with intracerebral hemorrhage. Neurology 1998;50:1933-1934.

25. Galluzzi S, Zanetti O, Binetti G, et al. Coma in a patient with Alzheimer's disease taking low dose trazodone and Ginkgo biloba. J Neurol Neurosurg Psych 2000;68:679–680.

26. Shader RI, Greenblatt DJ. Phenelzine and the dream machine—ramblings and reflections. J Clin Psychopharmacol 1985;5:65.

27. Jones BD, Runikis AM. Interaction of ginseng with phenelzine. J Clin Psychopharmacol 1987;7:201–202.

28. Janetzky K, Morreale AP. Probable interaction between warfarin and ginseng. Am J Health-Syst Pharm. 1997;54:692–693.

29. Zhu M, Chan KW, Ng LS, et al. Possible influences of ginseng on the pharmacokinetics and pharmacodynamics of warfarin in rats. J Pharm Pharmacol 1999;51:175–180.

30. McRae S. Elevated serum digoxin levels in a patient taking digoxin and Siberian ginseng. Can Med Assoc J 1996;155:293–295.

31. Awang DVC. Siberian ginseng toxicity may be case of mistaken identity. Can Med Assoc J 1996;155:1237.

32. Kane GC, Lipsky JJ. Drug-grapefruit juice interactions. Mayo Clin Proc 2000;75:933–942.

33. Libersa CC, Brique SA, Motte KB, et al. Dramatic inhibition of amiodarone metabolism induced by grapefruit juice. Br J Clin Pharmacol 2000;49:373–378.
34. Almeida JC, Grimsley EW. Coma from the health food store: Interaction between kava and alprazolam. Ann Intern Med 1996; 125:940–941.
35. Schelosky L, Raffauf C, Jendroska K, Poewe W. Kava and dopamine antagonism. J Neurol Neurosurg Psych 1995;58:639–640.
36. de Klerk GJ, Nieuwenhuis MG, Beutler JJ. Hypokalaemia and hypertension associated with use of liquorice flavoured chewing gum. BMJ 1997;314:731–732.
37. Chandler RF. *Glycyrrhiza glabra*. In De Smet PAGM, Keller K, Hänsel R, Chandler RF (eds). Adverse Effects of Herbal Drugs. Vol. 3, Berlin, Springer, 1997, pp. 67–87.
38. Walker BR, Edwards CRW. Licorice-induced hypertension and syndromes of apparent mineralocoriticoid excess. Endocrinol Metab Clin North Am 1994; 23:359–377.
39. Shintani S, Murase H, Tsukagoshi H, Shiigai T. Glycyrrhizin (licorice)-induced hypokalemic myopathy: report of 2 cases and review of the literature. Eur Neurol 1992;32:44–51.
40. Chen M-F, Shimada F, Kato H, et al. Effect of oral administration of glycyrrhizin on the pharmacokinetics of prednisolone. Endocrinol Japon 1991;38:167–174.
41. Dandekar UP, Chandra RS, Dalvi SS, et al. Analysis of a clinically important interaction between phenytoin and Shankhapushpi, an ayurvedic preparation. J Ethnopharmacol 1992;35:285–288.
42. Roots I, Johne A, Schmider J, et al. Interaction of a herbal extract from St. John's wort with amitriptyline and its metabolites. Clin Pharmacol Therap 2000;67:159(Abstract).
43. Irefin S, Sprung J. A possible cause of cardiovascular collapse during anesthesia: long-term use of St. John's wort. J Clin Anesth 2000;12:498–499.
44. Breidenbach T, Hoffmann MW, Becker T, et al. Drug interaction of St John's wort with ciclosporin. Lancet 2000;355:1912.
45. Ruschitzka F, Meier PJ, Turina M, et al. Acute heart transplant rejection due to Saint John's wort. Lancet 2000;355:548–549.
46. Johne A, Brockmöller J, Bauer S, et al. Pharmacokinetic interaction of digoxin with an herbal extract from St. John's wort (*Hypericum perforatum*). Clin Pharmacol Ther 1999;66:338–345.
47. Piscitelli SC, Burstein AH, Chaitt D, et al. Indinavir concentrations and St. John's wort. Lancet 2000;355:547–548.
48. Yue Q-Y, Bergquist C, Gerden B. Safety of St John's wort (*Hypericum perforatum*). Lancet 2000;355:576–577.
49. Ernst E. Second thoughts about safety of St John's wort. Lancet 1999;354:2014–2016.
50. Lantz MS, Buchalter E, Giambanco V. St. John's wort and antidepressant drug interactions in the elderly. J Geriatr Psych Neurol 1999;12:7–10.
51. Gordon JB. SSRIs and St. John's wort: possible toxicity? Am Fam Physician 1998;57:950, 953.
52. Prost N, Tichadou L, Rodor F, et al. Interaction millepertuis-venlafaxine [St. John's wort-venlafaxine interaction]. Presse Med 2000;29:1285–1286 [English translation]
53. Nebel A, Schneider BJ, Baker RK, Kroll DJ. Potential metabolic interaction between St. John's wort and theophylline. Ann Pharmacother 1999;33:502.

54. Mustapha A, Yakasai IA, Aguye IA. Effect of *Tamarindus indica* L. on the bioavailability of aspirin in healthy human volunteers. Eur J Drug Metab Pharmacokin 1996;21:223–226.
55. De Smet PAGM. Yohimbe alkaloids—general discussion. In De Smet PAGM (ed): Adverse Effects of Herbal Drugs. Vol. 3. Berlin, Springer, 1997, pp. 181–205.
56. Shannon M. Yohimbine. Ped Emerg Care 2000;16:49–50.

references for "Potential Effects & Interactions" section

1. Brinker F. Herb Contraindications and Drug Interactions. 2nd ed. Sandy, Oregon, Eclectic Medical Publications, 1998.
2. McGuffin M, Hobbs C, Upton R, Goldberg A (eds). American Herbal Products Association's Botanical Safety Handbook. Boca Raton, CRC Press, 1997.
3. Newall CA, Anderson LA, Phillipson JD. Herbal Medicines: A Guide for Health-Care Professionals. London, The Pharmaceutical Press, 1996.
4. Schulz V, Hänsel R, Tyler VE. Rational Phytotherapy. A Physician's Guide to Herbal Medicine, 4th ed. Berlin, Springer, 2001.
5. Blumenthal M. Interactions between herbs and conventional drugs: introductory considerations. HerbalGram 2000;49:52–63.
6. Potential herb-drug interactions. The Review of Natural Products. St. Louis, Facts and Comparisons, Dec. 2000.
7. Blumenthal M (ed). The Complete German Commission E Monographs: Therapeutic Guide to Herbal Medicines. Boston, MA, Integrative Medicine Communications, 1998.
8. Mills S, Bone K. Principles and Practice of Phytotherapy: Modern Herbal Medicine. NY, Churchill Livingstone, 2000.
9. DeSmet PAGM, D'Arcy PF. Drug interactions with herbal and other non-orthodox remedies. In: Mechanisms of Drug Interactions (Handbook of Experimental Pharmacology, Vol. 122). Berlin, Springer, 1996, pp. 327–352.
10. Heck AM, DeWitt BA, Lukes AL. Potential interactions between alternative therapies and warfarin. Am J Health-Syst Pharm 2000;57:1221–1230.
11. Potential Coumadin interactions with herbal products. Information provided by DuPont Pharmaceuticals, December 1999.
12. Okazaki K, Nakayama S, Kawazoe K, Takaishi Y. Antiaggregant effects on human platelets of culinary herbs. Phytother Res 1998;12:603–605.
13. DeSmet PAGM. Toxicological outlook on the quality assurance of herbal remedies. In DeSmet PAGM (ed). Adverse Effects of Herbal Drugs. Vol. 1. Berlin, Springer, 1992, pp 1–72.
14. Hoult JRS, Payá M. Pharmacological and biochemical actions of simple coumarins: natural products with therapeutic potential. Gen Pharmacol 1996; 27:713–722.
15. Roundtree R. Diuretics: herbs or drugs? Herbs for Health 2000;Sept–Oct: 26–27.
16. Heron S, Yarnell E. Recurrent kidney stones: a naturopathic approach. Altern Complement Ther 1998;Feb:60–67.
17. Herbal diuretics. Review of Natural Products. St. Louis, MO, Facts and Comparisons, Nov. 1998.
18. Priya D, Kochar MS. Herbs and hypertension. Veterans Health Syst J 2000;5:58–64.

19. Austin S, Yarnell E, Gaby A, Brown D. Clinical applications of complementary and alternative medicine: hypertension (Part 2: Nutritional supplements and botanicals). Healthnotes Rev Complement Intregr Med 2000;7:151–159.

20. Yarnell E. Southwestern and Asian botanical agents for diabetes mellitus. Altern Complement Ther 2000;Feb:7–11.

21. Brown DJ, Gaby A, Reichert RG, Yarnell E. Phytotherapeutic and nutritional approaches to diabetes mellitus. Quarterly Rev Natural Med 1998;Winter: 329–351.

22. Ernst E. Plants with hypoglycemic activity in humans. Phytomed 1997;4:73–78.

23. Anon. Phytoestrogens. Med Letter 2000;42:17–18.

24. Zava DT, Dollbaum CM, Blen M. Estrogen and progestin bioactivity of foods, herbs, and spices. Proc Soc Exp Biol Med 1998;217:369–378.

25. Ernst E. Harmless herbs? A review of the recent literature. Am J Med 1998;104:170–178.

26. Yarnell E. Misunderstood "toxic" herbs. Alternat Complement Med 1999; Feb:6–11.

27. Yarnell E. Botanical hepatotoxicity: A critical review and update. Healthnotes Rev Complement Integr Med 2000;7:119–124.

II: Herb Evaluations

Introduction

An overwhelming volume of herbal information is available in the medical and popular literature. Although much is biased and confusing, a considerable amount of high-quality data has become available, especially in the last few years. The intent of the following "snapshots" is to provide practicing clinicians with a concise summary of the best evidence-based information available, in a practical and readable format. We obtained this information by searching several online databases (including Medline and the Cochrane Library), scientific herbal medicine textbooks and resources, and reference lists of all articles found. The resulting data has been reviewed, analyzed, and synthesized to produce the following summations, which are organized into specific sections:

Rating: Each herb's leading indication is given a *Benefit Rating* of one to three leaves, and a *Safety Rating* indicated by a plus or minus sign. These ratings are based on the evidence presented, and are meant to denote only an estimate of the herb's demonstrated efficacy and safety (see table).

Beneath the rating are bulleted key points, which include the most common usages and most important highlights of the efficacy and safety data. This box is followed by a brief description of the plant, including the Latin binomial name, common names, and other pertinent characteristics.

Uses: Includes the principal current uses of the herb, especially those promoted for popular products sold in North America

Herb Ratings

Benefit Rating

🐝 🐝 🐝 = Convincing evidence of clinical benefit is demonstrated in multiple randomized, controlled trials.

🐝 🐝 = Clinical benefit is suggested by controlled clinical trials, but results are conflicting or the evidence is not convincing or conclusive.

🐝 = There is minimal to no evidence of clinical benefit from controlled clinical trials.*

Safety Rating**

[+] = Safe and well tolerated, with minimal to no adverse effects, based on both controlled clinical trials *and* widespread experience

[–] = Significant adverse effects, interactions, or risks that are well-characterized for certain populations or clinical situations

---

* Herbal medicines in this category may be ineffective, or simply lack appropriate studies to demonstrate potential benefits.

** No [+] or [–] rating indicates lack of sufficient evidence to place in either category (e.g., insufficient or limited safety data; *or* well-tolerated based on widespread experience but not documented in controlled trials, *or* vice-versa; or theoretical risks or cautions that are poorly characterized or documented).

and Europe. This section also briefly summarizes other traditional uses and historical details of interest.

Pharmacology: Lists the most frequently reported or well-known chemical constituents; many apparently minor or inactive components are not mentioned. Relevant, available pharmacologic information that is pertinent to humans is reviewed. Animal and *in vitro* data that may be relevant are summarized as much as possible. Reputable textbooks, review articles, and other secondary literature sources that have already reviewed this data are often cited, especially for *in vitro* and animal data. The primary literature is cited, whenever possible, for human pharmacologic studies.

Clinical Trials: Special emphasis is given to primary literature references and high-quality systematic reviews and meta-analyses. Generally, the most clinically relevant studies with the highest methodologic quality are discussed. Attempts were made to locate difficult-to-find foreign articles and to read English translations when available; only when this was not possible was information summarized from abstracts or other sources.

Adverse Effects, Interactions, Cautions: These sections summarize adverse effects and other potential risks. Emphasis is placed on the primary clinical literature and systematic reviews, although opinions of leading herbal medicine authorities are included when pertinent. Evidence-based information is distinguished from anecdotes, generalizations, and hypotheses as much as possible. In general, it is recognized that herbal remedies should be avoided in pregnant or breast-feeding women, unless there is good evidence of safety.

Preparations & Doses: Summarizes information from published clinical trials as well from herbal pharmacopoeias. It is recognized that there may be a wide range of doses for crude herbs, as well as for the many different extract formulations. As a consequence, dosing recommendations can vary considerably. Because each herbal product is unique, brand names of the products demonstrated to be effective in controlled clinical trials are included, especially if they are marketed in the U.S. (Note that the manufacturer's names appears in parentheses after the product name.) Traditional liquid-dosage forms, such as tinctures and fluid extracts, are not emphasized, unless they have been specifically studied in clinical trials (see chapter "Understanding Herbal Dosage Forms"). Also, doses are described for adults only; evidence-based recommendations for pediatric use are poorly established and are not included.

Summary Evaluation: Presents a synopsis of the clinically relevant evidence regarding efficacy and safety, as just discussed. Recommendations for using herbs that are particularly beneficial (or negative recommendations for those that are potentially harmful) are made with confidence for a limited number of herbs. However, it is understood that the evidence can be interpreted differently by individual practitioners. Clinicians must decide whether reported results are valid and pertain to particular patients. Some practitioners may require rigorous evidence of efficacy, while others may only require convincing evidence of minimal harm. Many other factors, such as cost, quality assurance, treatment options (both herbal and orthodox), the patient's medical condition, the acceptability of herbal therapies, and one's philosophy regarding employment of the placebo effect, will influence the decision made by practitioner and patient. Use your own experience and judgment to determine the acceptability of the conclusions presented here.

Aloe Gel (*Aloe vera*)

rating: 🐾 🐾 +

> - Used topically for abrasions, burns, and other dermatologic disorders; mixed results in controlled clinical trials
> - Used orally for diabetes, ulcers, AIDS; may be of some value in diabetes
> - Appears safe and well tolerated

The succulent, cactus-like *Aloe vera* plant, one of over 300 Aloe species, was previously known as *Aloe barbadensis* and *Aloe vulgaris*. Aloe gel is a clear viscous liquid obtained from the inner portion of the long, fleshy leaves.

Uses: Topically, aloe gel is commonly used for minor abrasions, burns, wounds, and a variety of dermatologic disorders. Aloe gel is a common household remedy in many cultures, and is an ingredient in numerous commercial skin lotions, sun blocks, and cosmetics. Therapeutic claims also have been made for oral ingestion of the gel, including benefits for diabetes, peptic ulcer, cancer, AIDS, and inflammatory bowel disease, and as a general tonic.[1,2]

Aloe gel is distinct from, and often confused with, the bitter yellow liquid derived from the outer rind of the leaf. This bitter exudate is variably referred to as aloe juice, sap, latex, or simply aloes; it contains anthraquinone glycosides that have strong laxative properties when taken orally.[3,4] Dried aloes is a powerful cathartic drug similar to senna and cascara, but has largely been superceded by gentler laxatives.

Pharmacology: Active chemical constituents from the gel include mucilaginous polysaccharides (e.g., glucomannans, acemannan), beta-sitosterol, lectins, fatty acids, and enzymes.[2,5] The polysaccharides and high water content make aloe gel an effective moisturizing agent or emollient, which accounts for its use in many cosmetics.

The activity of aloe gel has been investigated in hundreds of *in vitro* and animal studies.[2,5–7] Although not all study results were positive in animal models, topical and injectable aloe gel have been found to inhibit acute inflammation, speed the healing of wounds and burns, increase wound strength, and enhance tissue survival in frostbite. The proposed cellular mechanisms for aloe gel's activity on wound healing are numerous, although the clinical effects are not necessarily correlated with these actions. Studies have demonstrated an increase in fibroblast and collagen proliferation, stimulation of new capillaries, and reduced thromboxane production. Although inflammation is reduced, immune stimulation (increased antigenic, macrophage, and natural killer cell activity) has also been demonstrated *in vitro* and in animal models, primarily with injectable acemannan, which is also used clinically.[5] In addition, the fresh gel (but not commercial preparations) inhibited tumor cell growth in vitro, and injectable acemannan also reduced tumor growth and mortality in animal models of cancer.[5]

Aloe extracts have *in vitro* antibacterial, antifungal, and antiviral activity, including activity against herpes and HIV viruses.[6,7] Oral administration of the gel in several animal studies has produced inconsistent results on blood glucose concentrations and gastric ulcers.[5] Hypoglycemic activity may be greater for the bitter aloe juice exudate.[5]

Clinical Trials: Many potential uses of aloe gel are based on case reports and uncontrolled trials. In a systematic review of the worldwide literature, only 10 controlled clinical trials of aloe vera gel were found; six were randomized controlled trials (RCTs) and four were double-blinded.[8]

• Topical Use—Two controlled trials have investigated the effects of aloe gel on wounds and burns; both trials compared aloe and standard dressings on opposite sides of the wound. After full-face dermabrasion of 18 patients for acne vulgaris, healing was reported to occur 72 hours faster on the side of the face with the aloe gel–saturated dressing (total healing time in the control group was about 10 days).[9] Similarly, in 27 patients with partial-thickness burns, healing was faster with the aloe dressing than the vaseline dressing (11.9 versus 18.2 days, respectively; $P < 0.002$).[10] Although both studies showed significant results, neither study was randomized or blinded.

In contrast, acemannan was not effective for open wounds from gynecologic surgery that required healing by secondary intention. In this unblinded RCT, open surgical wounds in 40 patients actually took *longer* to heal using the aloe gel extract (83 days) compared to standard care (53 days).[11] For prevention of radiation-induced skin injury in women receiving radiation for breast cancer, two RCTs from the same investigators (one double-blinded with 194 patients) found that a 98% aloe vera gel was no more effective than placebo or standard care.[12] In two double-blind RCTs for the treatment of aphthous ulcers, one found no consistent benefits using different gels containing a 0.125% aloe extract,[13] and the other found faster healing times with an acemannan hydrogel product compared to a placebo (5.89 vs. 7.80 days; P = 0.003).[14] In an unblinded RCT of 30 patients with uninfected pressure ulcers, an acemannan hydrogel dressing was equivalent to, but no more effective than, a moist saline gauze applied daily,[15].

Positive results were best documented in double-blinded RCTs for seborrheic dermatitis, psoriasis, and genital herpes. In 44 adult patients with seborrheic dermatitis, clinical resolution or substantial improvement was significantly more frequent with a 30% aloe extract emulsion than a bland aqueous control cream, as assessed by patients (62% vs. 25%; P = 0.03) and dermatologists (58% vs. 15%; P = 0.009).[16] In 60 patients with mild-moderate psoriasis, a 0.5% aloe cream helped heal plaques in 83% of patients in 4 weeks, compared to 7% using placebo.[17] In a study of 120 male patients with first-onset genital herpes, mean duration of healing was 4.8 days for a 0.5% aloe extract cream, 7 days for a 0.5% aloe vera gel, and 14 days for a placebo cream. The percentages of "cured" patients were 70%, 45%, and 7.5%, respectively, at 2 weeks.[18] A similar study by the same investigators in 60 patients showed almost identical results.[19] Note that the three studies for psoriasis and herpes (with rather remarkable results) were all performed by the same research group.

• Oral Use—Ingesting 10–20 ml of aloe vera daily was reported to reduce triglycerides and total and LDL cholesterol compared to placebo in 60 patients over 3 months. However, it is not clear if this study (published in abstract form) was randomized or blinded.[8]

One tablespoon b.i.d. of aloe vera gel extract was reported to reduce blood glucose levels (from 250 to 141 mg/dl) compared to placebo (unchanged) in 72 new-onset diabetics after 42 days.[20] A similar study by the same group found identical benefits in treated diabetics.[21] Triglyceride levels also decreased significantly, without a change in total cholesterol. However, these studies are difficult to accept. Both were single-blinded and not randomized, and in the treated diabetic control group, glibenclamide (glyburide) 20 mg/day had no effect on blood glucose when used alone.

Although preliminary studies of acemannan initially suggested benefits in AIDS patients, a well-designed double-blind RCT in 63 patients given an oral dose of 1600 mg/day for 1 year found no effects on CD_4 counts or viral loads.[22]

Adverse Effects: Topically applied aloe gel is generally well tolerated, with occasional reports of stinging sensation, mild itching, or hypersensitivity reactions.[8,23,24] There are no reported adverse effects with oral ingestion of the gel.

Interactions: There are no recognized drug interactions with topical or oral administration of aloe gel.

Cautions: Unlike pure aloe vera gel, total leaf extracts (sometimes referred to as aloe "juice") or contaminated gel products may contain anthraquinones from the bitter sap. Excessive oral ingestion of anthraquinones can result in severe intestinal cramping, diarrhea, hypokalemia, and other toxicities of laxative abuse.[3,4] While topical application by pregnant or lactating women is considered safe, oral consumption should be avoided due to lack of data.[2]

Preparations & Doses: The gel is usually applied topically 2–4 times daily or as needed. When using the fresh plant, a leaf can be cut and the gel of the inner leaf applied directly to the injury. Pure aloe gel is available commercially for topical use, but more cosmetically acceptable products are also available; these are typically marketed in percentage strengths such as 0.5% (i.e., 0.5 g of 100% gel is contained in 100 ml or g of lotion, cream, or other preparation). Recommended oral doses of aloe gel (in concentrations up to 100%) vary widely; typical oral doses of liquid products are 30 ml 1–3 times daily. The gel is also marketed in solid extract forms. Careful processing of the gel is necessary to avoid contamination with anthraquinones, and stabilization is needed to reduce degradation of the active components, which occurs quickly. The International Aloe Science Council certifies products with some assurance of quality (http://www.iasc.org).

Summary Evaluation

Although widely applied as an easy-to-use household remedy, objective evidence that aloe gel can enhance the healing of abrasions and burns is limited. Nevertheless, simple emollient and occlusive properties may be soothing. Consistent healing benefits were not demonstrated in studies of open surgical wounds and in studies examining prevention of radiation-induced dermatitis, aphthous ulcers, and pressure sores. Benefits have been reported for seborrheic dermatitis, psoriasis, and genital herpes, but these results need verification. Oral administration of acemannan is not effective for AIDS. Benefits have been reported for diabetes, but claims for the oral use of aloe gel for any indication have not been confirmed in reliable, controlled studies.

references

1. Goldberg A: Aloe: Aloe spp. Botanical Series 315. Austin, TX, American Botanical Council, 1999.
2. Kemper KJ, Chiou V: Aloe vera (*Aloe vera*), revised July 29, 1999. The Longwood Herbal Task Force. Accessed February 7, 2001 at http://www.mcp.edu/herbal/default.htm
3. World Health Organization: WHO Monographs on Selected Medicinal Plants. Vol. 1. Geneva, WHO, 1999.
4. European Scientific Cooperative on Phytotherapy: Aloe capensis: Cape aloes. Monographs on the Medicinal Uses of Plant Drugs. Exeter, UK, ESCOP, July 1997.
5. Reynolds T, Dweck AC: Aloe vera leaf gel: A review update. J Ethnopharmacol 68:3–37, 1999.
6. Boon H, Smith M: The Botanical Pharmacy: The Pharmacology of 47 Common Herbs. Kingston, Ontario, Quarry Press, 1999.
7. Klein AD, Penneys NS: Aloe vera. J Am Acad Dermatol 18:714–720, 1988.
8. Vogler BK, Ernst E: Aloe vera: A systematic review of its clinical effectiveness. Br J Gen Pract 49:823–828, 1999.
9. Fulton JE: The stimulation of postdermabrasion wound healing with stabilized aloe vera gel-polyethylene oxide dressing. J Dermatol Surg Oncol 16:460–467, 1990.
10. Visuthikosol V, Sukwanarat Y, Chowchuen B, et al: Effect of aloe vera gel to healing of burn wound a clinical and histologic study. J Med Assoc Thai 78:403–408, 1995.
11. Schmidt JM, Greenspoon JS: Aloe vera dermal wound gel is associated with a delay in wound healing. Obstet Gynecol 78:115–117, 1991.
12. Williams MS, Burk M, Loprinzi CL, et al: Phase III double-blind evaluation of an aloe vera gel as a prophylactic agent for radiation-induced skin toxicity. Int J Radiation Oncol Biol Phys 36:345–349, 1996.
13. Garnick JJ, Singh B, Winkley G: Effectiveness of a medicament containing silicon dioxide, aloe, and allantoin on aphthous stomatitis. Oral Surg Oral Med Oral Pathol Oral Radiol Endod 86:550–556, 1998.
14. Plemons JM, Rees TD, Binnie WH, et al: Evaluation of acemannan in the treatment of recurrent aphthous stomatitis. Wounds 6(2):40–45, 1994.
15. Thomas DR, Goode PS, LaMaster K, Tennyson T: Acemannan hydrogel dressing versus saline dressing for pressure ulcers: A randomized, controlled trial. Adv Wound Care 11:273–276, 1998.

16. Vardy DA, Cohen AD, Tchetov T, et al: A double-blind, placebo-controlled trial of an *Aloe vera* (*A. barbadensis*) emulsion in the treatment of seborrheic dermatitis. J Dermatol Treat 10:7–11, 1999.

17. Syed TA, Ahmad SA, Holt AH, et al: Management of psoriasis with *Aloe vera* extract in a hydrophilic cream: A placebo-controlled, double-blind study. Trop Med Intl Health 1:505–509, 1996.

18. Syed TA, Cheema KM, Ahmad SA, Holt AH: *Aloe vera* extract 0.5% in hydrophilic cream versus aloe vera gel for the management of genital herpes in males. A placebo-controlled, double-blind, comparative study. J Eur Acad Dermatol Venereol 7:294–295,1996.

19. Syed TA, Afzal M, Ahmad SA, et al: Management of genital herpes in men with 0.5% *Aloe vera* extract in hydrophilic cream: A placebo-controlled double-blind study. J Dermatol Treat 8:99–102, 1997.

20. Yongchaiyudha S, Rungpitarangsi V, Bunyapraphatsara N, Chokechaijaroenporn O: Antidiabetic activity of *Aloe vera* L. juice. I. Clinical trial in new cases of diabetes mellitus. Phytomed 3:241–243, 1996.

21. Bunyapraphatsara N, Yongchaiyudha S, Rungpitarangsi V, Chokechaijaroenporn O: Antidiabetic activity of *Aloe vera* L. juice. II. Clinical trial in diabetes mellitus patients in combination with glibenclamide. Phytomed 3:245–248, 1996.

22. Montaner JSG, Gill J, Singer J, et al: Double-blind placebo-controlled pilot trial of acemannan in advanced human immunodeficiency virus disease. J Acquired Imm Defic Synd Hum Retrovirol 12:153–157, 1996.

23. Morrow D, Rapaport MJ, Strick RA: Hypersensitivity to aloe. Arch Dermatol 116:1064–1065, 1980.

24. Hogan DJ: Widespread dermatitis after topical treatment of chronic leg ulcers and stasis dermatitis. Can Med Assoc J 138:336–338, 1988.

American Ginseng
(*Panax quinquefolius*)
rating: 🐜🐜

> - Similar to Asian ginseng; considered a tonic or adaptogen (balancing agent) to enhance health and combat stress or disease
> - Mild attenuation of post-prandial glycemia, but no benefit for enhancing physical performance
> - No apparent adverse effects based on limited data

The American ginseng plant, *Panax quinquefolius*, is similar in appearance and is in the same botanic genus as Asian ginseng (*Panax ginseng*). First described in the early 18th century in Eastern Canada, *P. quinquefolius* was primarily harvested for export to China. American ginseng is also referred to as North American, Canadian, or Wisconsin ginseng, referring to primary areas of harvest or cultivation, although it is now grown in many areas of the world. The root is used medicinally.

Uses: Ginsengs are marketed in the U.S. to boost energy, relieve stress, improve concentration, and enhance physical or cognitive performance. Most ginsengs are believed to act as general restoratives, tonics, or adaptogens, which have nonspecific strengthening properties to restore the body's balance, enhance stamina, and increase resistance to stress and disease.

In traditional Chinese medicine (TCM), Asian and American ginsengs are used to restore vital energy (*qi* or *chi*) in the body. However, American ginseng is considered to have more cooling or calming (*yin*) qualities, as opposed to Asian ginseng's more heating or stimulating (*yang*) properties. According to TCM theory, American ginseng is used to calm the ailing respiratory or digestive systems and as therapy for diabetes or "thirsty" syndromes, and may be preferred in warmer climates.

Native Americans traditionally employed American ginseng to help with childbirth and fertility and to strengthen mental powers, and for a variety of ailments such as respiratory disorders, headaches, and fevers.[1-3]

Pharmacology: American ginseng shares similar chemical constituents with Asian ginseng.[4–6] The roots of both species contain triterpene saponins or ginsenosides. Over 28 ginsenosides have been isolated from American ginseng, and there are minor differences between the two species. The Rb-1 ginsenoside is more abundant in American ginseng, and Rg-1 is relatively deficient. Rf is absent in *P. quinquefolius*.

Based on animal and *in vitro* experiments using isolated ginsenosides, the Rb-1 ginsenoside is considered to have more "depressant" activity than Rg-1 (CNS-depressant, anticonvulsant, antipyretic, hypotensive, ulcer protectant properties), while Rg-1 is considered more "stimulating" (slight CNS-stimulation at low doses, hypertensive, antifatigue, increases ulcers).[6] The herbal and Chinese scientific communities use these contrasting activities to help explain the balanced or adaptogenic properties of the whole root, or sometimes to explain the opposing *yin* and *yang* properties of the two Panax species.[1]

Few experiments have specifically used *P. quinquefolius* root preparations. American ginseng extracts have been shown to induce hypoglycemia when administered by intraperitoneal injection to mice, but not with orally administered ginsenoside fractions.[7,8] Oral, powdered root preparations administered chronically to male rats enhanced sexual arousal as measured by copulatory behavior. Testosterone and LH levels and androgen-dependent tissue weights were unaffected, but prolactin levels decreased significantly.[9]

In another rat study, oral administration did not affect initial learning or memory tasks, but did facilitate task behavior in memory-compromised animals with anticholinergic-induced amnesia. Choline uptake was increased in brain synaptosomes, and *P. quinquefolius* was hypothesized to have central cholinergic effects in this model.[10]

In *in vitro* studies, American ginseng extracts have been found to have antioxidant properties[11,12]; to inhibit growth of cancer cells and potentiate the activity of chemotherapeutic drugs[13]; and to inhibit thrombin-induced endothelin release.[14] None of these pharmacologic activities have been correlated with clinical effects.

Clinical Trials: There are few controlled clinical trials using American ginseng products.[15] In one randomized, double-blind, placebo-controlled crossover study of eight athletic volunteers, a noncommercial American ginseng extract in a daily dose of 8 or

16 mg/kg for 7 days failed to enhance physical performance as measured by a cycle ergometer.[16] There were no significant differences compared to placebo in any of the outcome measures, which included oxygen uptake, heart rate, time to exhaustion, lactate and glucose concentrations, and rating of perceived exertion.

In a series of randomized, single-blind, placebo-controlled studies by the same investigators, a single dose of American ginseng (Chai-Na-Ta Corp) was found to reduce post-prandial glycemia by about 10–20%.[17–19] Effects were not found to be dose dependent. In healthy subjects, 1–3 g doses reduced glycemia when given at least 40 minutes before a glucose load.[17,18] In type-II diabetics, 3–9 g doses were tested and found to reduce glycemia when given with, or up to 2 hours prior to, a glucose load.[17,19]

Adverse Effects: No significant adverse effects have been reported in the few clinical trials, and there are no case reports of clinical toxicities. Due to similar chemical constituents, American ginseng has the potential to cause any of the side effects possible with Asian ginseng, which appear to be uncommon and idiosyncratic (see page 84).

Interactions: No drug interactions are recognized.

Cautions: One American ginseng product has been shown to mildly blunt the hyperglycemic effect of food[17–19]; this may theoretically be detrimental in a tightly controlled or labile diabetic. Unlike Asian ginseng products, adulteration or contamination of American ginseng has not yet been reported. Safety has not been established during pregnancy or breast feeding.

Preparations & Doses: American ginseng is available in multiple forms, from whole root products to a variety of more concentrated formulations and extracts in capsules, tablets, liquids, teas, and foods. The crude root is usually taken in doses of 1–2 g/day, but up to 9 g or more is used in traditional Chinese medicine. Many formulations contain concentrated extracts or preparations standardized to ginsenosides, usually as 100–200 mg of extract per dose.

--------- **Summary Evaluation** ---------

American ginseng, like Asian and Siberian ginseng, is traditionally used as a tonic or adaptogen to enhance health and combat stress or disease. Few clinical trials have been conducted. In one well-designed study, American ginseng did not enhance physical performance. In another series of studies, single doses of one product mildly attenuated post-prandial glycemia; whether this effect is reproducible and beneficial for diabetics awaits chronic dosing trials. There are no well-documented adverse effects of American ginseng.

references

1. Foster S: American Ginseng: *Panax quinquefolius*. Austin, TX, American Botanical Council, Botanical Series #308, 1996.
2. Okrent N: Ginseng-Part 1. Townsend Letter for Doctors (Feb/March):162–168, 1994.
3. Okrent N: Ginseng-Part 2. Townsend Letter for Doctors (April):304–309, 1994.
4. Awang DVC: The anti-stress potential of North American ginseng (*Panax quinquefolius* L.). J Herbs Spices Med Plants 6(2);87–91, 1998.
5. Newall CA, Anderson LA, Phillipson JD: Herbal Medicines: A Guide for Health-Care Professionals. London, The Pharmaceutical Press, 1996.
6. Shibata S, Tanaka O, Shoji J, Saito H: Chemistry and pharmacology of *Panax*. In Wagner H, Hikino H, Farnsworth NR (eds): Economic and Medicinal Plant Research. Vol 1. Orlando, FL, Academic Press, 1985, pp 217–284.
7. Oshima Y, Sato K, Hikino H: Isolation and hypoglycemic activity of quinquefolans A, B, and C, glycans of Panax quinquefolium roots. J Natural Prod 50:188–190, 1987.
8. Martinez B, Staba EJ: The physiological effects of Aralia, Panax and Eleuterococcus on exercised rats. Japan J Pharmacol 35:79–85, 1984.
9. Murphy LL, Cadena RS, Chavez D, Ferraro JS: Effect of America ginseng (*Panax quinquefolium*) on male copulatory behavior in the rat. Physiol Behav 64:445–450, 1998.
10. Sloley BD, Pang PKT, Huang B-H, et al: American ginseng extract reduces scopolamine-induced amnesia in a spatial learning task. J Psychiatry Neurosci 24:442–452, 1999.
11. Kitts DD, Wijewickreme AN, Hu C: Antioxidant properties of a North American ginseng extract. Molec Cell Biochem 203:1–10, 2000.
12. Li J-P, Huang M, Teoh H, Man RYK: Interactions between *Panax quinquefolium* saponins and vitamin C are observed in vitro. Molec Cell Biochem 204:77–82, 2000.
13. Duda RB, Zhong Y, Navas V, et al: American ginseng and breast cancer therapeutic agents synergistically inhibit MCF-7 breast cancer cell growth. J Surg Oncol 72:230–239, 1999.
14. Yuan C-S, Attele AS, Wu JA, et al: *Panax quinquefolium* L. inhibits thrombin-induced endothelin release *in vitro*. Am J Chinese Med 27:331–338, 1999.
15. Vogler BK, Pittler MH, Ernst E: The efficacy of ginseng. A systematic review of randomised clinical trials. Eur J Clin Pharmacol 55:567–575, 1999.
16. Morris AC, Jacobs I, McLellan TM, et al: No ergogenic effect of ginseng ingestion. Int J Sport Nutr 6:263–271, 1996.
17. Vuksan V, Sievenpiper JL, Koo VYY, et al: American ginseng (*Panax quinquefolius* L.) reduces postprandial glycemia in nondiabetic subjects and subjects with type 2 diabetes mellitus. Arch Intern Med 160:1009–1013, 2000.

18. Vukson V, Sievenpiper JL, Wong J, et al: American ginseng (*Panax quinque-folius* L.) attenuates postprandial glycemia in a time-dependent but not dose-dependent manner in healthy individuals. Am J Clin Nutr 73:753–758, 2001.

19. Vuksan V, Stavro MP, Sievenpiper JL, et al: Similar postprandial glycemia reductions with escalation of dose and administration time of American ginseng in type 2 diabetes. Diabetes Care 23:1221–1226, 2000.

Ashwagandha (*Withania somnifera*)
rating: 🐾

> - Indian herbal equivalent of ginseng; used for stress, arthritis, and many other conditions
> - Efficacy not adequately established in clinical trials
> - Appears to be safe and well tolerated, based on limited data

Ashwagandha, a traditional Indian (Ayurvedic) medical herb, is thought of as "Indian ginseng." It is often marketed simply as "Withania" and is also called winter cherry or Dunal. The berries, fruits, and roots have been used traditionally. In Western herbal medicine, most preparations are made from the root of the shrub.

Uses: As is the case with ginseng, ashwagandha has been employed for numerous conditions in traditional Asian therapies, and for additional disorders in contemporary herbal practice.[1-3] A major traditional use of the herb is in "balancing life forces," which may be regarded as an adaptogenic or anti-stress tonic effect. Thus, ashwagandha is considered to be a general promoter of health, or a "rasayana" that promotes rejuvenation according to traditional Ayurvedic practice.

Purported anti-inflammatory benefits have led to use in tuberculosis, liver disease, rheumatic disorders, and skin problems. The herb's "panacea" reputation has expanded its repertoire to include therapy for weakness, stress, sexual debility, aging symptoms, and anemia, among many other conditions. It is claimed to be effective in infections, particularly those caused by fungi. The Latin species name is a tribute to its supposed effectiveness in promoting somnolence and improving sleep. Recently, AIDS and cancer have been added to the list of its proposed immunostimulant uses,[3] although clinical evidence is lacking.

Pharmacology: Much of the pharmacologic literature on ashwagandha is in foreign journals; or consists of older reports or studies carried out on rodents; or employs techniques that are difficult to evaluate. Over 35 active chemicals have been identified in the herb, including steroidal lactones (such as withanolides and withaferins), alkaloids (such as somniferine, scopoletin, withanine, and anaferine), saponins, and glycosides.[2] Additional chemicals of possible importance include choline, beta-sitosterol, flavonoids, tannins, an essential oil called ipuranol, a crystalline alcohol called withaniol, and several acylsterylglucosides or sitoindosides.[3,4]

Several specific withanolides and withaferins have been shown to have antineoplastic effects in animals.[1,4] Withaferins have shown anti-inflammatory, antioxidant, and antimicrobial actions.[1] Withanolide-D and withaferin-A appear to contribute immunoactive effects.[2] Somniferine is a hypnotic, while scopoletin is a smooth muscle relaxant in guinea pigs.[5] The adaptogenic properties of the characteristic glycosides (sitoindosides VII and VIII) and other derivatives of Withania are sometimes explained as resulting from a state of "nonspecific increase in resistance," resulting in enhancement of survival when under stress[2]; however, this concept fails to convey any insights into its action.

Clinical Trials: There are few controlled clinical trials that confirm the multiple claims that are made for ashwagandha. Many of the published studies only evaluate multiple-herb preparations. In one double-blinded, cross-over clinical trial of osteoarthritis, 42 patients were randomized to 3 months on uncertain doses of ashwagandha combined with other herbs or to a placebo. The herbal combination was reported to significantly reduce pain ($p < 0.001$) and disability ($p < 0.05$).[6,7] In another randomized, double-blind, placebo-controlled trial on 182 patients with rheumatoid arthritis over 16 weeks, an Ayurvedic herbal mixture of four plants, including ashwagandha, was reported to cause an improvement in symptoms, but the benefit was statistically insignificant.[8,9] Ashwagandha alone has not yet been evaluated in any clinical studies in rheumatic disorders.[7]

Several other reports of clinical findings have been published in Indian journals of Ayurvedic medicine, and these have been summarized without full details.[5] In one double-blind, 60-day study, 58 children were given 2 g/day of ashwagandha or a placebo. The treated group showed significant increases in mean corpuscular hemoglobin and serum albumin, but no other significant changes. The authors concluded that the herb is a growth promoter with antianemic activity, but the details of the study are inadequate for such a conclusion.

A 1-year, double-blind trial in 101 adults also reported an increase in hemoglobin ($p < 0.001$) and red blood count ($p < 0.02$) with 3 g/day of ashwagandha root compared to placebo.

Improvements were also reported in sexual performance and in seated stature, along with less greying of the hair, less loss of nail calcium, decreased cholesterol, and a fall in erythrocyte sedimentation rate.[5] Such provocative findings are difficult to interpret, and cannot be accepted unless equivalent findings are obtained in additional carefully structured studies that are reported in peer-reviewed journals.

Adverse Effects: Based on a long history of traditional use, ashwagandha appears to be well tolerated without significant adverse effects.[1,2] There is little data from clinical studies. It is claimed anecdotally that large doses of ashwagandha products or the berries may cause gastrointestinal irritation.[2]

Interactions: As a potential sedative-hypnotic, it may theoretically potentiate other sedatives; this has not been reported or studied, and such effects are unlikely to be significant.

Cautions: The herb has not been studied in nursing or pregnant women, but it has been anecdotally reported to have abortifacient properties.[10] Like echinacea, its potential immunostimulant effect may be contraindicated in patients with autoimmune disorders; this has not been reported or studied, and significant effects are unlikely.

Preparations & Doses: A typical daily dose is 3–6 g of powdered root,[5] but up to 30 g/day of the herb has been advocated by commercial herbalists. Pill extracts are also available, as are tinctures and numerous herbal mixtures.

Summary Evaluation

Ashwagandha is promoted for many different uses. It is taken to improve immune function and as a rejuvenator, aphrodisiac, and tonic for general health. It is inappropriately promoted by some marketers as a treatment for serious diseases such as multiple sclerosis, cancers, and AIDS. It is often employed as a sedative and antiarthritic for self-therapy. However, its value has not been adequately established for any of the numerous clinical conditions to which it has been applied.

---

references

1. Schauss AG, Milholland RBR, Munson S. Therapeutic applications of *Withania somnifera* (ashwagandha)—A popular Ayurvedic botanical medicine. Natural Med J 1(10):16–19, 1998.

2. Mishra LC, Singh BB, Dagenais S. Scientific basis for the therapeutic use of *Withania somnifera* (ashwagandha): A review. Altern Med Rev 5:334–336, 2000.

3. Ashwaganda. Accessed June 1, 2001 at www.holistic-online.com/Herbal-Med

4. Withania. In DerMarderosian A (ed): The Review of Natural Products. St. Louis, MO, Facts and Comparisons, 2001, pp 631–632.

5. Mills S, Bone K. Principles and Practice of Phytotherapy: Modern Herbal Medicine. Edinburgh, UK, Churchill Livingstone, 2000.

6. Kulkarni RR, Patki PS, Jog VP, et al. Treatment of osteoarthritis with a herbomineral formulation: A double-blind, placebo-controlled cross-over study. J Ethnopharmacol 33:91–95, 1991.

7. Ernst E, Chrubasik S. Phyto-anti-inflammatories. A systematic review of randomized, placebo-controlled, double-blind trials. Rheum Dis Clin North Am 26:13–27, 2000.

8. Chopra A. Ayurvedic medicine and arthritis. Rheum Dis Clin North Am 26:133–144, 2000.

9. Chopra A, Patwardhan B, Lavin P, et al. A clinical study of an herbal (Ayurvedic) formulation in rheumatoid arthritis. Arthritis Rheum 39(Suppl): S283 [abstract], 1996.

10. Tierra M. Ashwagandha. Accessed June 1, 2001 at www.planetherbs.com

Asian Ginseng (*Panax ginseng*)
rating: 🐾🐾

> - Considered to be an adaptogen, or tonic, to enhance health and combat stress or disease
> - Controlled trials have reported potential benefits, with many studies offering contrasting results.
> - Adverse effects appear to be rare.

Asian, Chinese, Korean, or "true" ginseng are all common names for *Panax ginseng*, one of the world's oldest known herbal medicines. The word *Panax*, of Greek derivation, means "all-cure" and gives rise to the word *panacea*. In Chinese, "ginseng" (*schin-seng*) refers to the human-shaped figure of the root, which is believed to suggest powerful properties. White ginseng refers to the unprocessed dried root, while red ginseng refers to the steamed root, which is red or caramel colored.

Uses: Ginseng has been used for thousands of years in Asian countries to boost energy, relieve stress, improve concentration, and enhance physical and cognitive performance. It is claimed to be a general restorative, tonic, or adaptogen, which restores the body's balance, enhances stamina, and increases resistance to stress and disease. Among many other claims, ginseng is also recommended as an aphrodisiac, for cardiovascular diseases, to prevent or treat cancers, and to prolong life.[1–3] In traditional Chinese medicine, ginseng is used to restore the vital life force (*qi* or *chi*) in the body. Asian ginseng is considered more stimulating or heating (*yang*), while American ginseng is considered more calming or cooling (*yin*).

Pharmacology: The triterpene saponins, commonly referred to as ginsenosides, are considered to be the main pharmacologic constituents of *P. ginseng*. At least 30 of these steroidal compounds have been described, based on their sugar side chains.[4] The most abundant or important ginsenosides are Rg-1, Rg-2, Rb-1, Rb-2, Rc, Rd, and Rf.[4,5] Like lipid-soluble steroid hormones, ginsenosides may insert into cell membranes and interact with membrane channels and proteins, or transverse the membrane to initiate genomic effects.[6] In addition, polysaccharides, polyacetylenes, and other non-saponin constituents of *P. ginseng* have pharmacologic activity.

Hundreds of *in vitro* and animal studies, mostly from the Asian and Russian literature, have investigated the biochemical and pharmacologic activities of *P. ginseng*, and numerous properties have been described.[3-9] For example, pharmacologic effects on the cardiovascular system (anti-ischemic, antiplatelet, vasodilatory), endocrine system (hypoglycemic, ACTH-stimulating), immune system (immunostimulatory, anti-inflammatory), and nervous system (CNS-stimulating and inhibiting) have been reported. Cytoprotective, cognitive, and anticarcinogenic activities are also alleged. Cytoprotective effects include resistance against ischemia, toxins, oxidation, and radiation.

Clinical Trials: Fifty-seven randomized controlled trials (RCTs) were found in a systematic review of the worldwide clinical literature, but many have significant methodologic flaws.[10] The Chinese and Russian literatures in particular are unreliable, as methodologic quality, flawed criteria, and publication bias are common concerns.[11,12] Therefore, double-blind RCTs in the American and Western European literature with statistically significant results are discussed here. Most of the best RCTs used a European proprietary product (G115, standardized to 4% ginsenosides) as either a mono-preparation or a combination product containing a mixture of vitamins and minerals (sometimes combined with deanol, or dimethylaminoethanol bitartrate).

• Physical Performance—Many controlled studies have been reviewed.[10,13] Eight double-blind RCTs evaluated chronic dosing of standardized ginseng products in volunteers on cycle ergometers.[10,13-15] Four trials found a significant decrease in heart rate and an increase in maximal oxygen uptake, whereas the other four trials found no improvement. Evaluation of these studies does not suggest that ginseng significantly improves physical performance.[10,13]

• Cognitive Functioning—In two separate RCTs, the G115 preparation increased arithmetic calculation ability (without affecting other cognitive skills),[16] while a different ginseng product enhanced abstract thinking and auditory reaction times (without affecting memory or concentration).[17] The combination G115 product improved cognitive functioning in middle-aged patients with mild memory impairments,[18] but failed to improve cognition in geriatric patients.[19] A combination ginseng/ginkgo preparation had equivocal effects on memory (beneficial effects after the morning dose, but detrimental effects after the afternoon dose).[20] Overall, these studies do not suggest consistent benefits in memory, concentration, and cognitive function.

• Quality of Life (QOL)—Several placebo-controlled trials have evaluated the G115 combination product on overall QOL (i.e., well-being) over several months. One research group found no overall benefits using two QOL questionnaires in 417 healthy adults,[21] and using three QOL scales measuring well-being and menopausal symptoms in 384 perimenopausal women.[22] Benefits were found in certain subsets of questions. Other RCTs also failed to find statistically beneficial effects for QOL, somatic symptoms, and activities of daily living, or mood and affect.[18,19,23,24] In contrast, beneficial effects were reported in two RCTs evaluating the G115 combination product in stressed or fatigued subjects. In a study of 232 patients diagnosed with "functional fatigue," a significant decrease in the fatigue score was seen after 6 weeks of treatment.[25] In 625 "stressed or fatigued" adults, QOL was significantly improved compared to the vitamin and mineral components alone.[26] Overall, no consistent benefit on QOL is discerned, although efficacy may be better in "fatigued" patients.

• Immune Function—Immunologic effects have been evaluated in three RCTs over 2- to 3-month study periods. In 20 healthy Thai students, no changes were found in total and differential leukocytes, or in lymphocyte subpopulations.[27] In contrast, G115 was reported to increase leukocyte activity, NK cell activity, and T-lymphocyte quantity and activity in 60 healthy adults.[28] In another RCT of 227 volunteers by the same investigators, G115 significantly decreased the incidence of colds and flu (13% in the ginseng group vs. 37% in the placebo group), and increased antibody titers.[29]

• Endocrine—In an 8-week RCT of 36 type II diabetics, 100 or 200 mg/day of a (presumably Asian) ginseng product improved fasting blood glucose levels and HgA1c levels (200-mg dose only) compared to placebo.[30] However, lack of reported data make these study results difficult to analyze. The G115 product did not affect glucose levels measured as a secondary endpoint in a separate trial of 60 healthy non-diabetics.[29] Significant increases in sperm count and sperm motility, as well as serum testosterone, FSH, and LH levels were reported in one uncontrolled study of 66 men.[31] However, controlled studies have failed to confirm these effects. No hormonal effects were found in an RCT of 384 perimenopausal women with hot flashes, based on estradiol levels, FSH levels, endometrial thickness, and vaginal cytology and pH [22]. Testosterone levels were also unaffected in a 3-month RCT of 90 men with primarily psychogenic erectile dysfunction. Although improvements were reported in subjective erectile functioning, this study did not appear to be double-blinded.[32]

• Miscellaneous—Ethanol consumed with 3 g of Korean ginseng decreased serum alcohol levels in one small study, presumably by increasing blood alcohol clearance.[33] In 24 patients with chronic non-viral hepatitis, a 3-month RCT found insignificant effects of the G115 combination product on liver testing.[34] In three epidemiologic studies from Korea, ginseng use was associated with a decreased risk of certain cancers (head and neck, gastrointestinal, liver, pancreas, and lung).[35] Epidemiologic studies cannot confirm causation, however, and all three studies were conducted by the same research group.

Adverse Effects: Side effects appear to be mild and uncommon, and are usually similar to placebo in controlled clinical trials.[2,10] Rare idiosyncratic reactions have been reported, such as Stevens-Johnson syndrome and cerebral arteritis.[36,37] Estrogen-like properties such as vaginal bleeding and mastalgia have been associated with ginseng use in isolated reports.[38,39] However, a cause and effect relationship is doubtful, as controlled clinical studies of standardized products have not demonstrated hormonal effects.[4,22,38] Many of these reactions are most likely due to adulteration or contamination by unrelated herb or drug products, which has been well described with many Asian herbal medicines.[38,40]

CNS-stimulation and a "ginseng abuse syndrome" (hypertension, nervousness, insomnia, skin eruptions, and morning diarrhea) were described in 10-20% of chronic ginseng users in an uncontrolled survey of psychiatric patients in 1979.[41] These adverse effects have not been observed in controlled studies, and this "syndrome" is probably nonexistent.[38] However, several Asian ginseng supplements have been reported to contain significant amounts of methylxanthines,[42] and CNS-stimulation has been reported with ginseng use in other psychiatric patients.[43,44]

Interactions: Asian ginseng appeared to inhibit the effects of warfarin in one patient, although no interaction could be detected in a rat model.[45,46] Ginseng combination products were loosely associated with stimulant or manic effects in two patients taking phenelzine, a monoamine oxidase inhibitor.[47,48] Overall, interactions do not appear to be a significant concern, but data is limited.

Cautions: Adulteration or contamination with drugs (e.g., steroids, stimulants, sedatives), pesticides, and heavy metals has been well described for many Asian herbal medicines,[38,40,49] and is a particular concern for pregnant and nursing women. Although caution in using ginseng during pregnancy and breast-feeding is advisable, in a survey of 88 women who consumed ginseng during pregnancy, reproductive outcome was no different than matched controls.[50] No mutagenic, carcinogenic, teratogenic, or adverse reproductive effects are seen in animal models.[4,5,38]

Preparations & Doses: Ginseng is commercially available as the whole or powdered root, in capsules and tablets, as teas, candies, and in many other forms. In traditional Chinese medicine, 10 g or more may be employed, usually in combination with other herbs. In Western herbal medicine, 1–2 g/day of a crude or powdered root preparation is commonly used.[2,9] Commercial extract products (standardized to 4% ginsenosides) are usually dosed as 100 mg b.i.d., which is equivalent to about 1 g/day of ginseng root.[2] The proprietary extract examined in many controlled trials (G115, standardized to 4% ginsenosides) is marketed in the U.S. as Ginsana, and the product combined with vitamins and minerals as Vitasana (Pharmaton Natural Health Products).

The American Botanical Council's Comprehensive Ginseng Evaluation Program recently analyzed 13 commercially available "standardized" Asian ginseng products for lot-to-lot consistency. Most products were reasonably consistent, but the ginsenoside content of a few products was more variable.[51]

Summary Evaluation

Asian ginseng is claimed to have multiple pharmacologic and clinical effects, most of which have not been established in rigorous controlled trials in the Western literature. Although some controlled studies have reported potential benefits, many others offer contrasting results and thus provide little convincing evidence. The overall evidence does not support claims that Asian ginseng can reliably improve physical performance, cognitive functioning, and quality of life. Beneficial effects on fatigue, diabetes, and viral URIs have been demonstrated in single or limited clinical trials, but in general, the efficacy of Asian ginseng is not established beyond a reasonable doubt for any indication. Side effects appear to be rare. Although millions of people have taken ginseng daily for years, suggesting that it is very benign, adulteration or contamination of Asian ginseng products with unwanted substances is concerning.

references

1. Foster S. Asian ginseng: *Panax ginseng*. American Botanical Council Botanical Series #303, 1996.
2. Blumenthal M, Goldberg A, Brinckmann J (eds). Herbal Medicine: Expanded Commission E Monographs. Newton, MA, Integrative Medicine Communications, 2000.
3. Huang KC. The Pharmacology of Chinese Herbs. 2nd ed. New York, CRC Press, 1999.
4. World Health Organization. WHO Monographs on Selected Medicinal Plants. Vol. 1. Geneva, WHO, 1999.
5. Newall CA, Anderson LA, Phillipson JD. Herbal Medicines: A Guide for Health-Care Professionals. London, The Pharmaceutical Press, 1996.
6. Attele AS, Wu JA, Yuan C-S. Ginseng pharmacology: multiple constituents and multiple actions. Biochem Pharmacol 1999;58:1685–1693.
7. Liu C-X, Xiao P-G. Recent advances on ginseng research in China. J Ethnopharmacol 1992;36:27–38.
8. Ong YC, Yong EL. Panax (ginseng)—Panacea or placebo? Molecular and cellular basis of its pharmacolgical activity. Ann Acad Med Singapore 2000;29:42–46.
9. Mills S, Bone K. Principles and Practice of Phytotherapy: Modern Herbal Medicine. Edinburgh, UK, Churchill Livingstone, 2000.
10. Vogler BK, Pittler MH, Ernst E. The efficacy of ginseng. A systematic review of randomised clinical trials. Eur J Clin Pharmacol 1999;55:567–575.
11. Vickers A, Goyal N, Harland R, Rees R. Do certain countries produce only positive results? A systematic review of controlled trials. Controll Clin trials 1998;19:159–166.
12. Tang J-L, Zhan S-Y, Ernst E. Review of randomised controlled trials of traditional Chinese medicine. BMJ 1999;319:160–161.
13. Bahrke MS, Morgan WP. Evaluation of the ergogenic properties of ginseng: an update. Sports Med 2000:29:113–133.
14. Pieralisi G, Ripari P, Vecchiet L. Effects of a standardized ginseng extract combined with dimethylaminoethanol bitartrate, vitamins, minerals, and trace elements on physical performance during exercise. Clin Therapeut 1991; 13:373–382.
15. Kolokouri I, Engels H-J, Cieslak T, Wirth JC. Effect of chronic ginseng supplementation on short duration, supramaximal exercise test performance. Med Sci Sports Exercise 1999;31(Suppl):S117(abstract).
16. D'Angelo L, Grimaldi R, Caravaggi, et al. A double-blind, placebo-controlled clinical study on the effect of a standarized ginseng extract on psychomotor performance in healthy volunteers. J Ethnopharmacol 1986;16:15–22.
17. Sorensen H, Sonne J. A double-masked study of the effects of ginseng on cognitive functions. Curr Therap Res 1996;57:959–968.

18. Neri M, Andermarcher E, Pradelli JM, Salvioli G. Influence of a double blind pharmacological trial on two domains of well-being in subjects with age associated memory impairment. Arch Gerontol Geriatr 1995;21:241–252.

19. Thommessen B, Laake K. No identifiable effect of ginseng (Gericomplex) as an adjuvant in the treatment of geriatric patients. Aging Clin Exp Res 1996; 8:417–420.

20. Wesnes KA, Faleni RA, Hefting NR, et al. The cognitive, subjective, and physical effects of a *Ginkgo biloba/Panax ginseng* combination in healthy volunteers with neurasthenic complaints. Psychopharmacol Bull 1997:33:677–683.

21. Wiklund I, Karlberg J, Lund B. A double-blind comparison of the effects on quality of life of a combination of vital substances including standardized ginseng G115 and placebo. Curr Therapeut Res 1994:55:32–42.

22. Wiklund ID, Mattson L-A, Lindgren R, Limoni C. Effects of a standardized ginseng extract on quality of life and physiological parameters in symptomatic postmenopausal women: a double-blind, placebo-controlled trial. Int J Clin Pharm Res 1999;19:89–99.

23. Ussher JM, Dewberry C, Malson H, Noakes J. The relationship between health related quality of life and dietary supplementation in British middle managers: a double blind placebo controlled study. Psychol Health 1995;10:97–111.

24. Smith K, Engels H-J, Martin J, Wirth JC. Efficacy of a standardized ginseng extract to alter psychological function characteristics at rest and during exercise stress. Med Sci Sports Exercise 1995(Suppl);27(5):S147(Abstract).

25. Le Gal M, Cathebras P, Struby K. Pharmaton capsules in the treatment of functional fatigue: a double-blind study versus placebo evaluated by a new methodology. Phytother Res 1996;10:49–53.

26. Caso Marasco A, Vargas Ruiz R, Salas Villagomez A, Begona Infante C. Double-blind study of a multivitamin complex supplemented with ginseng extract. Drugs Exptl Clin Res 1996;22:323–329.

27. Srisurapanon S, Ribal S, Siripol R, et al. The effect of standardized ginseng extract on peripheral blood leukocytes and lymphocyte subsets: A preliminary study in young healthy adults. J Med Assoc Thai 1997;80(Suppl. 1):S81–S85.

28. Scaglione F, Ferrara F, Dugnani S, et al. Immunomodulatory effects of two extracts of *Panax ginseng* C.A. Meyer. Drugs Exptl Clin Res 1990;16:537–542.

29. Scaglione F, Cattaneo G, Alessandria M, Cogo R. Efficacy and safety of the standardized ginseng extract G115 for potentiating vaccination against common cold and/or influenza syndrome. Drugs Exptl Clin Res 1996;22: 65–72.

30. Sotaniemi EA, Haapakoski E, Rautio A. Ginseng therapy in non-insulin-dependent diabetic patients. Diabetes Care 1995;18:1373–1375.

31. Salvati G, Genovesi G, Marcellini L, et al. Effects of *Panax ginseng* C.A. Meyer saponins on male fertility. Panminerva Med 1996;38:249–254.

32. Choi HK, Seong DH, Rha KH. Clinical efficacy of Korean red ginseng for erectile dysfunction. Int J Impotence Res 1995;7:181–186.

33. Lee FC, Ko JH, Park JK, Lee JS. Effects of Panax ginseng on blood alcohol clearance in man. Clin Exp Pharmacol Physiol 1987;14:543–546.

34. Zuin M, Battezzati PM, Camisasca M, et al. Effects of a preparation containing a standardized ginseng extract combined with trace elements and multivitamins against hepatotoxin-induced chronic liver disease in the elderly. J Int Med Res 1987;15:276–281.

35. Shin HR, Kim JY, Yun TK, et al. The cancer-preventive potential of *Panax ginseng:* a review of human and experimental evidence. Cancer Causes Control 2000;11:565-576.

36. Dega H, Laporte J-L, Frances C, et al. Ginseng as a cause for Stevens-Johnson syndrome? Lancet 1996;347:1344.

37. Ryu S-J, Chien Y-Y. Ginseng-associated cerebral arteritis. Neurology 1995; 45:829–830.

38. Sonnenborn U, Hansel R. Panax ginseng. In De Smet PAGM (ed): Adverse Effects of Herbal Drugs. Vol. 1. Berlin, Springer, 1992, pp. 179–192.

39. Palop-Larrea V, Gonzálvez-Perales JL, Catalán-Oliver C, et al. Metrorrhagia and ginseng. Ann Pharmacother 2000;34:1347–1348.

40. Ko RJ. Adulterants in Asian patent medicines. N Engl J Med 1998;339:847.

41. Siegel RK. Ginseng abuse syndrome: problems with the panacea. JAMA 1979;241:1614–1615.

42. Vaughan MA, Doolittle RL, Gennett T, Levesque M. Physiological effects of ginseng may be due to methylxanthines. Med Sci Sports Exercise 1999; 31(May Suppl):S121(Abstract 470).

43. Wilkie A, Cordess C. Ginseng—a root just like a carrot? J Royal Soc Med 1994;87:594–595.

44. Gonzalaz-Seijo JC, Ramos YM, Lastra I. Manic episode and ginseng: report of a possible case. J Clin Psychopharmacol 1995;15:447–448.

45. Janetzky K, Morreale AP. Probable interaction between warfarin and ginseng. Am J Health-Syst Pharm. 1997;54:692–693.

46. Zhu M, Chan KW, Ng LS, et al. Possible influences of ginseng on the pharmacokinetics and pharmacodynamics of warfarin in rats. J Pharm Pharmacol 1999;51:175–180.

47. Shader RI, Greenblatt DJ. Phenelzine and the dream machine—ramblings and reflections. J Clin Psychopharmacol 1985;5:65.

48. Jones BD, Runikis AM. Interaction of ginseng with phenelzine. J Clin Psychopharmacol 1987;7:201–202.

49. Keane FM, Munn SE, du Vivier AWP, Higgins EM. Analysis of chinese herbal creams prescribed for dermatological conditions. WJM 1999;170:257–259.

50. Chin RKH. Ginseng and common pregnancy disorders. Asia Oceana J Obstet Gyn 1991;17:379–380.

51. Hall T, Lu Z-Z, Yat PN, et al. Ginseng evaluation program. Part one: Standardization phase. HerbalGram 2001;52:27–47.

52. Cardinal BJ, Engels H-J. Ginseng does not enhance psychological well-being in healthy young adults: Results of a double-blind, placebo-controlled, randomized clinical trial. J Am Diet Assoc 2001;101:655–660.

Astragalus
(*Astragalus membranaceous*)
rating: 🐾

- Traditional Chinese herb for improving immunity; advocated for many diseases
- No reliable and controlled clinical trials in the Western literature
- Appears safe and well tolerated based on traditional use of large dosages

---

The astragalus species that is obtained from China is *A. membranaceous*, also known as Mongolian milk vetch, or by its Chinese name, huang qi. It is quite different from other species of Astragalus, known as locoweeds, which contain large amounts of selenium and other potential toxins, and from the Middle Eastern plant, *A. gummifer*, which is the source of gum tragacanth.

Uses: In Chinese traditional medicine, the root of A. membranaceous is a popular and potent tonic used for numerous specific indications, especially infections.[1,2] It is thought to improve depressed immunity, and therefore it has been recommended for the treatment of AIDS and other viral diseases, and as an adjuvant in cancer therapy. The herb is now advocated for a wide variety of illnesses, including the common cold, influenza, respiratory insufficiency, diabetes, hypertension, liver disease, cardiac ischemia, heart failure, vascular insufficiency, and nephritis.[2-4]

Pharmacology: The important constituents include numerous triterpene saponins, known as astragalosides and related compounds such as soyasaponins.[1] A number of polysaccharides, such as astragalans I-IV, have been isolated.[3] Important flavonoids include quercetin and kaempferol; among its many other constituents are isoflavonoids, sugars, amino acids, and linoleic acid.[1-3] It is unclear which of the numerous constituents are of therapeutic value. However, the polysaccharides and saponins have been suggested to be the major agents.[3,5]

The polysaccharide fractions of the root extract have been reported to have *in vitro* effects that suggest an immune-enhancing capability.[6,7] There is some evidence that astragalus can potentiate the effect of interferon against viruses and can increase IgA and IgM in nasal secretions in humans.[4] Animal experiments have shown that extracts of astragalus can restore the immune properties of cancer patient T-cells *in vitro*.[6] A more recent rat study does not confirm earlier reports that astragalus extract can prevent myelosuppression by cyclophosphamide.[7]

Clinical Trials: Almost all of the clinical studies on astragalus are in Chinese medical books or journals and are therefore not readily evaluated. In an open study on 1000 subjects,[8] it is alleged that a 2-month prophylactic course of the herb in a dosage of 8 g/day in combination with interferon was correlated with a significant reduction in colds compared to placebo or interferon alone.[9]. Benefits in humans for a wide variety of chronic and serious disorders also have been reported. For example, it is asserted that astragalus increases serum IgM, IgE, and cAMP; enhances left ventricular function and cardiac output in patients with angina pectoris; improves hemorrhagic indices in patients with systemic lupus erythematosus; increases survival in lung cancer when combined with conventional therapy; improves leukopenia; improves liver function in chronic viral hepatitis; and so on.[3,4,9]

However, none of these reports are evaluable, and the testing applied as well as the observations made by investigators do not conform to standard methods used in Western medicine. In general, these studies were uncontrolled or unblinded, and no reliable clinical studies in support of these indications have been reported in the English-language peer-reviewed literature. Thus, there is only very equivocal evidence to support the numerous clinical claims that are made for astragalus, particularly as an immune system restorative or as an immune modulator for use in the treatment of cancer.

Adverse Effects: Herbalists regard astragalus as very safe based on its reputation as a valued traditional medication.[1] It is unlikely that astragalus has any serious toxicity, although there is a lack of reliable clinical data.

Interactions: There are no recognized drug interactions.

Cautions: Astragalus can be obtained in combination mixtures, in which other agents may have a potential for toxicity.

Preparations & Doses: Sliced astragalus root is often used to make teas, soups, or decoctions. The usual daily dose varies from 2 to 30 g or more of the dried root[1]; although large doses appear to be safe, 8–15 g/day seems to be more reasonable.[3,10] Some products contain standardized extracts, packaged in unit doses. Capsules containing 150–500 mg are commonly marketed, to be taken as often as 8 or 9 times a day[10]; tinctures and fluid extracts are also available. In traditional Chinese medicine, it is usual to take astragalus in combination with other herbs.

--------- **Summary Evaluation** ---------

A. membranaceous is a popular Chinese herb that has long been used as a tonic. Increasing claims suggest that it is of value as an immune restorative to fight viral diseases, as a treatment for cancer, and as a cure for other disorders. However, the scientific evidence of clinical effectiveness is of unclear quality, and has not been validated outside the Asian literature. Thus, actual benefits are not substantiated. The fact that large doses can be taken with no reported toxicity suggests that astragalus has minimal pharmacologic potency.

references

1. Leung A, Foster S: Encyclopedia of Common Natural Ingredients Used in Food, Drugs, and Cosmetics, 2nd ed. New York, John Wiley & Sons, 1996.
2. Chang H, But P: Pharmacology and Applications of Chinese Materia Medica. Vol. 2. Singapore, World Scientific, 1987.
3. Upton R (ed): Astragalus root. American Herbal Pharmacopeia and Therapeutic Compendium. Santa Cruz, CA, American Herbal Pharmacopeia, 1999.
4. Bone K: Clinical Applications of Ayurvedic and Chinese Herbs. Warwick, Australia, Phytotherapy Press, 1996.
5. Miller AL: Botanical influences on cardiovascular disease. Altern Med Rev 3:422–431, 1998.
6. Chu DT, Wong WL, Mavligit GM: Immunotherapy with Chinese medicinal herbs II. Reversal of cyclophosphamide-induced immune suppression by administration of fractionated *Astragalus membranaceous* in vitro. J Clin Lab Immunol 25:125–129, 1988.
7. Khoo KS, Ang PT: Extract of *Astragalus membranaceous* and *Lingustrum lucidum* does not prevent cyclophosphamide-induced myelosuppression. Singapore Med J 36:387–390, 1995.
8. Peng J, Wu S, Zhang L, et al: Inhibitory effects of interferon and its combination with antiviral drugs on adenovirus multiplication. Chung-kuo I Hsueh K'o Hsueh Yuan Hsueh Pao 6:116–119, 1984. [Chinese]
9. Mills S, Bone K: Principles and Practice of Phytotherapy: Modern Herbal Medicine. Edinburgh, UK, Churchill Livingstone, 2000.
10. McCaleb RS, Leigh E, Morien K: The Encyclopedia of Popular Herbs. Roseville, CA, Prima Health, 2000.

Bilberry (*Vaccinium myrtillus*)
rating: 🐾 🐾

> - Used for vision and peripheral vascular disorders, and as an antioxidant
> - Positive European clinical trials are promising, but most indications require better study. Benefit for night vision has not been demonstrated.
> - No significant adverse effects

Bilberry is related to the American blueberry. Bilberries and other closely related members of the *Vaccinium* genus are also referred to as European blueberries, bog blueberries, whortleberries, and huckleberries.

Use: Bilberry fruit extracts are currently marketed in the U.S. as "vision" and "capillary" herbal supplements. In World War II, there were rumors that British Royal Air Force aviators experienced increased night vision after eating bilberry jam. This led to support for treating poor night vision and a variety of ophthalmic and microvascular disorders—including myopia, glaucoma, cataracts, diabetic retinopathy, and retinal degeneration, as well as capillary fragility, varicose veins, venous insufficiency, and hemorrhoids—with European bilberry extracts. Bilberry contains antioxidants that are also used as herbal supplements in anti-aging diets. Traditionally, bilberry leaves and fruit have been employed for their astringent and antiseptic properties to treat diarrhea, dyspepsia, infections, and burns, and also for diabetes, scurvy, and other disorders.[1-3]

Pharmacology: The berries are rich in flavonoids, the most well defined being the anthocyanins (also called anthocyanosides), which are the pigments that impart the intense indigo blue color to the ripe fruit[4,5]. Anthocyanins and other polyphenolic flavonoids are effective antioxidants and free radical scavengers.[5-7] They have significant biochemical and physiologic effects on cells and tissues; these effects are related to their antioxidant properties, activity on specific enzymes, and regulation of extracellular matrix protein synthesis and degradation.[1,8-10] In experimental studies, anthocyanins have been reported to increase the endothelium barrier effect and reduce capillary permeability,[8] inhibit edema,[9] and protect microvessels from cholesterol-induced atherosclerosis.[10] Anthocyanins also inhibit the synthesis and secretion of elastase and collagenase (proteases important in extracellular matrix remodeling and vascular permeability) and may stimulate rhodopsin regeneration in the retina.[1]

Anti-platelet activity of anthocyanins and bilberry extracts has been demonstrated *in vitro* and in rodents, in which extremely large oral doses prolong the bleeding time.[1] In humans, a standardized oral dose of a bilberry extract (480 mg/day of Myrtocyan, containing 36% anthocyanins) affected platelets such that ADP- and collagen-induced aggregation was inhibited[11]; increased bleeding times have not been reported, however. In animal studies, anthocyanins also have been reported to reduce plasma glucose and triglyceride levels in rats with induced diabetes,[12] increase lipoprotein catabolism,[12] protect against carbon tetrachloride induced-hepatotoxicity,[13] and have anti-tumor cell activity *in vitro*.[14,15]

Clinical Trials: Benefits of bilberry extracts (sometimes combined with beta-carotene or vitamin E) on ophthalmic and other microvascular disorders have been reported in numerous studies.[1,2] Almost 40 such trials have been published, primarily in the Italian and French literature; most used proprietary extracts containing 25–36% anthocyanins, such as Tegens or Myrtocyan. Few well-designed randomized, controlled trials have been published in peer-reviewed English-language journals; only controlled trials are reviewed here.

• Ophthalmic Uses—Improvements in night vision and quicker adaptation to darkness were originally reported in several studies from the 1960s, which have been reviewed by others.[1,2] Two placebo-controlled trials found statistically significant benefits in subjects after a single dose of bilberry extract, but not after multiple doses.[2] A double-blind study in 40 healthy subjects reported an enhanced pupillary light reflex with a single dose of bilberry anthocyanins; however, a similar percentage of subjects had enhanced reflexes in the placebo group.[16] In addition, more recent crossover trials that were randomized, double-blind, and placebo-controlled have failed to find any effect on night vision tests in healthy volunteers. One trial used a single dose and another used multiple small doses of anthocyanins (24–48 mg/day; Strix, Sweden) combined with beta-carotene.[17,18] Negative results were also verified with larger doses in a recent, well-designed, U.S. study; no significant differences were found on night vision testing in 15 healthy male subjects given an extract or placebo t.i.d. for 3 weeks.[19] This double-blind crossover trial used 480 mg/day of a product containing 25% anthocyanins, a dose similar to that used in the European trials.

Other studies have reported ophthalmic benefits such as improved visual perception in myopia and glaucoma, and improved retinopathy in patients with diabetes, hypertension, and other disorders.[1,2] Only three trials were appropriately controlled. Two reportedly double-blind, placebo-controlled trials evaluated the progression of diabetic retinopathy in 36 and 40 patients, over 1 and 12 months, respectively.[20,21] Patients taking Tegens 160 mg b.i.d. exhibited improvements or stabilization in ophthalmoscopic or fluorangiographic examinations compared to placebo. Although the first study was randomized, the second study was not, nor was the data analyzed statistically. Bilberry products were also reported to halt the progression of mild senile cataracts in a double-blind and placebo-controlled trial of 50 patients, but details are not available in English.[22]

• Peripheral Vascular and Other Disorders—Bilberry extracts have been evaluated in many studies for ulcerative dermatitis, chronic venous insufficiency, varicose veins, hemorrhoids, bleeding and other postoperative complications, and dysmenorrhea. Of these studies, only four are placebo-controlled; none are published in English-language journals; and all used the Myrtocyan product. These studies have been summarized by others,[1] although study methods have not been adequately assessed.

In one double-blind trial of 47 patients with various peripheral vascular disorders, treatment with 480 mg/day for 30 days was associated with significant improvements in subjective symptoms, such as paraesthesia and pain. In a single-blind, 30-day trial of 60 patients with venous insufficiency, treatment with 480 mg/day was also associated with a significant reduction in the severity of edema and subjective symptoms (pressure, paraesthesia, and cramps). In a double-blind trial, 30 patients with chronic primary dysmenorrhea were treated with 320 mg/day for 3 days before and during menses, which resulted in a significant improvement of symptoms over the 2-month treatment period. Lastly, in a single-blind study of 181 operative patients, pre-treatment with 160–320 mg/day for 10 days was reported to decrease intra- and postoperative bleeding and prevent onset of subsequent hemor-rhagic complications.

Adverse Effects: There are no significant adverse effects of bilberry extracts reported in the clinical trials.[1] Myrtocyan was well tolerated in a European post-marketing surveillance study of 2295 patients, in which 94 subjects (4.1%) reported side effects that in-cluded mainly gastrointestinal, skin, or nervous system complaints.[1]

Interactions: There are no documented drug interactions.

Cautions: Bilberry anthocyanins have antiplatelet effects in animal and human studies, but effects do not appear to be clini-cally significant with usual doses; bleeding problems and relevant drug interactions have not been reported in clinical trials or case reports. One study reported less intraoperative bleeding and he-morrhagic complications with bilberry pre-treatment.[1] Bilberry's safety during pregnancy and lactation has not been established. Consumption of 160–480 mg/day of anthocyanins during the last 3 months of pregnancy had no adverse effects on standard serum laboratory values.[23]

Preparations & Doses: Specific standardized European ex-tracts used in the clinical trials usually contained 25–36% antho-cyanins, and were given as 160–480 mg/day (40–120 mg/day anthocyanins) in two to three divided doses.[1] The concentrated extract in one of these products, Tegens (containing 25% antho-cyanins), is also marketed in the U.S. as Bilberry Extract by Enzymatic Therapy/PhytoPharmaca, and Bilberry Extract by Solaray.[24] Many other preparations containing concentrated an-thocyanins are also available on the U.S. market in encapsulated and other forms. Bilberry leaves and dried fruits are employed in traditional herbal medicine, usually as a decoction or extract.

———————— **Summary Evaluation** ————————

Numerous European clinical trials, supported by pharmacologic studies, suggest that anthocyanin-rich bilberry extracts with an-tioxidant properties may provide benefits in a variety of oph-thalmic and peripheral vascular disorders. Improvement of diabetic retinopathy, cataracts, chronic venous insufficiency, and dysmenorrhea are supported by placebo-controlled studies in the European literature, although many of these studies have not been adequately evaluated. In view of bilberry's apparent safety, there is little harm in patients and consumers trying this herb in conjunction with standard medical therapies for these indications. However, controlled studies of good methodologic quality are limited, and none of these indications have been proven beyond a reasonable doubt. Although often promoted to improve night vision based on early European studies, recent well-designed clinical trials have failed to verify this effect, which also raises doubts about the validity of other claims for bilberry.

references

1. Morazzoni P, Bombardelli E: *Vaccinium myrtillus* L. Fitoterapia 67:3–29, 1996.
2. Barrette E-P: Bilberry fruit extract for night vision. Alternative Medicine Alert, Atlanta GA, American Health Consultants 2(Feb.):20–21, 1999.
3. Blumenthal M, Goldberg A, Brinckmann J (eds): Herbal Medicine: Expanded Commission E Monographs. Newton, MA, Integrative Medicine Communications, 2000.
4. Rice-Evans CA, Miller NJ, Bolwell PG, et al: The relative antioxidant activities of plant-derived polyphenolic flavonoids. Free Rad Res 22:375–383, 1995.
5. Tsuda T, Shiga K, Ohshima K, et al: Inhibition of lipid peroxidation and active oxygen radical scavenging effect of anthocyanin pigments isolated from *Phaseolus vulgaris* L. Biochem Pharmacol 52:1033–1039, 1996.
6. Bagchi D, Garg A, Krohn RL, et al: Oxygen free radical scavenging abilities of vitamins C and E, and a grape seed proanthocyanidin extract *in vitro*. Res Commun Mol Pathol Pharmacol 95:179–189, 1997.
7. Laplaud PM, Lelubre A, Chapman MJ: Antioxidant action of *Vaccinium myrtillus* extract on human low-density lipoproteins *in vitro:* initial observations. Fundam Clin Pharmacol 11:35–40, 1997.
8. Mian E, Curri SB, Lietti A, Bombardelli E: Anthocyanosides and the walls of the microvessels: Further aspects of the mechanism of action of their protective effect in syndromes due to abnormal capillary fragility. Minerva Med 68:3565-3581, 1977. [English abstract]
9. Lietti A, Cristoni A, Picci M: Studies on *Vaccinium myrtillus* anthocyanosides. I. Vasoprotective and anti-inflammatory activity. Arzneimittelforschung 26:829–832, 1976. [English abstract]
10. Kadar A, Robert L, Miskulin M, et al: Influence of anthocyanoside treatment on the cholesterol-induced atherosclerosis in the rabbit. Paroi Arterielle 5:187–205, 1979.
11. Pulliero G, Montin S, Bettini V, et al: *Ex vivo* study of the inhibitory effects of *Vaccinium myrtillus* anthocyanosides on human platelet aggregation. Fitoterapia 60:69–74, 1989.
12. Cignarella A, Nastasi M, Cavalli E, Puglisi L: Novel lipid-lowering properties of *Vaccinium myrtillus* L. leaves, a traditional antidiabetic treatment, in several models of rat dyslipidaemia: A comparison with ciprofibrate. Thromb Res 84:311–322, 1996.
13. Mitcheva M, Astroug H, Drenska D, et al: Biochemical and morphological studies on the effects of anthocyanins and vitamin E on carbon tetrachloride induced liver injury. Cell Mol Biol 39:443–448, 1993.

14. Kamei H, Kojima T, Hasegawa M, et al: Suppression of tumor cell growth by anthocyanins *in vitro*. Cancer Invest 13:590–594, 1995.
15. Bomser J, Madhavi DL, Singletary K, Smith MA: *In vitro* anticancer activity of fruit extracts from *Vaccinium* species. Planta Med 62:212–216, 1996.
16. Vannini L, Samuelly R, Coffano M, Tibaldi L: Study of the pupillary reflex after anthocyanoside administration. Bolletino Di Oculistica Anno 65(Suppl.6): 569–577, 1986. [English translation]
17. Levy Y, Glovinsky Y: The effect of anthocyanosides on night vision. Eye 12:967–969, 1998.
18. Zadok D, Levy Y, Glovinsky Y: The effect of anthocyanosides in a multiple oral dose on night vision. Eye 13:734–736, 1999.
19. Muth ER, Laurent JM, Jasper P: The effect of bilberry nutritional supplementation on night visual acuity and contrast sensitivity. Altern Med Rev 5:164–173, 2000.
20. Perossini M, Guidi G, Chiellini S, Siravo D: Diabetic and hypertensive retinopathy therapy with *Vaccinium myrtillus* anthocyanosides (Tegens) double-blind placebo-controlled clinical trials. Ann Ottal Clin Ocul 113:1173–1190, 1987. [English translation]
21. Repossi P, Malagola R, De Cadilhac C: The role of anthocyanosides on vascular permeability in diabetic retinopathy. Ann Ottal Clin Ocul 113:357–361, 1987. [English translation]
22. Bravetti GO, Fraboni E, Maccolini E: Preventive medical treatment of senile cataract with vitamin E and *Vaccinium myrtillus* anthocianosides: Clinical evaluation. Ann Ottalmol Clin 115:109–116, 1989. [English abstract]
23. Teglio L, Mazzanti C, Tronconi R, Guerresi E: *Vaccinium myrtillus* anthocyanosides (Tegens) in the treatment of venous insufficiency of lower limbs and acute piles in pregnancy. Quad Clin Obstet Ginecol 42:221–231, 1987. [English translation]
24. Tyler VE: A guide to clinically tested herbal products in the U.S. market. Healthnotes Rev Complem Integr Med 7:279–287, 2000.

Black Cohosh
(*Cimicifuga racemosa*)
rating: 🐾 🐾

- Commonly used for menopausal symptoms, but appears to lack estrogenic effects
- Benefits found in European clinical trials, but most studies not of high quality
- Standardized preparations generally safe and well-tolerated

---

Black cohosh (*C. racemosa* or *Actaea racemosa*) is a North American native and a member of the buttercup family. Common names include bugbane, bugwort, black snakeroot, and squaw root. Its rhizomes and roots are used medicinally. Black cohosh should not be confused with blue or white cohosh, which are unrelated plants.

Uses: Black cohosh is most commonly used for symptoms associated with menopause.[1,2] Introduced into Germany in the 1950s, it has been actively promoted as an alternative to estrogen, since it is believed to have estrogen-like benefits without the unpleasant or harmful side effects. Black cohosh has been adopted for a variety of menstrual, menopausal, and reproductive maladies, and was an essential ingredient in Lydia Pinkham's Vegetable Compound, a popular patent remedy for "female complaints." The herb has also been used traditionally for rheumatism and inflammatory conditions.

Pharmacology: Constituents include triterpene glycosides (thought to be markers of biologic activity), caffeic acid, and isoferulic acid.[2,3] Remifemin, a proprietary extract standardized to the triterpene glycoside 27-deoxyactein, is the preparation most studied by German investigators. Other triterpene glycosides include actein and cimicifugoside.

Investigators have sought to determine whether black cohosh is a phytoestrogen, an herb that binds to estrogen receptors and has estrogenic properties—but results are contradictory.[2,3] Early animal studies found that black cohosh induced estrus and increased uterine weight in rats and mice, suggesting estrogenic effects. Methanol extracts of the herb were also reported to bind to estrogen receptors and to selectively reduce luteinizing hormone (LH) in animals.[4–6] These extracts were thought to contain formononetin, an isoflavone that binds to estrogen receptors. However, isoflavones are usually found in legumes (such as soybeans and red clover), not in plants related to black cohosh, and a recent study failed to find formononetin in commercial ethanol extracts such as Remifemin.[7]

In several older studies in menopausal women, usual doses of Remifemin were associated with estrogen-like vaginal epithelial stimulation and reduced LH levels.[2,6,8,9] However, results were confounded by lack of study blinding, small groups, or lack of baseline hormone measurements; more recent pharmacologic studies contradict these results. In a well-controlled animal study, commercial ethanolic black cohosh extracts did not produce estrogenic effects on the uteri or vagina of rats and mice.[10] In a randomized, double-blind study in 152 menopausal women, daily doses of 40 mg or 127 mg of Remifemin for 6 months reportedly had no effect on LH, follicle-stimulating hormone, sex hormone–binding globulin, prolactin, estradiol, or vaginal cytology.[11] A randomized double-blind trial in women with breast cancer also found no effects on LH or follicle stimulating hormone (FSH) with 40 mg/day of Remifemin over 2 months.[12] In addition, several in vitro studies of whole black cohosh extracts (including Remifenin) failed to demonstrate binding to, or stimulation of, estrogen receptors.[2,13–15]

Clinical Trials: Black cohosh was reported to benefit thousands of patients in early case series and uncontrolled studies.[2,3] The benefits included relief from menopausal symptoms, menstrual irregularities, and other instabilities thought to be associated with "hormone imbalances." In the 1980s, there were six European trials of Remifemin that reported benefits for the treatment of menopausal symptoms using objective outcome measurement tools.[8,9,16–19] However, only three studies were controlled, and only one of these was randomized and blinded.[2,3]

In the only European double-blind, randomized, controlled trial (RCT), 80 menopausal women were randomized to 80 mg of Remifemin daily, 0.625 mg of conjugated estrogens for 21 days/month, or a placebo.[8] After 12 weeks, the black cohosh preparation was statistically superior to both estrogen and placebo, as evaluated by a standardized symptom index (measuring hot flashes and other typical symptoms) and a separate standardized anxiety scale. Of the 16 patients who self-discontinued treatment, only one was from the black cohosh group, 12 were from the estrogen group (for "ineffectiveness"), and three were from the placebo group. Because estrogen had no more effect than placebo in this study, the results of this trial are questionable.

The other two controlled studies each included 60 women with natural or surgical menopause. Remifemin was found to have similar benefits to 0.625 mg of conjugated estrogens or 2 mg of diazepam in one study, and to 1 mg of estriol, 1.25 mg conjugated estrogens, or 1 mg of an estrogen-gestagen combination in the other study.[9,18] However, neither trial was blinded; thus the results cannot be adequately interpreted.

In contrast to the European studies, a recent well-designed U.S. double-blind RCT failed to find beneficial effects for Remifemin in women with daily hot flashes who had completed primary treatment for breast cancer. In 85 women (69 completed the study) evaluated at 30 and 60 days, both hot flashes and general menopausal symptoms were reduced equally well by black cohosh and placebo. Changes in blood levels of FSH and LH also did not differ in the two groups.[12]

Adverse Effects: Black cohosh is well-tolerated. In the controlled studies of Remifemin lasting up to 6 months, mild gastric discomfort, weight gain, and headache were reported in a few patients. A single case of unexplained nocturnal seizures in a patient taking black cohosh, chaste tree berry, and evening primrose oil has been reported,[20] but a cause-and-effect relationship with black cohosh is doubtful. Occasional statements in the literature that large doses of black cohosh may cause dizziness, stiffness, and trembling can be traced to old homeopathic provings, and are probably not pertinent to modern use of the herb.[2]

Interactions: There are no known drug interactions.

Cautions: Based on older studies suggesting estrogen-like properties, some feel that black cohosh is contraindicated for patients with breast cancer or other potential hormone-sensitive conditions. Although absolute risks are unknown, recent evaluations have not validated estrogenic activity, and this herb can probably be used in these conditions with relative safety. Black cohosh is not recommended during pregnancy and lactation due to inadequate evaluation.[1,3] In addition, there are isolated reports of a premature birth and a malformed infant associated with maternal black cohosh use.[21,22] A severely poor neurologic outcome in a full-term baby was associated with a combination of black cohosh and blue cohosh taken orally to induce labor, although a cause-and-effect relationship is doubtful.[23,24]

The German Commission E Monograph recommends limiting the duration of black cohosh use to 6 months; however, this appears to be based on lack of prolonged studies, and not on documented or potentially harmful effects.[1,2]

Preparations & Doses: There are many preparations of black cohosh available on the market. Remifemin, the standardized German product used in all of the clinical trials, is available in the U.S. as a tablet or liquid extract (distributed by GlaxoSmithKline). Twenty mg of herbal extract is contained in one tablet or 20 drops, standardized to the triterpene glycosides (i.e., 27-deoxyactein). The dose for menopausal symptoms used in the European clinical trials was 80 mg/day, administered as 40 mg (2 tablets or 40 drops) b.i.d. The manufacturer of Remifemin now states that half this dose, or 20 mg b.i.d., is equivalent to the dose used previously. This change is due to an internal manufacturer's trial in 1996 in which both doses reportedly had equivalent effects; dosing recommendations by the German manufacturer were changed to reflect the lowest effective dose.[25]

Dosing of traditional herbal preparations is roughly 0.5–1 g of dried rhizome or root, taken 3–4 times daily, usually as a decoction, tincture, or extract.[3]

--- **Summary Evaluation** ---

Benefits for menopausal symptoms are suggested by empiric use and some clinical studies; however, clinical effects have not been adequately proven due to lack of high-quality clinical trials. One well-designed U.S. clinical trial found effects comparable to placebo in breast cancer survivors experiencing hot flashes. Based on recent investigations indicating a lack of direct estrogenic activity, harmful effects are unlikely in patients with breast cancer or other hormone-sensitive conditions. Note that black cohosh has not been shown to have other demonstrated benefits (e.g., prevention of osteoporosis) seen with conventional hormone replacement therapy.

references

1. Blumenthal M, Goldberg A, Brinckmann J (eds). Herbal Medicine: Expanded Commission E Monographs. Newton, MA, Integrative Medicine Communications, 2000.

2. Foster S. Black cohosh: *Cimicifuga racemosa:* A literature review. HerbalGram 45:35–50, 1999.

3. Mills S, Bone K. Principles and Practice of Phytotherapy: Modern Herbal Medicine. Edinburgh, UK, Churchill Livingstone, 2000.

4. Jarry H, Harnischfeger G. Untersuchungen zur endokrinen wirksamkeit von inhaltsstoffen aus *Cimicifuga racemosa:* 1. Einfluss auf die serumspiegel von hypophysenhormonen ovariektomierter ratten. [Studies on the endocrine effects of the contents of *Cimicifuga racemosa:* 1. Influence on the serum concentration of pituitary hormones in ovariectomized rats.] Planta Med 51:46–49 [English abstract], 1985.

5. Jarry H, Harnischfeger G, Düker E. Untersuchungen zur endokrinen wirksamkeit von inhaltsstoffen aus *Cimicifuga racemosa:* 2. In vitro-bindung von inhaltsstoffen an östrogenrezeptoren. [Studies on the endocrine effects of the contents of *Cimicifuga racemosa:* 2. In vitro binding of compounds to estrogen receptors.] Planta Med 51:316–319 [English abstract], 1985.

6. Düker E-M, Kopanski L, Jarry H, Wuttke W. Effects of extracts of *Cimicifuga racemosa* on gonadotropin release in menopausal women and ovariectomized rats. Planta Med 57:420–424, 1991.

7. Struck D, Tegtmeier M, Harnischfeger G. Flavones in extracts of *Cimicifuga racemosa*. Planta Med 63:289, 1997.

8. Stoll W. Phytotherapeutikum beeinflusst atrophisches vaginalepithel: Doppelblindversuch *Cimicifuga* vs östrogenpräparat. [Phytopharmacon influences atrophic vaginal epithelium: Double blind study—*Cimicifuga* vs estrogenic substances.] Therapeutikon 1: 23–31 [English translation], 1987.

9. Lehmann-Willenbrock VE, Riedel H-H. Klinische und endokrinologische untersuchungen zur therapie ovarieller ausfallserscheinungen nach hysterektomie unter belassung der adnexe. [Clinical and endocrinologic examinations concerning therapy of climacteric symptoms following hysterectomy with remaining ovaries.] Zent Bl Gynäkol 110:611–618 [English translation], 1988.

10. Einer-Jensen N, Zhao J, Andersen KP, Kristoffersen K. Cimicifuga and Melbrosia lack oestrogenic effects in mice and rats. Maturitas 25:149–153, 1996.

11. Liske E, Wustenberg P. Therapy of climacteric complaints with *Cimicifuga racemosa:* Herbal medicine with clinically proven evidence. Menopause 5:250 [abstract], 1998.

12. Jacobson JS, Troxel AB, Evans J, et al. Randomized trial of black cohosh for the treatment of hot flashes among women with a history of breast cancer. J Clin Oncol 19:2739–2745, 2001.

13. Zava DT, Dollbaum CM, Blen M. Estrogen and progestin bioactivity of foods, herbs, and spices. Proc Soc Exp Biol Med 217:369–378, 1998.

14. Liu J, Burdette JE, Xu H, et al. Evaluation of estrogenic activity of plant extracts for the potential treatment of menopausal symptoms. J Agric Food Chem 49:2472–2479, 2001.

15. Dixon-Shanies D, Shaikh N. Growth inhibition of human breast cancer cells by herbs and phytoestrogens. Oncol Rep 6:1383–1387, 1999.

16. Daiber W. Klimakterische beschwerden: ohne hormone zum erfolg! [Climacteric complaints: Success without using hormones!] Arztl Prax 35:1946–1947 [English translation], 1983.

17. Vorberg G. Therapie klimakterischer beschwerden. [Treatment of menopausal complaints.] Z Allgeneinmed 60:626–629 [English translation], 1984.

18. Warnecke G. Beeinflussung klimakterischer beschwerden durch ein pytotherapaeutikum. [Influencing menopausal symptoms with a phytotherapeutic agent.] Die Medizinis Welt 36:871–874, 1985.

19. Pethö A. Klimakterische beschwerden: Umstellung einer hormonbehandlung auf ein pflanzliches gynmkologikum möglich? [Menopausal complaints: Changeover of a hormone treatment to a herbal gynecological remedy practicable?] Arztl Praxis 38:1551–1553 [English translation], 1987.

20. Shuster J. Black cohosh root? Chasteberry tree? Seizure! Hosp Pharm 31:1553–1554, 1996.

21. Newall CA, Anderson LA, Phillipson JD. Herbal Medicines: A Guide for Health-Care Professionals, London, The Pharmaceutical Press, 1996.

22. Mellin GW. Drugs in the first trimester of pregnancy and the fetal life of Homo sapiens. Am J Obst Gynec 90:1169–1180, 1964.

23. Gunn TR, Wright IMR. The use of black and blue cohosh in labour. NZ Med J 109:410–411, 1996.

24. Baillie N, Rasmussen P. Black and blue cohosh in labour. NZ Med J 110:20–21, 1997.

25. Remifemin scientific brochure [English translation]. Salzgitter, Germany, Schaper & Brümmer GmbH & Co. KG, December 1997

Black Currant and Borage Oil
(*Ribes nigrum* and *Borago officinalis*)
rating: 🐾 🐾

> - Rich sources of gamma-linolenic acid, used for a variety of inflammatory conditions
> - Modest but favorable effects for patients with rheumatoid arthritis; mixed results in patients with dermatitis
> - Well tolerated based on controlled clinical trials

Several parts of the black currant (*Ribes nigrum*) and borage (*Borago officinalis*) plants are used medicinally. Black currant berries are also called quinsy berries, and borage seed oil is also called starflower oil. The plant oils are derived from the berries or seeds.

Uses: Historically, the leaves of black currant and borage plants have been used for various rheumatic and inflammatory conditions, and as herbal diuretics. Black currant has also been used for diarrhea, while borage has also been used as an antipyretic, expectorant, and general tonic. Currently, both plant oils are employed as rich sources of gamma-linolenic acid (GLA). Along with evening primrose oil, these GLA-containing oils are used for chronic inflammatory and other conditions such as eczema, rheumatic disorders, mastalgia, premenstrual syndrome, and diabetic neuropathy.[1–4] Patients with these disorders are thought to be unable to sufficiently convert their dietary essential fatty acids to GLA, a precursor of anti-inflammatory eicosanoids[5]; thus, supplementation with GLA-rich plant oils is considered beneficial.

Pharmacology: The richest plant source of GLA is borage seed oil (about 23%), followed by black currant oil (15–20%) and evening primrose oil (7–10%).[1,5] The borage plant also contains small amounts of pyrrolizidine alkaloids (highest in the leaves and stems), mucilages, saponins, and tannins.[6] Black currant contains flavonoids, proanthocyanidins, and tannins,[4] and the oil is also rich in alpha-linoleic acid; this can be converted in the body to eicosapentanoic acid, which is also found in fish oils.

The metabolic pathway of GLA has been well established in humans and other animals.[5,7] Dietary linoleic acid (LA), an essential fatty acid, is converted to GLA by a rate-limiting enzymatic step. GLA is then rapidly converted to dihomo-gammalinolenic acid (DGLA), which is further metabolized to 1-series prostaglandins (PGs, such as PGE_1) and 3-series leukotrienes (LTs), which have anti-inflammatory properties, and to arachidonic acid (AA) in limited amounts. AA is converted by cyclo-oxygenases and lipoxygenases to pro-inflammatory mediators such as the 2-series prostaglandins (e.g., PGE_2), the 4-series leukotrienes (e.g., LTB4), and platelet activating factor.

LA → GLA → DGLA → 1-series PG, 3-series LT (anti-inflammatory)
\ → AA → 2 series PG, 4 series LT (pro-inflammatory)

GLA supplementation has been shown to attenuate the *in vitro* inflammatory response by enriching cells with DGLA, the immediate precursor of PGE_1, without increasing synthesis of AA.[5] DGLA or another metabolite, 15-hydroxy-DGLA, appears to inhibit the AA pathway to its inflammatory byproducts, further inhibiting inflammation, and also has direct immune modulating effects on T-lymphocytes. A variety of anti-inflammatory effects from GLA supplementation has been demonstrated in animals and humans.

Most pharmacologic studies used evening primrose oil as the source of GLA. However, borage oil (and to a lesser extent, black currant oil) supplementation in humans has similarly been found to increase cellular DGLA concentrations, and to have immunomodulatory activity by altering cytokine production.[8–12]

Based on an elevated ratio of PGE_1 to pro-aggregatory eicosanoids, GLA is expected to reduce platelet aggregation. Controlled studies in humans have reported varying results, however, with most studies reporting an increase or no change in aggregation.[1] Bleeding time data has not been evaluated.

Clinical Trials:

• Dermatitis—Atopic dermatitis and infantile seborrheic dermatitis have been the subject of several GLA supplementation studies from Germany. Small placebo-controlled studies of borage or black currant oil with doses providing up to 600 mg/day of GLA reported both positive[13–15] and negative[16,17] results. The largest and most rigorous study of borage oil (providing 690 mg/day GLA) failed to find a significant benefit in the intention-to-treat group. This was a randomized, double-blind, placebo-controlled trial of 160 patients with atopic dermatitis, in which 6 months of supplementation was no more effective than placebo.

Subgroup analysis found benefits in specific populations.[18,19] Similarly, while early trials of atopic dermatitis using evening primrose oil reported benefits, more recent and better controlled trials have been disappointing. Thus, while the doses used were relatively low, clear benefits with GLA-containing oils for atopic dermatitis have not been demonstrated.

• Rheumatoid Arthritis—In patients with rheumatoid arthritis, chronic low doses of evening primrose oil (providing 540 mg/day GLA) have shown conflicting results in two separate trials [7]. Larger doses of GLA from borage or black currant oil were generally more successful in three double-blind, randomized, controlled trials from the same research group, all lasting 6 months. In the two trials using borage oil (n = 37 and 56), daily doses provided 1.4 g and 2.8 g of GLA, respectively.[20,21] Both of these trials found modest but statistically significant improvements overall, along with improvements in specific signs and symptoms such as joint tenderness, swelling, and pain assessments at 6 months.

In the higher-dose study, patients in the treatment group were 6.5 times more likely than placebo to experience meaningful improvement at 6 months, and the placebo group was 3.4 times more likely to experience deterioration.[21] Statistically significant improvements were not seen at interval checks prior to 6 months.

In the trial using black currant oil (providing 2 g/day GLA) in 34 subjects, the investigators found no improvements in global assessment, pain, swelling, or stiffness, but the joint tenderness score improved statistically compared to placebo (soybean oil).[22]

Adverse Effects: GLA-containing plant oils are well tolerated in clinical trials lasting up to 1 year. A few cases of diarrhea or soft stools, belching, and abdominal bloating have been reported.[5]

Interactions: There are no recognized drug interactions.

Cautions: Although controversial, there is concern that borage oil may contain small amounts of toxic pyrrolizidine alkaloids (PAs), which are found in the leaves and stems of the plant. Unsaturated PAs found in other plants are known to cause severe veno-occlusive hepatotoxicity in animals and humans, and carcinogenic and mutagenic effects in animal models.[23] There are no reports of hepatotoxicity with borage plants or products, probably due to the very low concentrations of these alkaloids, and the seeds and oil of borage may contain insignificant amounts.[24] However, without official quality standards and regulations, American consumers have no way of knowing the PA content of borage oil supplements.

Additionally, data regarding the use of black currant and borage oils during pregnancy and lactation is lacking.

Preparations & Doses: Most GLA-containing oils are manufactured in capsule (or softgel) form; they are also available as pure bottled liquid. Capsules may contain about 1000–1300 mg or more of oil (170–300 mg GLA, depending on the plant source). To attain daily GLA supplementation of at least 1–2 g, the dose found to be effective in most controlled studies, 3–12 capsules/day are needed, depending on the product. More traditional preparations of the leaf parts include infusions and tinctures.[6]

Summary Evaluation

Black currant and borage oils are the richest known plant sources of GLA, an omega-6 fatty acid and precursor to anti-inflammatory eicosanoids. Preliminary results from studies of inflammatory skin disease such as atopic dermatitis were hopeful, but generally poor results were found in larger or better-quality trials. Larger doses benefited patients with rheumatoid arthritis in limited trials; this herbal remedy may be helpful in some of these patients. A practical limitation to the use of GLA-containing plant oils is the large number of capsules needed for adequate dosing, and the long onset of action (several months) before clinical benefits are observed.

references

1. Barre DE. Potential of evening primrose, borage, black currant, and fungal oils in human health. Ann Nutr Metab 45:47–57, 2001.
2. Blumenthal M (ed). The Complete German Commission E Monographs: Therapeutic Guide to Herbal Medicines. Boston, MA, Integrative Medicine Communications, 1998.
3. Borage. Lawrence Review of Natural Products. St. Louis, MO, Facts and Comparisons, August 1992.
4. European Scientific Cooperative on Phytotherapy. *Ribis nigri folium:* Black currant leaf. Monographs on the Medicinal Uses of Plant Drugs. Exeter, UK, ESCOP, July 1997.
5. Fan Y-Y, Chapkin RS. Importance of dietary gamma-linolenic acid in human health and nutrition. J Nutr 128:1411–1414, 1998.
6. Newall CA, Anderson LA, Phillipson JD. Herbal Medicines: A Guide for Health-care Professionals. London, Pharmaceutical Press, 1996.
7. Belch JJF, Hill A. Evening primrose oil and borage oil in rheumatologic conditions. Am J Clin Nutr 71(Suppl):352S–356S, 2000.
8. Thijs C, van Houwelingen A, Poorterman I, et al. Essential fatty acids in breast milk of atopic mothers: Comparison with non-atopic mothers, and effect of borage oil supplementation. Eur J Clin Nutr 54:234–238, 2000.

9. Fisher BAC, Harbige LS. Effect of omega-6 lipid-rich borage oil feeding on human function in healthy volunteers. Biochem Soc Transactions 25:343S, 1997.

10. Barre DE, Holub BJ, Chapkin RS. The effect of borage oil supplementation on human platelet aggregation, thromboxane B2, prostaglandin E1 and E2 formation. Nutr Res 13:739–751, 1993.

11. Pullman-Mooar S, Laposata M, Lem D, et al. Alteration of the cellular fatty acid profile and the production of eicosanoids in human monocytes by gamma-linolenic acid. Arthr Rheum 33:1526–1533, 1990.

12. Wu D, Meydani M, Leka LS, et al. Effect of dietary supplementation with black currant seed oil on the immune response of healthy elderly subjects. Am J Clin Nutr 70:536–543, 1999.

13. Bahmer FA, Schafer J. Treatment of atopic dermatitis with borage seed oil (Glandol)-A time series analytic study. [German; Medline abstract] Kinderarztl Prax 60(7):199–202, 1992.

14. Buslau M, Thaci D. Atopic dermatitis: Borage oil for systemic therapy. [Cochrane Library abstract] Z Dermatol 182:131–132,134–136, 1996.

15. Andreassi M, Forleo P, Di Lorio A, et al. Efficacy of gamma-linolenic acid in the treatment of patients with atopic dermatitis. J Internat Med Res 25:266–274, 1997.

16. Rilliet A, Queille C, Saurat J-H. Effects of gamma-linolenic acid in atopic dermatitis. Dermatologica 177:257, 1988.

17. Borreck S, Hildebrandt A, Forster J. [Gamma-linolenic-acid-rich borage seed oil capsules in children with atopic dermatitis. A placebo-controlled double-blind study]. [German; Medline abstract] Klin Padiatr 209(3):100–104, 1997.

18. Henz BM, Jablonska S, Van de Kerkhof PCM, et al. Double-blind, multicentre analysis of the efficacy of borage oil in patients with atopic eczema. Br J Dermatol 140:685–688, 1999.

19. Kapoor R, Klimaszewski A. Efficacy of borage oil in patients with atopic eczema (correspondence). Br J Dermatol 143:200–201, 2000.

20. Leventhal LJ, Boyce EG, Zurier RB. Treatment of rheumatoid arthritis with gammalinolenic acid. Ann Intern Med 119:867–873, 1993.

21. Zurier RB, Rossetti RG, Jacobson EW, et al. Gamma-linolenic acid treatment of rheumatoid arthritis. Arthr Rheum 39:1808–1817, 1996.

22. Levanthal LJ, Boyce EG, Zurier RB. Treatment of rheumatoid arthritis with blackcurrant seed oil. Br J Rheumatol 33:847–852, 1994.

23. Westendorf J. Pyrrolizidine alkaloids-General discussion. In: De Smet PAGM (ed): Adverse Effects of Herbal Drugs. Vol 1. Berlin, Springer-Verlag, 1992, pp193–226.

24. De Smet PAGM. Safety of borage seed oil. Can Pharm J 124:5, 1991.

Capsicum Peppers (*Capsicum* spp.)
rating: 🌶🌶

- Capsicum peppers are the source of capsaicin, which is used for the topical treatment of arthritis, neuralgia, and other painful syndromes.
- Precise value is difficult to evaluate; results are mixed in controlled trials.

The *Capsicum* peppers vary considerably in shape, size, color, and pungency, with over 20 different species. The very pungent, hot-tasting peppers, indigenous to more tropical habitats, are often called chile, chili, or Cayenne pepper, whereas the milder European varieties are known as sweet peppers, bell peppers, or paprika. *Capsicum* peppers are distinct from black pepper (*Piper nigrum*), a vine native to India that is the source of peppercorns, mainly used as a condiment spice.

Uses: Various members of the *Capsicum* pepper family have been used traditionally in Central and South America and in Asia to treat many diseases.[1,2] Common indications include cardiovascular, circulatory, and respiratory problems; bowel disorders; wounds; burns; joint pains; and headaches.[3] Currently, extracts of *Capsicum* species are commonly employed for local analgesia in acute and chronic pain syndromes, and capsaicin is available in a variety of pharmaceutical products. Pepper extracts are also used in sprays for defense against wild animals, humans, and garden pests.

Pharmacology: Peppers contain over 125 volatile oils, as well as glycosides and vitamins.[1,3] The main component of capsicum peppers is the glycoside capsaicinoid, or capsaicin (N-vanillyl-8-methyl-6-[E]-nonenamide).[4,5] This chemical is related to eugenol (a major component of cloves) and vanillin (a major component of vanilla). Pure capsaicin and the related dihydrocapsaicin are extraordinarily pungent; they can be detected in a dilution of 1 in 17 million.[5,6] The "hotness" of peppers is measured on the Scoville Organoleptic scale. Sweet bell peppers usually have zero Scoville units; habañeros measure over 200,000 units; and pure capsaicin rates over 15,000,000 units.[4] The capsaicinoids are insoluble in water but readily dissolve in alcohol and vegetable oils.

A great deal is known about capsaicin. This molecule has proved to be a valuable tool for evaluating physiological mechanisms of cough, bronchospasm, and mucus production in humans and animals.[9] However, its most important use is as a treatment for pain. Capsaicin is a lipophilic vanilloid that acts on receptors in the peripheral terminals of the nocioceptors that respond to painful stimuli. The stimulated receptor opens specific cation channels, resulting in transmission of sensory input through unmyelinated C-fibers. The transmitted impulse produces release of a neuropeptide, substance P, from sensory nerves that mediate pain.[9] It has been shown that repeated or prolonged stimulation by capsaicin—which initially causes pain—gradually inactivates the nocioceptors and sensory nerve fibers, and they eventually degenerate. Pain may return, however, as receptors and nerve fibers regenerate over several weeks.[10]

Clinical Trials: An accepted value of capsaicin is its use as a topical rubefacient, counter-irritant, and analgesic for various forms of arthritis,[11,12] and it is considered to be beneficial for neuropathic pain syndromes, such as fibromyalgia, peripheral neuropathy, causalgia, post-mastectomy pain, and trigeminal neuralgia.[10,15,16] There is also some evidence supporting its use for pruritic disorders such as psoriasis, and for circulatory impairment that causes cold extremities.[7,11]

In spite of the acceptance of capsaicin as a pharmaceutical drug, there is controversy about its clinical value for pain relief. A meta-analysis evaluated 13 randomized, double-blind, placebo-controlled trials of capsaicin for painful conditions in a total of 991 patients.[13] For diabetic neuropathy, of four trials totaling 309 patients, only two trials showed significant benefit. For osteoarthritis, of three trials totaling 382 patients, only one trial using either 0.025% or 0.075% capsaicin showed significant benefit. For post-herpetic neuralgia and for post-mastectomy pain, single small trials found no significant benefits. For psoriasis, four trials totaling 245 patients were analyzed, and significant improvement was found in all trials. However, despite being of some benefit, topical capsaicin does not offer the most effective treatment when used in a concentration of 0.025% or 0.075%, although these are the strengths commonly marketed.[13,14]

In one other meta-analysis of different treatments for post-herpetic neuralgia, the authors could only find 11 published and one unpublished randomized controlled trials.[15] Of these, two could be analyzed for the effect of capsaicin; the pooled results showed a significant benefit, but blinding difficulties may have affected the findings.[16]

In evaluating other potential uses of capsaicin, one controlled trial failed to support claims that intranasal capsaicin is effective for migraine or cluster headaches.[17] Capsaicin has been used by urologists who instill it intravesically to treat neurogenic hypereflexia of the bladder; a review of eight open and two placebo-controlled trials suggested that it may offer benefits.[18]

Adverse Effects: People who are not conditioned to using peppers in large amounts will find oral or topical exposure to be unpleasant. Topical use causes increased pain for the first few days of use; patients must be counseled about this effect. Oral intake of peppery preparations can lead to gagging, coughing, inability to speak, dyspnea, and vomiting. Some patients with dyspepsia may find oral capsaicin increases discomfort and can induce gastroenteritis, diarrhea, and proctitis. Smaller doses of enteric capsules can prevent these dose-dependent consequences of capsaicin ingestion. It is still unclear whether peppery products can cause stomach ulcers, and some studies have found chili peppers to be protective.[11]

Interactions: ACE inhibitor pretreatment may enhance the cough induced by inhaled capsaicin; one patient on an ACE inhibitor only coughed when she applied topical capsaicin to her extremities.[6] Oral capsicum pepper was found to enhance the absorption characteristics of a sustained release form of theophylline in a European controlled study.[7] These reports have not been confirmed.

Cautions: Topical solutions, extracts, and creams should not be allowed to contact the eyes or broken skin because they could cause intense irritation. If capsaicin gets onto the fingers, the hands should be washed with soapy water to avoid inadvertently bringing capsaicin into or around the eyes. Some individuals are allergic to peppers. Alveolitis can occur in paprika packers who inhale its dust, and asthma or chronic cough can be precipitated in susceptible individuals who work with pepper products.[19] Pepper remedies should always be used with caution if the tolerance of the patient is unknown. Small doses or concentrations should be initiated, and increases made as indicated and tolerated.

Preparations & Doses: Oral dosages of 30–120 mg of cayenne pepper or 1–2 mg of the oleoresin up to three times a day are usually recommended,[13] although larger doses may be tolerated. Oral products are usually available as capsules. Capsaicin can be used in topical products; commercial creams that are well known (e.g., Zostrix) contain 0.025% or 0.075% capsaicin. Some patients tolerate and require higher concentrations, which they can make themselves. Cayenne powder can be mixed into vegetable oil or a topical cream to give concentrations of 0.1% to 0.5% for application several times a day.[7] If tolerated, higher concentrations up to 5% can be tried. In all cases, small or dilute amounts should be used initially, because excessive amounts will irritate the skin and cause pain.

Summary Evaluation

Capsicum peppers, which contain capsaicinoids, are of importance as research tools and as medications. Topical capsaicin creams and oils produce a sense of warmth and burning; repeated applications cause less discomfort, and the analgesic effect becomes predominant. Such application to painful muscle, skin, or joint areas has been shown to be therapeutic. Capsicum products are well accepted in orthodox medical practice for treating arthritic, musculoskeletal, and neuropathic pain, although clinical trial results are mixed. Other potential uses, such as for treating sinusitis and bronchitis, have not been studied and have not gained equal recognition. A major problem is that the pungent, burning qualities make sham treatment or double-blind assessment impossible.

references

1. Andrews J: Peppers. The Domesticated Capsicums. Austin, University of Texas Press, 1984.
2. Cichewitz RH, Thorpe PA: The antimicrobial properties of chile peppers (*Capsicum* species) and their use in Mayan medicine. J Ethnopharmacol 52:61–70, 1996.
3. Blumenthal M, Goldberg A, Brinckman J (eds): Herbal Medicine. Expanded Commission E Monographs. Newton, MA, Integrative Medicine Communications, 2000.
4. Mike's Pepper Garden. Accessed March 22, 2001 at http://www.edgein.home.mindspring.com/index.html
5. Bruneton J: Pharmacognosy, Phytochemistry, Medicinal Plants. Secaucus, NY, Lavoisier Publishing, 1995.
6. Hakas JF Jr. Topical capsaicin induces cough in patient receiving ACE inhibitor. Ann Allergy 1990;65:322–323.

7. Bouraoui A, Toumi A, Bouchacha S, et al. Influence de l'alimentation épicée et piquante sur l'absorption de la théophylline [Influence of spiced and pungent food on the absorption and bioavailability of theophylline]. Therapie 1986;41:467–471.

8. Reference deleted.

9. Baron R: Capsaicin and nocioception: From basic mechanisms to novel drugs. Lancet 356:785–786, 2000.

10. Nolano M, Simone DA, Wendelschafer-Crabb G, et al: Topical capsaicin in humans: Parallel loss of epidermal nerve fibers and pain sensation. Pain 81:135–145, 1999.

11. Newall CA, Anderson LA, Phillipson JD: Herbal Medicines: A Guide for Health Care Professionals. London, The Pharmaceutical Press, 1996.

12. Towheed TE, Hochberg MC: A systematic review of controlled trials of pharmacological therapy in osteo-arthritis of the knee, with an emphasis on trial methodology. Semin Arthritis Rheum 26:755–770, 1997.

13. Zhang WY, Li Wan Po A: The effectiveness of topically applied capsaicin. A meta-analysis. Eur J Clin Pharmacol 46:517–522, 1994.

14. McQuay HJ, Moore RA: An Evidence-Based Resource for Pain Relief. Oxford, Oxford University Press, 1998. See also Oxford Pain Internet Site: Topical capsaicin for pain relief. Accessed January 2, 2001 at http://jr2.ox.ac.uk/Bandolier

15. Volmink J, Lancaster T, Gray S, Silagy C: Treatments for postherpetic neuralgia: A systematic review of randomized controlled studies. Fam Pract 13: 84–91, 1996.

16. Yaphe J, Lancaster T: Postherpetic neuralgia. In Clinical Evidence. Vol. 3. London, BMJ Publishing Group, 2000, pp 358–365.

17. Marks DR, Rappoport A, Padla D, et al: A double-blind placebo-controlled trial of intranasal capsaicin for cluster headache. Cephalgia 13:114–116, 1993.

18. De Sèze M, Wiart L, Fernière J, et al: Intravesical instillation of capsaicin in urology: A review of the literature. Europ Urol 36:267–277, 1999.

19. Blanc P, Liu D, Juarez C, Boushey H: Cough in hot pepper workers. Chest 99:27–32, 1991.

Cat's Claw (*Uncaria tomentosa*)

rating: 🐾

- An Amazon rainforest herb promoted for a myriad of health benefits
- Claims based primarily on traditional use and laboratory investigations
- No well-documented side effects, but data limited
- Caution advised for patients with autoimmune disorders

Cat's claw, also known as uña de gato, belongs to the genus *Uncaria* and is indigenous to the Amazon rainforest and other tropical areas of South and Central America. *Uncaria* plants are woody vines with characteristic curved thorns, which resemble cat claws, on their stems. The species most widely used for medicinal purposes in Western countries is *Uncaria tomentosa*, but a related species, *U. guianensis*, is also employed. Other species are popular in Asia.

Uses: Cat's claw preparations have been employed by native populations of the upper Amazon basin for generations to treat a myriad of health problems. The Peruvian Ashàninka Indians view the vine as "life giving." Cat's claw is traditionally used to treat arthritis and rheumatism, ulcers and other disorders of the gastrointestinal tract, asthma, wounds, gonorrhea, dysentery, and tumors; to help recover from childbirth; and as a contraceptive (in large doses).[1–3] In North America and Europe, cat's claw is currently promoted for similar uses, with an emphasis on stimulating the immune system to treat disorders such as cancer, viral diseases (including AIDS), gastrointestinal illnesses, and inflammatory disorders.[1–3] Anecdotal reports abound describing the healing properties of cat's claw preparations for many serious or chronic medical conditions.

Pharmacology: Active chemical constituents from the roots, bark, and other parts of the plant include pentacyclic and tetracyclic oxindole alkaloids, quinovic acid glycosides, polyhydroxylated triterpenes, and several steroidal components (such as beta-sitosterol).[4,5] Peruvian Indian healers can reportedly identify plants that have the most healing properties, which may be of a specific botanic chemotype that contains more pentacyclic (rather than tetracyclic) alkaloids.[4,5] These constituents, as well as whole extracts, have been investigated in a variety of experiments to assess their proposed immunomodulatory, anti-inflammatory, and anticancer properties.

Contrasting effects on the immune/inflammatory system are found *in vitro*. Aqueous bark extracts inhibit the inflammatory response by suppressing TNF-alpha production.[6] In contrast, higher concentrations induce IL-1 and IL-6 production, at least in rat alveolar macrophages.[7] Although isolated pentacyclic oxindole alkaloids enhance phagocytic activity and affect the proliferation of human lymphocytes, the tetracyclic alkaloids antagonize this activity on lymphocytes.[4,5,8] In animal studies, extracts are reported to increase induced lymphocyte proliferation in splenocytes, increase peripheral white blood cell (WBC) counts, and enhance recovery of chemotherapy-induced leukopenia.[9,10] Quinovic acid glycosides reduce an experimental inflammatory response, and oral administration attenuates indomethacin-induced intestinal inflammation in animal models.[11,12]

Preliminary investigations of cat's claw extracts have demonstrated potential anticancer activity. Specific extracts appear to have cytoprotective antioxidant properties, and enhance repair of DNA breaks in irradiated rats.[6,9] They inhibit specific leukemia and lymphoma cell lines by inducing apoptosis and cell death.[4,13]

Among miscellaneous *in vitro* studies, extracts have been found to inhibit stomatitis virus, to noncompetitively bind to estrogen receptors, and to inhibit the cytochrome P450 3A4 isozyme.[14–16] Tetracyclic oxindole alkaloids and other constituents from *Uncaria* species used in Asia are reported to have CNS (sedative, anticonvulsant) and cardiovascular (hypotensive, antithrombotic) properties in animal models.[5] These effects have not been studied in South American species of *Uncaria*.

Pharmacologic studies in humans are limited. In both a case report and a randomized, double-blind study of 24 subjects, smokers given *U. tomentosa* reportedly had decreased mutagenic activity of their urine.[5,17] In another study, four healthy volunteers took a 350-mg capsule of a purified water-soluble extract (called C-MED-100) daily for 6 weeks.[9] An increase in WBCs was reported, but this was not clinically significant (mean increase from 6.6 to 7.18×10^3).

Clinical Trials: No complete clinical trials have been published. One uncontrolled clinical trial has been partially described in a review article.[4] Thirteen subjects with HIV infection who refused other therapies were given 20 mg/day of a *U. tomentosa* root extract (containing 12 mg/g of pentacyclic oxindole alkaloids) for a period ranging from 2.2 to 5 months. The total leukocyte count and T4/T8 ratio were not altered. The relative and absolute lymphocyte count increased slightly (from 24% to 33.7%), which was statistically significant. In a double-blind, randomized, controlled trial that was unpublished but reported in company literature, 40 patients with rheumatoid arthritis were given three 20-mg capsules daily of Krallendorn (by Immodal Pharmaka), a popular European cat's claw extract, or placebo for 6 months.[18] Two of three primary outcomes were reportedly improved in the treatment group, including objective evaluations of number and severity of tender joints ($p < 0.05$).

Adverse Effects: Cat's claw is generally considered to be safe and well tolerated, although data is limited. No side effects were reported in the few human studies, and no adverse effects were found in rodent toxicity studies.[4,5,18] Screening laboratory analyses were not affected in the 6-month clinical trial in rheumatoid arthritis patients.[18] Mild lymphocytosis, erythrocytosis, constipation, diarrhea, and hyperuricemia have been anecdotally reported by European researchers.[5,18]

Interactions: In one *in vitro* study, cat's claw inhibited activity of the 3A4 isozyme of cytochrome P450, a common drug metabolizing enzyme.[16] This has not been validated *in vivo*, and no drug interactions have been reported.

Cautions: Based on *in vitro* studies, European researchers believe that products containing the tetracyclic oxindole alkaloids (TOAs) may be detrimental or can attenuate the beneficial immunologic effects of the pentacyclic alkaloids.[4,5] They recommend that these products not be used for transplant patients, or for other conditions in which "immune-stimulation" may be detrimental. A case report of reversible acute renal failure (possibly due to allergic interstitial nephritis) was associated with ingestion of a cat's claw supplement in a patient with systemic lupus erythematosus (SLE).[19] Although this may represent an idiosyncratic reaction, it would be prudent for patients with SLE to avoid this herb, and caution should be advised to other patients with autoimmune disorders.

Because of cat's claw's traditional use as a contraceptive, it is not recommended during pregnancy. Its safety while breast feeding is not known.

Preparations & Doses: Traditionally, cat's claw vine bark is boiled in water and the decoction is drunk daily. Commercial preparations are available from a number of Peruvian, European, and U.S.-managed companies. Preparations are usually available in 200- to 500-mg capsules of *U. tomentosa*, although concentrated extracts are available. Some manufacturers standardize their product to contain a specific amount of oxindole alkaloids and polyphenols, and advertise that they are free of TOAs. Krallendorn (by Immodal Pharmaka, Austria), one of the original cat's claw products evaluated and used in Europe, is marketed in the U.S. as Saventaro (by Enzymatic Therapy/PhytoPharmica). It is a standardized root extract and stated to be free of TOAs. The suggested dose is one 20-mg capsule t.i.d. for the first 10 days, then one capsule daily thereafter, although in the clinical trial of rheumatoid arthritis patients the t.i.d. dose was administered for 6 months.

Dosage recommendations vary widely among different products and are generally empirical. Tea preparations are also available, predominantly used for treating gastrointestinal ailments such as gastritis, peptic ulcer disease, colitis, diverticulitis, hemorrhoids, and "leaky bowel syndrome."[3]

-------------------- **Summary Evaluation** --------------------

The current popularity of cat's claw is based primarily on traditional use, anecdotes, and preliminary *in vitro* and animal studies. Reported clinical benefits have not been objectively evaluated in published peer-reviewed studies, and the plethora of positive claims is most likely exaggerated. Extracts and chemical constituents have active pharmacologic properties *in vitro* and in animal experiments that warrant clinical investigation, but there is little objective evidence that cat's claw preparations reliably benefit any medical disorder. Cat's claw appears to be safe for most people (without autoimmune disorders), and it has no known side effects.

references

1. Cat's claw (Una de gato). The Lawrence Review of Natural Products. St. Louis, MO, Facts and Comparisons, April 1996.

2. Anon. Una de gato "Cat's claw". Raintree Tropical Plant Database. Accessed Sept. 26, 2000 at www.rain-tree.com/catclaw.htm

3. Jones K. The herb report: Uña de gato—Life-giving vine of Peru. Am Herb Assoc Newsletter 10(3):4, 1994.

4. Keplinger K, Laus G, Wurm M, et al. *Uncaria tomentosa* (Willd.) DC—Ethnomedicinal use and new pharmacological, toxicological and botanical results. J Ethnopharmacol 64:23–34, 1999.

5. Reinhard K-H. *Uncaria tomentosa* (Willd.) D.C.: Cat's claw, Una de Gato, or Saventaro. J Altern Complem Med 5:143–151, 1999.

6. Sandoval M, Charbonnet RM, Okuhama NN, et al. Cat's claw inhibits TNF-alpha production and scavenges free radicals: Role in cytoprotection. Free Radical Biol Med 29:71–78, 2000.

7. Lemaire I, Assinewe V, Cano P, et al. Stimulation of interleukin-1 and –6 production in alveolar macrophages by the neotropical liana, *Uncaria tomentosa* (Una de Gato). J Ethnopharmacol 64:109–115, 1999.

8. Wagner H, Kreutzkamp B, Jurcic K. The alkaloids of *Uncaria tomentosa* and their phagocytosis-stimulating action. Planta Med 5:419–423, 1985.

9. Sheng Y, Bryngelsson C, Pero RW. Enhanced DNA repair, immune function and reduced toxicity of C-MED-100, a novel aqueous extract from *Uncaria tomentosa*. J Ethnopharmcol 69:115–126, 2000.

10. Sheng Y, Pero RO, Wagner H. Treatment of chemotherapy-induced leukopenia in a rat model with aqueous extract from *Uncaria tomentosa*. Phytomed 7:137–143, 2000.

11. Aquino R, De Simone F, Pizza C. Plant metabolites. Structure and in vitro antiviral activity of quinovic acid glycosides from *Uncaria tomentosa* and *Guettarda platypoda*. J Nat Prod 52: 679–685, 1989.

12. Sandoval-Chacon M, Thompson JH, Zhang X-J, et al. Anti-inflammatory actions of cat's claw: The role of NF-KB. Aliment Pharmacol Ther 12:1279–1289, 1998.

13. Sheng Y, Pero RW, Amiri A, Bryngelsson C. Induction of apoptosis and inhibition of proliferation in human tumor cells treated with extracts of *Uncaria tomentosa*. Anticancer Res 18:3363–3368, 1998.

14. Aquino R, De Feo V, De Simone F, et al. Plant metabolites. New compounds and anti-inflammatory activity of *Uncaria tomentosa*. J Nat Prod 54:453–459, 1991.

15. Salazar EL, Jayme V. Depletion of specific binding sites for estrogen receptor by *Uncaria tomentosa*. Proc West Pharmacol Soc 41:123–124, 1998.

16. Budzinski JW, Foster BC, Vandenhoek S, Arnason JT. An *in vitro* evaluation of human cytochrome P450 3A4 inhibition by selected commercial herbal extracts and tinctures. Phytomed 7:273–282, 2000.

17. Rizzi R, Re F, Bianchi A, et al. Mutagenic and antimutagenic activities of *Uncaria tomentosa* and its extracts. J Ethnopharmacol 38:63–77, 1993.

18. Summary and Assessment of Clinical Examinations of Krallendorn Products. IMMODAL Pharmaka GmbH, Austria, 1999.

Chamomile (*Matricaria recutita*)
rating: 🐝🐝 +

- Traditionally used for skin inflammation, colic or dyspepsia, and anxiety
- Limited clinical studies; results conflicting and inconclusive
- Generally safe and well tolerated; occasional allergic reactions

---

A number of plants have "chamomile" as part of their common name. For medicinal use, German chamomile (*Matricaria recutita*) is by far the most popular, but Roman chamomile (*Chamaemelum nobile*) is also used. These plants belong to the Asteraceae family. The flower heads are the primary plant parts used in herbal medicine.

Uses: German and Roman chamomile have been employed medicinally for centuries, dating back to Egyptian and Roman eras. Chamomile is most often adopted as an anti-inflammatory, antispasmodic, and calming agent. It is used topically to treat inflammatory skin and mucous membrane disorders, or orally for minor colicky digestive problems and anxiety or nervousness.[1–3] It is also extensively used as a beverage, food additive, and flavoring agent, and in cosmetic, bath, and hair products.

Pharmacology: Constituents of chamomile considered to be most pharmacologically active include the terpenoids (e.g., alpha-bisabolol and bisabolol oxide derivatives, farnesene, matricine, and chamazulene). These constituents are derived from the essential oil obtained from the flower head of the plant.[1] Other important constituents that are more hydrophilic include the flavonoids (e.g., apigenin and luteolin), coumarins, and a mucilage.[1,3]

In vitro, chamomile constituents can inhibit the inflammatory mediators of the arachidonic acid cascade such as 5-lipoxygenase and cyclo-oxygenase.[3] Flavonoid compounds reportedly have *in vitro* anti-inflammatory effects similar to low-dose indomethacin.[1] Numerous animal studies have also evaluated the anti-inflammatory effects of chamomile.[3] In one study, mice exposed to an inflammatory skin agent had a reduction in edema and inflammation when treated with an extract of chamomile compared to placebo.[4]

Sedative and antispasmodic activities also have been demonstrated.[3] The flavonoid apigenin appears to bind to central benzodiazepine receptors.[5] The essential oil of chamomile reduced experimentally induced spasm of pig small intestine, resulting in decreased tonus and peristalsis compared to placebo.[6] The terpenoid (-)-alpha-bisabolol was noted to inhibit the development of stomach ulceration following treatment of rats with indomethacin, stressful stimuli, or alcohol.[7]

Clinical Trials:

• Topical Uses—Most clinical trials have reported benefits with topical applications of chamomile for the treatment of mucositis and dermatitis. Many are uncontrolled or open studies, and results are not well substantiated in randomized controlled trials (RCTs). For example, a chamomile oral rinse was used during head and neck radiation and/or chemotherapy in an uncontrolled series of 98 patients. With a prophylactic chamomile rinse, only 1 of 20 patients receiving radiation therapy developed mucositis, and 10 of 46 patients receiving chemotherapy developed mucositis.[8] However, in a relatively large, double-blind RCT, 164 patients receiving chemotherapy were given chamomile or placebo mouthwash t.i.d. for 14 days. No differences were noted between the treatment and placebo groups.[9] In another double-blind RCT, 48 women who had surgery for local breast cancer applied chamomile cream or almond ointment to the affected breast during radiation therapy.[10] Neither agent prevented radiation-induced skin changes, and there was no significant difference between the two treatments.

For inflammatory skin disorders, topically administered chamomile appears to have very mild effects. In an open comparative trial of 161 patients with an inflammatory dermatosis, a German chamomile cream was found to have similar efficacy to low-potency (0.25%) hydrocortisone.[11] In a partially double-blind RCT of 72 patients with eczema, a chamomile cream was more effective than a 0.5% hydrocortisone cream, but the effects were also no different from a placebo (vehicle) cream.[12] In a double-blind placebo-controlled trial, a chamomile extract was reported to decrease weeping in surgical wounds after dermabrasion of tattoos ($P < 0.05$).[3]

• Oral Uses—The antispasmodic and gastrointestinal effects of combination products have been evaluated in a few controlled trials. In a double-blind RCT of 68 healthy, full-term infants with colic, a multi-herb tea containing German chamomile (with vervain, licorice, fennel, and lemon balm) was administered for 7 days. Colic symptom scores were significantly improved in the treated group compared to placebo ($P < 0.05$), and more babies had their colic eliminated (57% vs. 26%) ($P < 0.01$).[13] In another double-blind RCT of 79 children with acute diarrhea also receiving usual rehydration, a combination chamomile extract and apple pectin preparation was compared with a placebo for 3 days. Faster resolution of diarrhea was reported with the chamomile-pectin therapy by at least 5 hours ($P < 0.05$)[14]; however, the active ingredient may have been the pectin component.

In a small, uncontrolled, but often quoted study from 1973, 12 hospitalized patients consumed two cups of chamomile tea during cardiac catheterization, and 10 of the 12 fell asleep during the procedure.[15] No controlled trials investigating chamomile's sedative effects have been published.

Adverse Effects: Chamomile is generally regarded as a mild and safe herb, and it is widely available in foods, beverages, and cosmetics. Excessive use has reportedly led to mild gastroparesis and emesis.[16] The only significant toxicity is an occasional allergic reaction, which may (rarely) lead to angioedema and anaphylaxis.[17-19] These cases primarily involved patients who had an allergy to ragweed or other plants in the Asteracea family.

Interactions: Theoretically, chamomile may enhance the effects of other sedatives. However, the popularity and common use of chamomile tea suggests that no relevant sedation occurs that necessitates a warning for users. Chamomile was reported to inhibit the *in vitro* activity of the 3A4 isozyme of cytochrome P450, a common drug-metabolizing enzyme.[20] This has not been validated *in vivo*, and there are no clinical drug interactions reported for chamomile.

Cautions: Safety during pregnancy or breast feeding has not been evaluated. Several animal studies have noted reduction in body weight at birth and increased abortions with high dosage administration.[16,21] Patients with a history of allergies to ragweed or other Asteracea plants (e.g., daisies, sunflowers, chrysanthemums) should avoid chamomile products.

Preparations & Doses: There is no universally accepted standardization of chamomile products. Traditional doses include

2–4 g of dried flower heads or an equivalent infusion (tea), tincture, or extract, usually taken t.i.d.[3] The majority of studies of German chamomile administered topically to both humans and animals involved the product Kamillosan, which is manufactured in Germany and available in the U.S. as Camillosan in Camocare skin care products (Abkit, Inc.).

Summary Evaluation

Chamomile has a long history of use as an anti-inflammatory, antispasmodic, and anxiolytic. Other than the treatment of infant colic in one study (with a combination product), there are few well-designed, controlled clinical trials to support these potential benefits. Based on empiric use and the relative safety of the herb, it is acceptable for patients to consider chamomile for the treatment of colic, mild skin or mucous membrane conditions, and anxiety. However, clinical benefits are likely to be small, and have not been proven beyond a reasonable doubt.

references

1. Chamomile. The Review of Natural Products. St. Louis, MO, Facts and Comparisons, May 2000.
2. Heneka N: *Chamomilla recutita*. Medicinal Plant Review. Aust J Med Herbalism 5:33–39, 1993.
3. Mills S, Bone K: Principles and Practice of Phytotherapy: Modern Herbal Medicine. Edinburgh, UK, Churchill Livingstone, 2000.
4. Jakovlev V, Isaac K, Thiemer K, et al: Pharmacological investigations with compounds of chamomile. II. New investigations on the antiphlogistic effects of (-)-alpha-bisabolol and bisabolol oxides. Planta Med 35:125–140, 1979.
5. Viola H, Wasowski C, Levi de Stein M, et al: Apigenin, a component of *Matricaria recutita* flowers, is a central benzodiazepine receptors-ligand with anxiolytic effects. Planta Med 61: 213–216, 1995.
6. Achterrath-Tuckermann U, Kunde R, Flaskamp E, et al: Pharmacological investigations with compounds of chamomile. V. Investigations on the spasmolytic effect of compounds of chamomile and Kamillosan on the isolated guinea pig ileum. Planta Med 39:38–50, 1980.
7. Szelenyi I, Isaac O, Thiemer K: Pharmacological experiments with compounds of chamomile. III. Experimental studies of the ulcerprotective effect of chamomile. Planta Med 35:218–227, 1979.
8. Carl W, Emrich LS: Management of oral mucositis during local radiation and systemic chemotherapy: A study of 98 patients. J Prosthet Dent 66:361–369, 1991.
9. Fidler P, Loprinzi CL, O'Fallon JR, et al: Prospective evaluation of a chamomile mouthwash for prevention of 5-FU-induced oral mucositis. Cancer 77:522–525, 1996.

10. Maiche AG, Grohn P, Maki-Hokkonen H: Effect of chamomile cream and almond ointment on acute radiation skin reaction. Acta Oncol 30:395–396, 1991.

11. Aertgeerts P, Albring M, Klaschka F, et al: Vergleichende pruufung von kamillosan crème gegenuber steroidalen externa in der erhaltungstherapie von ekzemerkrankungen. Z Hautkr 60:270–277, 1985.

12. Patzelt-Wenczler R, Ponce-Pöschl E: Proof of efficacy of Kamillosan cream in atopic eczema. Eur J Med Res 5(4):171–175, 2000.

13. Weizman Z, Alkrinawi S, Goldfarb D, et al: Efficacy of herbal tea preparation in infantile colic. J Pediatr 122:650–652, 1993.

14. De IMS, Bose-O'Reilly S, Heinisch M, Harrison F: Doppelblind-vergleich zwischen einem apfelpektin/Kamillenextrakt-präparat und plazebo bei kindern mit diarrhoe [Double-blind comparison of a preparation of pectin/chamomile extract and placebo in children with diarrhea]. Arzneim-Forsch/Drug Res 47:1247–1249, 1997. [Abstract]

15. Gould L, Reddy RCV, Gomprecht RF: Cardiac effects of chamomile tea. J Clin Pharmacol 13:475–479, 1973.

16. Mann C, Staba EJ: The chemistry, pharmacology, and commercial formulations of chamomile. In Craker LE, Simon JE (eds): Herbs, Spices, and Medicinal Plants: Recent Advances in Botany, Horticulture, and Pharmacology. Vol 1. Phoenix, AZ, Oryx Press, 1986, pp 235–280.

17. Jensen-Jarolim E, Reider N, Fritsch R, Breiteneder H: Fatal outcome of anaphylaxis to camomile-containing enema during labor: A case study. J All Clin Immunol 102:1041–1042, 1998.

18. Fott C, Nettis E, Panebianco R, et al: Contact urticaria from *Matricaria chamomilla*. Contact Dermat 42:360–361, 2000.

19. Hausen BM: Sesquiterpene lactones—*Chamomilla recutita*. In De Smet PAGM (ed): Adverse Effects of Herbal Drugs. Vol. 1. Berlin, Springer, 1992, pp 243–248, 263.

20. Budzinski JW, Foster BC, Vandenhoek S, Arnason JT: An *in vitro* evaluation of human cytochrome P450 3A4 inhibition by selected commercial herbal extracts and tinctures. Phytomed 7:273–282, 2000.

21. Newall CA, Anderson LA, Phillipson JD: Herbal Medicines: A Guide for Health-Care Professionals. London, The Pharmaceutical Press, 1996.

Chaste Tree (*Vitex agnus-castus*)
rating: 🐾 🐾 🐾

> - Used for a variety of menstrual-related disorders
> - Best clinical evidence is for treatment of PMS and cyclical mastalgia
> - Well tolerated with minimal side effects; use caution with dopaminergic drugs

The dried fruit or berry of the chaste tree is often referred to as Monk's pepper or chasteberry; it was historically thought to reduce libido or promote chastity. Chaste tree is also commonly referred to as vitex.

Uses: Standardized extracts of the chaste tree berry are popular in Europe, and now in North America, for a variety of women's problems primarily related to the menstrual cycle.[1–4] These disorders include menstrual cycle irregularities, the premenstrual syndrome (PMS), cyclic breast pain, dysfunctional uterine bleeding, and infertility. Historically, vitex has also been used for inflammatory conditions, diarrhea, flatulence, insufficient lactation, and menstruation induction.

Pharmacology: The major herbal constituents of the berry include terpenoids (e.g., vitexilactone), flavonoids (e.g., casticin), iridoid glycosides (e.g., agnuside and aucubin), and a volatile oil.[1,2] Small amounts of compounds related to androgenic steroids have been reported to be isolated from leaves and flowers,[5] but these plant parts generally are not used medicinally.

Studied primarily in Germany since the 1950s, hydro-alcoholic extracts of the herb have well-established central dopaminergic activity *in vitro* and *in vivo* (binding to dopamine$_2$ receptors), which inhibits pituitary prolactin secretion in animal studies.[1,2,6–8] Although traditionally used to increase lactation, large doses in lactating rats significantly reduced milk production in one study, presumably due to the drop in prolactin secretion.[4] Effects on prolactin in humans are complex and not well elucidated. While some studies demonstrate mild reductions in prolactin secretion (or prolactin levels), some show no changes or even increases.[1,9] Opioid and estrogen receptors are also bound *in vitro*,[6,10] although the estrogenic effect is significantly weaker than other known phyto-estrogens (e.g., red clover isoflavones).[10]

Several European trials suggest that vitex corrects deficient progesterone levels in women with "corpus luteum insufficiency" or "latent hyperprolactinemia," in which low progesterone levels predominate in the 2nd (luteal) phase of the menstrual cycle.[1,4,11] The mechanism of this effect is thought to be due to a reduction of prolactin secretion (especially in women with an absolute or relative hyperprolactinemia) or by an enhanced release of pituitary gonadotrophins. However, the actual pharmacologic activity is not well characterized. Clinical trials have not found consistent effects on progesterone and/or prolactin levels, and have found no effect on gonadotropins.[1,9,11–14]

Clinical Trials: Vitex has been reported to correct symptoms of menstrual and related disorders in over 30 European clinical trials during the last 50 years. Beneficial effects have been described for patients with PMS, mastalgia, irregular menstrual cycles, dysfunctional uterine bleeding, infertility, decreased lactation, and acne.[1–3] Most of these studies are uncontrolled or unblinded, including many large post-market surveillance studies. In this review, only double-blind randomized controlled trials (RCTs) are described; several are only available in German-language journals, and are reviewed in secondary sources.[1,2]

• Premenstrual Syndrome—Three double-blind RCTs, each lasting 3 months (or three menstrual cycles), have evaluated different vitex preparations for the symptoms of PMS. In one trial using 1800 mg/day of powdered vitex tablets, little difference was found between the vitex and placebo groups in the 217 women completing the trial.[15] The other two RCTs used standardized European commercial extract products. In 175 women, 4 mg/day of a vitex preparation (Agnolyte) was similar in effect to 200 mg/day of vitamin B_6 (both decreased symptoms by almost 50%); however, there was no placebo control.[16] In a recent RCT of 178 women using 20 mg/day of an extract product (Ze440), a significantly better response rate (> 50% reduction of symptoms) was demonstrated in the vitex vs. the placebo group (52% vs. 24%, respectively). Self-assessment of symptoms also improved significantly on a validated symptom scale compared to placebo (P < 0.001).[17]

• Cyclic Breast Pain—Cyclic mastalgia is often associated with the PMS complex of symptoms. Three double-blind, controlled trials have reported beneficial results with a standardized

European preparation, Mastodynon (vitex combined with several homeopathic herbs), using drops and/or tablets. In a trial of 160 women with premenstrual mastalgia, vitex was reported to provide good symptomatic relief more often than placebo (74.5% vs. 36.8%, respectively), and was equivalent to a progestational agent, lynestranol (82.1%).[18] Two similar RCTs, each lasting three menstrual cycles (n = 97 and 104 women), also reported almost identical, statistically significant reductions in symptoms compared to placebo.[13,19]

• Other—A double-blind RCT of 96 infertile women (66 were available at the final analysis) found that 30 drops of Mastodynon b.i.d. for 3 months was associated with twice the number of pregnancies (21%) compared to placebo (10%). These results were not statistically significant.[14] Controlled trials have reported benefits for insufficient lactation[20] and for acne,[1] but these older studies were not adequately randomized, controlled, or blinded.

Adverse Effects: Vitex appears to be very well tolerated. Reported side effects in the clinical studies are rare and transient (often similar in frequency to placebo), and primarily include mild gastrointestinal complaints, allergic reactions, or headaches.[1–4,17] A single case of unexplained nocturnal seizures in a patient taking chaste tree berry, black cohosh, and evening primrose oil has been reported[21]; a cause-and-effect relationship with vitex is doubtful.

Interactions: There are no reported interactions with vitex. Due to its potential effects on dopamine and prolactin, it is relatively contraindicated with other drugs that are dopamine agonists or antagonists (e.g., bromocriptine, metoclopramide, anti-Parkinson's drugs).

Cautions: Use during pregnancy and lactation should generally be avoided, although vitex has been employed to enhance fertility and stimulate lactation. In a case report of a woman undergoing unstimulated *in vitro* fertilization treatment, a combination herbal preparation containing vitex was associated with folliculogenesis and increased FSH, LH, and progesterone levels. In addition, the patient complained of symptoms suggestive of mild ovarian hyperstimulation syndrome.[22]

Preparations & Doses: Vitex preparations and doses vary considerably; only the standardized European products have been demonstrated to be effective. In the German clinical trials, small doses of standardized extract preparations (Agnolyte, Mastodynon, and Straton) are equivalent to about 30–40 mg of dried or crude herb, and are usually administered each morning.[2] Agnolyte is marketed in the U.S. as Femaprin (Nature's Way), and is usually given as one 4-mg tablet or 40 drops of extract per day. Herbalists in Britain and other English-speaking countries tend to use much larger doses of noncommercial preparations, equivalent to about 500–2000 mg/day of dried herb, often in liquid extracts and tinctures.[2,4] A more recent European product (Ze440; available as a 20-mg extract) is equivalent to about 120–240 mg of crude herb.[17]

Summary Evaluation

Vitex may affect the endocrine and reproductive systems by decreasing prolactin via dopaminergic stimulation, although these pharmacologic properties are not fully characterized in humans. Uncontrolled trials and decades of use in Europe suggest beneficial effects for a wide variety of menstrual-related disorders. Well-designed, randomized, controlled trials are limited, but do support beneficial effects for the treatment of PMS (one trial) and cyclic mastalgia (three trials). Because vitex appears safe and well tolerated, and there are few effective treatments for these conditions, it is reasonable for women with these disorders to give vitex a therapeutic trial. There is insufficient evidence to make recommendations for other indications.

references

1. Upton R (ed). Chaste tree fruit: *Vitex agnus-castus*. American Herbal Pharmacopoeia and Therapeutic Compendium. Santa Cruz, CA, American Herbal Pharmacopoeia, 2001.
2. Mills S, Bone K. Principles and Practice of Phytotherapy: Modern Herbal Medicine. Edinburgh, UK, Churchill Livingstone, 2000.
3. Blumenthal M, Goldberg A, Brinckmann J (eds). Herbal Medicine: Expanded Commission E Monographs. Newton, MA, Integrative Medicine Communications, 2000.
4. Christie S, Walker AF. *Vitex agnus-castus* L.: (1) A review of its traditional and modern therapeutic use; (2) current use from a survey of practitioners. Eur J Herbal Med (Phytotherapy) 3(3):29-45, 1997–1998.
5. Chaste Tree. The Review of Natural Products. St. Louis, MO, Facts and Comparisons, February 1998.
6. Meier B, Berger D, Hoberg E, et al. Pharmacological activities of *Vitex agnus-castus* extracts *in vitro*. Phytomed 7:373–381, 2000.
7. Winterhoff H. *Vitex agnus-castus* (Chaste Tree): Pharmacological and clinical data. In Lawson LD, Bauer R (eds): Phytomedicines of Europe: Chemistry and Biological Activity. ACS Symposium Series 691. Washington DC, American Chemical Society, 1998, pp 299–308.

8. Gardiner P. The Longwood Herbal Task Force. Chasteberry (*Vitex agnus castus*). Revised May 11, 2000. Accessed January 18, 2001 at www.mcp. edu/herbal/default.htm

9. Merz P-G, Gorkow C, Schrödter A, et al. The effects of a special Agnus castus extract (BP1095E1) on prolactin secretion in healthy male subjects. Exp Clin Endocrinol Diabetes 104:447–453, 1996.

10. Liu J, Burdette JE, Xu H, et al. Evaluation of estrogenic activity of plant extracts for the potential treatment of menopausal symptoms. J Agric Food Chem 49:2472–2479, 2001.

11. Milewicz A, Gijdel E, Sworen H, et al. *Vitex agnus castus*-extrakt zur behandlung von regeltempoanomalien infolge latenter hyperporlaktinämie. Arzneim-Forsch/Drug Res 43:752–656 [English abstract], 1993.

12. Neumann-Kühnelt B, Stief G, Schmiady H, Kentenich H. Investigations of possible effects of the phytotherapeutic agent agnus castus on the follicular and corpus luteum phases. Human Reprod 8(Suppl 1):110 [Abstract], 1993.

13. Wuttke W, Splitt G, Gorkow C, Sieder C. Behandlung zyklusabhängiger brustschmerzen mit einem Agnus castus haltigen arzneimittel. [Treatment of cyclical mastalgia with a medication containing Agnus castus: results of a randomised, placebo-controlled, double-blind study.] Geburtshilfe Frauenheilkunde 57:569–574 [English abstract], 1997.

14. Gerhard I, Patek A, Monga B, et al. Mastodynon for female infertility. Randomized, placebo-controlled, clinical double-blind study. Forsch Komplementärmed 5:272–278, 1998. [German. Reviewed in Reichert R: Treatment of female fertility disorders using vitex. Healthnotes Rev Complem Integr Med 7:100–101, 2000.]

15. Turner S, Mills S. A double-blind clinical trial on a herbal remedy for premenstrual syndrome: A case study. Complem Ther Med. 1:73–77, 1993.

16. Lauritzen C, Reuter HD, Repges R, et al. Treatment of premenstrual tension syndrome with *Vitex agnus castus:* Controlled, double-blind study versus pyridoxine. Phytomed 4:183–189, 1997.

17. Schellenber R, for the study group. Treatment for the premenstrual syndrome with agnus castus fruit extract: Prospective, randomised, placebo-controlled study. BMJ 322:134–137, 2001.

18. Kubista E, Müller G, Spona J. Behandlung der mastopathie mit zyklischer mastodynie: klinische ergebnisse und hormonprofile. [Treatment of mastopathy associated with cyclic mastodynia: Clinical results and hormonal profiles.] Gynäk Rdsch 26:65–79, 1986. [English abstract, and reviewed in reference 1].

19. Halaska M, Beles P, Gorkow C, Sieder C. Treatment of cyclical mastalgia with a solution containing a *Vitex agnus castus* extract: Results of a placebo-controlled, double-blind study. Breast 8:175–181, 1999.

20. Mohr H. Clinical investigations of means to increase lactation. Dtsch Med Wschr 79:1513–1516, [English translation], 1954.

21. Shuster J. Black cohosh root? Chasteberry tree? Seizure! Hosp Pharm 31:1553–1554, 1996.

22. Cahill DJ, Fox R, Warkle PG, Harlow CR. Multiple follicular development associated with herbal medicine. Human Reprod 9:1469–1470, 1994.

Chondroitin*

rating: 🐾 🐾 🐾

> - Evidence supports use of oral chondroitin in osteoarthritis
> - Benefit of combining with glucosamine has not been well studied
> - Generally well tolerated, with only mild gastrointestinal side effects

Chondroitin sulfate (galactosaminoglucuronoglycan sulfate) refers to a group of polysulfated glycosaminoglycans such as chondroitin-4-sulfate, chondroitin-6-sulfate, and others. Structurally, the chondroitin molecule resembles heparanoids; it is actually a minor component of danaparoid sodium (a mixture of heparan sulfate, dermatan sulfate, and chondroitin sulfate in a 21:3:1 ratio).[1] It is commonly prepared from bovine or porcine cartilage sources.

Uses: Chondroitin sulfate is marketed for use alone and in combination with glucosamine for musculoskeletal and joint pain. It has been primarily studied for osteoarthritis. Injectable forms are FDA-approved as viscoelastic agents for ophthalmic surgery.

Pharmacology: Chondroitin sulfate is a mucopolysaccharide that the body uses in the synthesis of cartilage. Its potential chondroprotective properties stem from its role as one of the "building blocks" for synthesis of new cartilage, as well as its inhibition of leukocyte elastase, an inflammatory enzyme that contributes to cartilage degradation.[2] *In vitro* models demonstrate stimulation of proteoglycan production and collagen and hyaluronic acid synthesis.[3,4] Animal studies have shown beneficial effects on serum lipids and atherogenesis, as well as antithrombogenic activity.[2] Because it is a large molecule, chondroitin is poorly absorbed; oral bioavailability is 8–18%.[5]

---

* *Editor's Note:* Although not an herb, chondroitin is a dietary supplement that is included here because of its current popularity.

Clinical Trials:

• Chondroitin Sufate Alone For Osteoarthritis (OA)—Numerous clinical trials of chondroitin have been conducted, and two recent meta-analyses of these trials have been published in peer-reviewed journals. The first meta-analysis examined only randomized, double-blind, controlled studies of oral chondroitin sulfate (CS) that met specific criteria for objective outcome measures.[6] Seven of 16 available trials were included in the analysis for a total of 372 patients with hip and knee OA. Assessment of pain scores using a visual analogue scale (VAS) revealed significant differences between CS and placebo groups. The mean VAS of pain decreased by 43% at 3 months and by 58% at study end (150–365 days) in the CS group, compared to 20% at both time points in the placebo group. In the six trials that used the Lequesne index (another validated OA symptom scale), pooled data represented a decrease of 49% for CS patients and < 20% for controls.

Accounting for standard deviations of results, 55–65% of CS patients would have greater benefit than placebo patients. All seven trials reported that the reduction in concomitant analgesic medication was significantly greater in the CS groups, although no patients were able to discontinue analgesics completely. Investigators postulated that CS in combination with analgesics is more effective than CS alone. Doses used in the seven studies ranged from 800 to 2000 mg/day, which did not correlate with differences in efficacy outcome measures.

The second meta-analysis included nine clinical trials with a total of 799 patients using chondroitin sulfate (two intramuscularly, seven oral).[7] This analysis took into account the varying outcome measures by calculating an overall effect size, which was 0.78 for chondroitin (a moderate effect). However, when influences such as trial size and trial quality were considered, the calculated effect sizes ranged from 0.3 (small effect) to 1.7 (very large effect). The investigators concluded that chondroitin does have efficacy in the treatment of OA, but that the efficacy is likely to be overestimated due to methodological flaws they identified in the existing trials. A problem common to both meta-analyses is that some trials included in the analyses were available only in abstract form, thereby limiting analysis of the quality of the trials.

Two more recent trials were not included in the meta-analyses. One was a randomized, double-blinded, placebo-controlled trial of 154 patients with knee OA, using CS 500 mg twice daily or placebo for 6 months. It showed a beneficial trend in pain reduction with CS, but the difference was not statistically significant .[8] A distinguishing characteristic of this trial was the use of CS from avian rather than bovine sources. This was done to conform to "new environmental guidelines"; presumably, use of an avian source would remove the possibility of transmission of bovine spongiform encephalitis.

The second was a randomized, double-blind comparison trial that examined the effects of 1 month of treatment with diclofenac sodium 150 mg/day versus 3 months of treatment with chondroitin sulfate 1200 mg/day. These protocols were followed by placebo, so that each group completed 6 months of treatment.[9] The investigators reported a greater lasting benefit from CS, as measured by decrease in an objective pain scale at 3 and 6 months. Chondroitin may have a long duration of effect, lasting well into the placebo period; however, comparison of treatments given for different time periods prevents firm conclusions.

• In Combination—One randomized, double-blind, placebo-controlled crossover study compared the efficacy of 8 weeks of treatment with a combination of glucosamine hydrochloride (1500 mg/day), CS (1200 mg/day), and manganese ascorbate (228 mg/day) versus placebo in active military personnel with degenerative joint disease of the knee or lower back.[10] Statistically significant improvements were seen in VAS and patient assessments of efficacy, but not in the Lequesne index, acetaminophen use, or physical examination scores. Because both chondroitin and glucosamine may exhibit benefits that last beyond the active treatment period, a major study limitation is the crossover design with no washout period.

For patients with temporomandibular joint syndrome, an uncontrolled case series of 50 patients treated with 3200 mg/day glucosamine HCl, 2400 mg/day CS, and 2000 mg/day ascorbic acid reported subjective decreases in perception of "joint noise," pain, and swelling.[11]

• Other Uses—One small, preliminary, crossover study examined intranasal chondroitin sulfate solution and placebo for the reduction of snoring.[12] Mean sleep time spent snoring was 31.3% with chondroitin vs. 46.5% with placebo, suggesting possible therapeutic benefit. Oral CS was reported to be of benefit in 120 patients with coronary heart disease over 6 years.[13] However, this was an uncontrolled and inadequate study, and no similar reports have been made in the last 30 years.

Adverse Effects: Gastrointestinal effects of mild epigastric pain, diarrhea, and constipation are the most commonly reported adverse events. However, in controlled trials, side effects were generally equal to or less frequent than those in placebo groups.[6]

Interactions: Although increased anticoagulation effects have been a concern because of the chemical structure resembling heparanoids, no problems have been documented in clinical studies, even at CS doses up to 10 g daily in patients on anticoagulant therapy.[5,13]

Cautions: Increased endogenous chondroitin sulfate levels were associated with poor outcomes and increased tumor progression in prostate cancer patients in one study.[14] Until more data is available, patients with prostate cancer or elevated prostate-specific antigen levels should consider this possible disadvantage of chondroitin use. Because chondroitin is prepared from bovine sources, there is a potential for viral transmission. Safety during pregnancy and lactation has not been determined.

Preparations & Doses: Doses of chondroitin sulfate used in osteoarthritis trials with positive results usually ranged from 800 to 1500 mg daily; the most common dose is 400 mg t.i.d. An optimum dosage has not been determined in dose-response studies.

———————— **Summary Evaluation** ————————

The evidence, although not definitive, is sufficient to support the use of chondroitin sulfate for symptoms of mild to moderate osteoarthritis. Like glucosamine, symptom reduction appears to be similar to that of analgesic doses of nonsteroidal anti-inflammatory drugs, with a more minimal adverse event profile. There is insufficient information at this point to determine if the combination of glucosamine sulfate and chondroitin sulfate provides additional or synergistic benefit over use of either product alone.

references
1. Chondroitin. The Review of Natural Products. St. Louis, MO, Facts and Comparisons, April 1998.
2. Abt L, Hammerly M (eds): AltMedDex System. Englewood, CO MICROMEDEX, Inc. (Edition expires 2001.)
3. Bassleer CT, Combal J-PhA, Bougaret S, Malaise M: Effects of chondroitin sulfate and interleukin-1β on human articular chondrocytes cultivated in clusters. Osteoarthr Cartilage 6:196–204, 1998.

4. de los Reyes GC, Koda RT, Lein EJ: Glucosamine and chondroitin sulfates in the treatment of osteoarthritis: A survey. Progress Drug Res 55:83–104, 2000.
5. Chondroitin. Natural Medicines Comprehensive Database. Accessed January 30, 2001 at http://www.naturaldatabase.com
6. Leeb BF, Schweitzer H, Montag K, Smolen JS: A meta-analysis of chondroitin sulfate in the treatment of osteoarthritis. J Rheumatol 27:205–211, 2000.
7. McAlindon TE, LaValley MP, Gulin JP, Felson DT: Glucosamine and chondroitin for treatment of osteoarthritis. A systematic quality assessment and meta-analysis. JAMA 283:1469–1475, 2000.
8. Uebelhart D, Knüssel O, Theiler R: Efficacy and tolerability of oral avian chondroitin sulfate in painful knee osteoarthritis. [Abstract] Schweiz Med Wochenschr 129:1174, 1999.
9. Morreale P, Manopulo R, Galati M, et al: Comparison of the anti-inflammatory efficacy of chondroitin sulfate and diclofenac sodium in patients with knee osteoarthritis. J Rheumatol 23:1385–1391, 1996.
10. Leffler CT, Philippi AF, Leffler SG, et al: Glucosamine, chondroitin, and manganese ascorbate for degenerative joint disease of the knee or low back: A randomized, double-blind, placebo-controlled pilot study. Military Med 164:85–91, 1999.
11. Shankland WE: The effects of glucosamine and chondroitin sulfate on osteoarthritis of the TMJ: A preliminary report of 50 patients. J Craniomandib Pract 16:230–235, 1998.
12. Lenclud C, Chapelle P, Van Muylem A, et al: Effects of chondroitin sulfate on snoring characteristics: A pilot study. Curr Therap Res—Clin Exper 59:234–243, 1998.
13. Morrison LM, Enrick N: Coronary heart disease: reduction of death rate by chondroitin sulfate A. Angiology 24:269–287, 1973.
14. Ricciardelli C, Quinn DI, Raymond WA, et al: Elevated levels of peritumoral chondroitin sulfate are predictive of poor prognosis in patients treated by radical prostatectomy for early-stage prostate cancer. Cancer Res 59:2324–2328, 1999.

Coenzyme Q10*

rating: 🐜🐜

> - Has antioxidant activity; clinical significance of this effect unknown
> - Clinical trial results for heart disease inconsistent; no strong indications of therapeutic value
> - Well tolerated with minimal adverse effects

Coenzyme Q10 is known by a variety of names, including CoQ, CoQ10, and ubiquinone. It is found in the mitochondria of many organ tissues such as the heart, kidney, and liver.[1] The name coenzyme Q10 refers to the coenzyme Q enzyme containing 10 isoprenoid subunits.[1] The reduced form of coenzyme Q10 is called ubiquinol and this form predominates in the systemic circulation. Most supplement companies obtain CoQ10 from plant sources.

Uses: CoQ10 has antioxidant properties, and it has been used primarily for cardiovascular conditions such as congestive heart failure (CHF), hypertension, ischemic heart disease, and cardiomyopathies. It is also used as a general antioxidant supplement.

Pharmacology: CoQ10 has been described as one of the most metabolically active molecules present in the body. It circulates in the blood in the reduced form, ubiquinol, and is involved in many cell processes (mitochondrial electron transport) and in the generation of adenosyl triphosphate (ATP), which powers processes that create energy.[1] It serves as an endogenous antioxidant, scavenging free radicals. CoQ10 may also have a protective action on cell membranes by inhibiting the action of phospholipase A_2.[2] All of these actions suggest that it has an important role in vital processes, including cardiac muscle performance. CoQ10 is structurally similar to menaquinone, also known as vitamin K_2.

Clinical Trials:

• Hypertension—Various clinical trials (open label and controlled studies), mostly published by the same research group,

---

* *Editor's Note:* Although not an herb, Coenzyme Q10 is a dietary supplement that is included because of its current popularity.

suggest that CoQ10 significantly decreases blood pressure in patients with mild-moderate hypertension. Statistically significant reductions in systolic and diastolic blood pressures (10 mmHg) were observed after 10 weeks; however, these studies were not blinded and lacked a placebo comparison group.[3–5] One randomized, double-blind, comparative trial and one randomized, placebo-controlled, crossover trial have suggested similar reductions in systolic and diastolic blood pressures.[6,7] In one of these trials, a reduction in systolic and diastolic blood pressure (7–10 mmHg) was observed after 8–10 weeks of CoQ10 therapy compared to placebo. These latter studies, however, suffer from inadequate treatment allocation and a lack of statistical power to detect differences. Thus, the clinical evidence for CoQ10's value in hypertension is inadequate.

• Congestive Heart Failure—Older studies suggested that CoQ10 was effective as adjunctive therapy in the treatment of CHF.[8,9] A meta-analysis of eight clinical trials concluded that, while more evidence was required, CoQ10 could play a useful role in the management of this condition.[10] Many of the clinical trials included in the meta-analysis lacked control groups, and used crude estimates of heart muscle function. Two recent, well-conducted clinical trials used objective assessments of heart muscle function in patients with CHF. One was a randomized, double-blind, placebo-controlled trial and the other was a randomized, double-blind, placebo controlled, crossover trial. In patients with CHF (NYHA III and IV), CoQ10, at a dose of 100–200 mg daily for 3–6 months, was not significantly more effective than placebo.[11,12] These trials used Swan-Ganz measurements as well as echocardiography to assess left ventricular function.

• Ischemic Heart Disease—Results from two randomized, double-blind, placebo-controlled trials found that CoQ10 supplementation improved a number of clinical measures in patients diagnosed with chronic stable angina or coronary artery disease, and in those patients who had a history of acute myocardial infarction.[13,14] These trials suggest improvements in the markers for atherosclerosis (lipoprotein (a) and HDL-cholesterol); in exercise tolerance; and in delaying the time to develop ischemic changes on electrocardiograph (ECG) tracings. Other improvements include a reduction in cardiac deaths and rate of reinfarction in those recovering from acute myocardial infarction, compared to placebo.[14] This trial suggests that the relative risk reduction of sudden cardiac death with CoQ10 is 27%; however, the absolute risk reduction of sudden cardiac death when compared to placebo is only 1.5%, suggesting a very small improvement in risk with CoQ10. Furthermore, these trials were of short duration (≤ 1 month), and clinical reliability is unknown.

• Cardiomyopathy—Two small crossover trials that were randomized, double-blind, and placebo-controlled assessed the effects of CoQ10 on moderate to severe cardiomyopathy.[15,16] In one trial, 25 patients with NYHA class I, II, and III received CoQ10 (100 mg daily) or placebo. At the end of 4 months, no statistically significant differences were observed in ventricular function, ejection fraction, and calculated cardiac output.[15] Additionally, no improvements in exercise tolerance or ECG tracings were observed. In the second trial, in 19 patients diagnosed with NYHA class III or IV cardiomyopathy, CoQ10 supplementation (100 mg daily) significantly improved cardiac function.[16] However, this study failed to account for any carry-over of effects in the crossover design.

Adverse Effects: CoQ10 is well tolerated. In clinical trials, nausea, anorexia, and gastrointestinal upset have rarely been reported. Some patients have experienced maculopapular rash and thrombocytopenia.[17,18] Other rare side effects include irritability, headache, and dizziness.[19,20]

Interactions: A decrease in endogenous levels of CoQ10 has been observed following administration of HMG-CoA reductase inhibitors.[21,22] The clinical significance of this effect is unknown. Patients beginning statin therapy should not require CoQ10 supplementation, as the benefits of statin therapy likely outweigh any potential risk associated with low CoQ10 levels. Given the chemical similarity between vitamin K and CoQ10, the potential exists for an interaction with warfarin. CoQ10 has decreased the effects of warfarin in various case reports.[23] Until more is known, CoQ10 should be used with caution or not at all in patients receiving warfarin therapy.

Cautions: *In vitro* studies suggested that CoQ10 may interfere with glucose regulation.[24] Randomized placebo-controlled trials in diabetics, however, have shown no effect on blood glucose or metabolic control.[25,26] Safety in pregnancy and lactation has yet to be determined.

Preparations & Doses: A minimum of 30 mg daily appears to be necessary to increase blood levels. The clinical significance of increasing blood levels is unknown.[12,16] For cardiac indications, typical doses are 100–150 mg daily in 2 or 3 divided doses. These doses increase baseline CoQ10 levels to 2–3 mcg/ml (normal in healthy adults is 0.7–1 mcg/ml).

—————————— **Summary Evaluation** ——————————

The value of CoQ10 shows promise in adequately controlled trials of ischemic heart disease, although trials are limited. Clinical trials for other cardiovascular disorders (heart failure, cardiomyopathy, and hypertension) are inadequate or provide mixed results, and do not currently support the use of CoQ10 for these indications. CoQ10 does have antioxidant activity, but the clinical significance of this effect is unknown.

references

1. Ernster L, Dallner G: Biochemical, physiological and medical aspects of ubiquinone function. Biochim Biophys Acta 1271:195–204, 1995.
2. Miyazaki Y, Nagai S, Hattori M, et al: The effect of coenzyme Q10 against the attack of phospholipase to myocardial membrane. Arzneim-Forsch 36:187–189, 1986.
3. Digiesi V, Cantini F, Oradei A, et al: Coenzyme Q10 in essential hypertension. Mol Aspects Med 15:S257–S263, 1994.
4. Langsjoen P, Langsjoen P, Willis R, et al: Treatment of essential hypertension with coenzyme Q 10. Mol Aspects Med 15:S265–S272, 1994.
5. Digiesi V, Cantini F, Bisi G, et al: Mechanism of action of coenzyme Q10 in essential hypertension. Curr Ther Res 51:668–671, 1992.
6. Digiesi V, Cantini F, Brodbeck B: Effect of coenzyme Q10 on essential arterial hypertension. Curr Ther Res 47:841–845, 1990.
7. Singh RB, Niaz MA, Rastogi SS, et al: Effect of hydrosoluble coenzyme Q10 on blood pressures and insulin resistance in hypertensive patients with coronary artery disease. J Hum Hyperten 13:203–208, 1999.
8. Morisco C, Nappi A, Argenziano L, et al: Noninvasive evaluation of cardiac hemodynamics during exercise in patients with chronic heart failure: Effects of short-term coenzyme Q10 treatment. Mol Aspects Med 15:S155–S163, 1994.
9. Morisco C, Trimarco B, Condorelli M: Effect of coenzyme Q10 therapy in patients with congestive heart failure: A long-term multicenter randomized study. Clin Investig 71:S134–S136, 1993.
10. Soja AM, Mortensen SA: Treatment of congestive heart failure with coenzyme Q10 illuminated by meta-analyses of clinical trials. Mol Aspects Med 18:S159–S168, 1997.
11. Khatta M, Alexander B, Krichten C, et al: The effect of coenzyme Q10 in patients with congestive heart failure. Ann Intern Med 132:636–640, 2000.
12. Watson PS, Scalia GM, Galbraith A, et al: Lack of effect of coenzyme Q on left ventricular function in patients with congestive heart failure. J Am Col Cardiol 33:1549–1552, 1999.

13. Singh RB, Niaz MA: Serum concentration of lipoprotein(a) decreases on treatment with hydrosoluble coenzyme Q 10 in patients with coronary artery disease: discovery of a new role. Int J Cardiol 68:23–29, 1999.

14. Singh RB, Wander GS, Rastogi A, et al: Randomized, double-blind, placebo-controlled trial of coenzyme Q 10 in patients with acute myocardial infarction. Cardiovasc Drugs Ther 12:347–353, 1998.

15. Permanetter B, Rossy W, Klein G, et al: Ubiquinone (coenzyme Q10) in the long-term treatment of idiopathic dilated cardiomyopathy. Eur Heart J 13:1528–1533, 1992.

16. Langsjoen PH, Vadhanavikit S, Folkers K: Response of patients in classes III and IV of cardiomyopathy to therapy in a blind and crossover trial with coenzyme Q10. Proc Natl Acad Sci USA 82:4240–4244, 1985.

17. Baggio E, Gandini R, Plancher AC, et al: Italian multicenter study on the safety and efficacy of coenzyme Q10 as adjunctive therapy in heart failure. Mol Aspects Med 15:S287–S294, 1994.

18. Matthews PM, Ford B, Dandurand RJ, et al: Coenzyme Q10 with multiple vitamins is generally ineffective in treatment of mitochondrial disease. Neurology 43:884–890, 1993.

19. Feigin A, Kieburtz K, Como P: Assessment of coenzyme Q10 tolerability in Huntington's disease. Mov Disord 11(3):321–323, 1996.

20. Lampertico M, Comis S: Italian multicenter study on the efficacy and safety of coenzyme Q10 as adjuvant therapy in heart failure. Clin Investig 71:S129–S133, 1993.

21. Mortensen SA, Leth A, Agner E, Rohde M: Dose-related decrease of serum coenzyme Q10 during treatment with HMG-CoA reductase inhibitors. Mol Aspects Med 18:S137–S144, 1997.

22. Human JA, Ubbink JB, Jerling JJ, et al: The effect of simvastatin on the plasma antioxidant concentrations in patients with hypercholesterolaemia. Clin Chim Acta 263:67–77, 1997.

23. Heck AM, DeWitt BA, Lukes AL: Potential interactions between alternative therapies and warfarin. Am J Health-Sys Pharm 57:1221–1230, 2000.

24. Lowe AG, Critchley AJ, Brass A: Inhibition of glucose transport in human erythrocytes by ubiquinone Q10. Biochim Biophys Acta 1069:223–228, 1991.

25. Henriksen JE, Andersen CB, Hother-Nielsen O, et al: Impact of ubiquinone (coenzyme Q10) treatment on glycaemic control, insulin requirement and well-being in patients with Type 1 diabetes mellitus. Diab Med 16:312–318, 1999.

26. Eriksson JG, Forsén TJ, Mortensen SA, et al: The effect of coenzyme Q10 administration on metabolic control in patients with type 2 diabetes mellitus. Biofactors 9:315–318, 1999.

Coltsfoot (*Tussilago farfara*)

rating: 🦌 –

> - A traditional soothing remedy for cough and other respiratory disorders
> - No clinical evidence of efficacy
> - Contains small amounts of hepatotoxic alkaloids; chronic use should be avoided

Coltsfoot was traditionally used as an antitussive cough medication, which explains its botanical name *Tussilago* (from *tussis*, coughing; *ago*, to chase) and its common name, cough-wort. It is similar to *Petasites vulgaris*, butterbur, which can be a dangerous toxic contaminant in coltsfoot products.[1] Both the flowers and the leaves of coltsfoot are gathered for herbal use.

Uses: Coltsfoot has been used as a candy and herbal remedy in different formulations for thousands of years. Oral preparations were advocated for use in cough and various respiratory diseases, and the smoke from burning coltsfoot leaves or from herbal cigarettes was also used for treating asthma and bronchitis.[2,3] Other former indications included diarrhea and slow metabolism, and coltsfoot has been employed as a blood purifier and as a diuretic.[4] It is relatively unique in having been selected by both traditional Western and Chinese herbalists for the same specific purpose—the treatment of cough.

Pharmacology: One of the main contents of coltsfoot leaves is a mucilage. This polysaccharide macromolecule forms a colloidal solution or a gel with water; this is said to coat the mucosa of the pharynx and have a demulcent effect.[5] Historically, there was a tendency to assume that the sticky quality of mucilages, which resemble mucus, signified their inherent value as throat soothers or expectorant agents, and thus there arose the suggestion that the herbal sources of such products were helpful in coughs. Another component, tussilagone, has been reported to stimulate the respiratory center and to increase blood pressure in animal models.[6]

Components of greater concern are the pyrrolizidine alkaloids—senkirkine, senecionine, and seneciphylline—which are present in small amounts. Of these, senkirkine and senecionine contain unsaturated necine bases; in animals, these have been reported to cause hepatoxic, carcinogenic, and possibly pneumotoxic effects.[7] European coltsfoot has smaller quantities of toxic compounds than some Chinese plants.

Coltsfoot also contains tannins, flavonoids, acids, bitters, and other constituents. Most of these have not been pharmacologically evaluated,[6] but an expectorant effect has been hypothesized to occur through stimulating gastric receptors to cause a vagal reflex in the lung that results in bronchial gland secretion.[8] Coltsfoot flower buds contain a compound (L-652,469) which has platelet-activating factor inhibitory properties,[6,9] but no clinical evaluation of this component has been made.

Clinical Trials: In spite of its long reputation as a "pectoral" for treating respiratory disease, there is no clinical trial evidence demonstrating that the herb itself or its components have any useful effect in treating cough or asthma.[3,10] It may be of empiric benefit for soothing sore throats, but there is no evidence that it is more effective than other syrupy drinks or candies. Since it is very difficult to prove that any drug is an effective expectorant,[8] it is not surprising that coltsfoot has never been demonstrated to possess this property. There is no clinical evidence to support claims that it has any clinically useful properties.

Adverse Effects: There are no known side effects with brief or occasional use.

Interactions: There are no recognized interactions with coltsfoot, although use with potential hepatotoxic agents should be avoided.

Cautions: Occasional reports have implicated the prolonged use of coltsfoot with the development of severe hepatic veno-occlusive disease; this is due to the hepatotoxic pyrrolizidine alkaloids.[4,7] Coltsfoot should be avoided by patients with liver disease and by those ingesting potentially hepatotoxic drugs and/or alcohol. Occasional concerns arise about the allergenicity and carcinogenicity of coltsfoot, but these claims have not been substantiated in humans.[7] It should not be taken by pregnant or breast-feeding women. Any use of coltsfoot should be restricted to a few days so as to decrease the risk of toxicity.

Preparations & Doses: Coltsfoot is commonly incorporated into candies and teas, which are particularly popular in France.[5] It is also available in many European countries as solutions, syrups, and tablets. A typical dose is 0.6–2 ml of a flower extract or up to 8 ml of a syrup.[6] Dosages of dried herb vary from 600 to 2000 mg t.i.d.[6]

Summary Evaluation

Coltsfoot has no clinically documented value as a respiratory remedy. As the herbal leaf and other components of coltsfoot have toxic effects and lack proven value, their use is discouraged. It is unlikely that small amounts given for a few days could cause significant harm. Nevertheless, safer herbs that may be more effective should be preferred for treatment of sore throats and coughs and for improving expectoration. Due to its potential toxicity, coltsfoot is not recommended by leading herbal authorities.[6,11]

references

1. McGuffin M, Hobbs C, Upton R, Goldberg A (eds): Botanical Safety Handbook. Boca Raton, FL, CRC Press, 1997.
2. Grieve M: A Modern Herbal. Harmondsworth, England, Penguin Books, 1984.
3. Ziment I: Historic overview of mucoactive drugs. In Braga PC, Allegra L (eds): Drugs in Bronchial Mucology. New York, Raven Press, 1989, pp 1–33.
4. Dailey A, Cupp. MJ: Coltsfoot. In: Cupp MJ (ed): Toxicology and Clinical Pharmacology of Herbal Products. Towata, NJ, Humana Press, 2000, pp 191–202.
5. Bruneton J: Pharmacognosy, Phytochemistry, Medicinal Plants. Secaucus, New York, Lavoisier Publishing Inc, 1995.
6. Newall CA, Anderson LA, Phillipson JD: Herbal Medicines. A Guide for Health Care Professionals. London, The Pharmaceutical Press, 1996.
7. Westendorf J: Pyrrolizidine Alkaloids—*Tussilago farfara*. In De Smet PAGM, et al (eds): Adverse Effects of Herbal Drugs. Vol. 1. New York, Springer-Verlag, 1992, pp 223–226.
8. Ziment I: Respiratory Pharmacology and Therapeutics. Philadelphia, WB Saunders Company, 1978.
9. Barnes PJ, Chung KF, Page CP: Platelet-activating factor as a mediator of allergic disease. J Allergy Clin Immunol 81:919–934, 1988.
10. Wade A (ed): Martindale. The Extra Pharmacopoeia, 27th ed. London, The Pharmaceutical Press, 1977.
11. Foster S, Tyler VE: Tyler's Honest Herbal. New York, The Haworth Herbal Press, 1999.

Comfrey (*Symphytum officinale*)

rating: 🐾 −

> - Previously used for wounds, lung disease, and other disorders
> - Contains hepatotoxic pyrrolizidine alkaloids
> - Not for systemic use

Comfrey, *Symphytum officinale*, is an herb that grows in temperate climates. It was long known in Europe under names such as boneset, blackwort, slippery root, and gum plant. It is in the same family as borage. Various species of comfrey are grown in different countries.

Uses: Comfrey is named from its ancient application in "bone-mending": the Latin, *con firma*, made firm; the Greek, *Symphytum*, to unite.[1] Traditionally, its roots and leaves have been used to treat broken bones and wounds. The mucilaginous root content was formerly promoted as an expectorant and antitussive, and to treat gastrointestinal disorders.[1,2] Comfrey is promoted in Ayurvedic and other herbal systems, with claims for benefit in disorders such as peptic ulcer. Comfrey also has been commonly used as a topical anti-inflammatory healing agent.[2] Although still a component in some cosmetics, comfrey is no longer readily available as an herbal remedy in the U.S. due to its toxic potential.

Pharmacology: Although the leaves are also used, the main therapeutic components are thought to be found in the roots. These include mucilage (fructans), tannins, allantoin, rosmarinic acid, sarracine, platyphylline, triterpenes, and sterols.[1–3] However, the most important constituents of the roots are the hepatotoxic pyrrolizidine alkaloids, such as intermedine and its acetylated derivatives—symphytine and the very toxic echimidine.[2,4,5] These compounds include an unsaturated necine base, which causes the pyrrolizidine alkaloids to be hepatotoxic. The non-toxic allantoin, mucilage, astringent tannins, and anti-inflammatory rosmarinic acid, however, could have a soothing effect on inflammatory skin disorders.[3]

Clinical Trials: No significant clinical trials have been reported in humans. There is insufficient evidence of comfrey's value to justify clinical studies.

Adverse Effects: The main toxic outcome of ingesting comfrey is liver disease, and several cases have been recorded of veno-occlusive disease of the liver, resulting in ascites and hepatic fibrosis.[5] Other toxicity may be seen, including a curare-like effect, adverse effects in pregnant women, and possibly carcinogenesis.[5] Presumably, individual patient factors affect susceptibility, but the dangers of the herb are unpredictable. Because of this, systemic use of comfrey has been banned in many countries, and the FDA discourages its use. Russian comfrey is said to be more toxic than the common comfrey of North America.[2]

Interactions: There are no recognized drug interactions.

Cautions: Comfrey should not be used orally or internally. Although it can be used topically, it should probably not be placed on broken skin.[6] All forms of comfrey should be avoided in pregnant and nursing women.

Preparations & Doses: Preparations of root and leaf parts are now less readily available. Tablets and other herbal extracts have been employed, but very dilute teas or decoctions are safer; however, internal use is not recommended. The herb is used in topical preparations including lotions, creams, salves, and poultices, and it is sometimes used as a gargle. Herbal authorities recommend that it can be employed externally for contusions, bruises, and sprains for up to 6 weeks during a year,[6,7] but such use is rarely justified.

Summary Evaluation

No evidence exists to support the clinical use of comfrey, and it has been found to have significant hepatotoxic effects. The topical use of comfrey products for skin diseases may be safe, provided the skin is not broken and the preparation is not used chronically. Oral administration of dilute teas may be safe, but in view of the potential serious toxicity and the lack of proven value, oral intake of comfrey should be avoided.

---

references

1. Chevalier A: The Encyclopedia of Medicinal Plants. New York, DK Publishing, 1996.
2. Foster S, Tyler VE: Tyler's Honest Herbalist, 4th ed. New York, The Haworth Herbal Press, 1999.
3. Bisset NG, Wichtl M (eds): Herbal Drugs and Phytopharmaceuticals. Boca Raton, CRC Press, 1994.

4. Bruneton J: Pharmacognosy, Phytochemistry, Medicinal Plants. Secaucus, NY, Lavoisier Publishing Inc, 1995.
5. Westendorf J: Pyrrolizidine alkaloids—*Symphytum* species. In De Smet PAGM, Keller K, Hänsel R, Chandler RF (eds): Adverse Effects of Herbal Drugs. Vol. 1. Berlin, Springer Verlag, 1992, pp 219–222.
6. Newall CA, Anderson LA, Phillipson JD: Herbal Medicines: A Guide for Health-Care Professionals. London, The Pharmaceutical Press, 1996.
7. McGuffin M, Hobbs C, Upton R, Goldberg A (eds): American Herbal Products Association's Botanical Safety Handbook. Boca Raton, CRC Press, 1997.

Cranberry (*Vaccinium macrocarpon*)
rating: 🐝 🐝 +

- Inhibits the adherence of **Escherichia coli** to urinary tract epithelial cells
- May help prevent (not treat) clinical urinary tract infections, but evidence is conflicting
- Safe and well tolerated

The cranberry plant, *Vaccinium macrocarpon*, is native to North America. Other related plants in the Vaccinium genus include blueberry and bilberry. The ripe fruit, which is extremely sour, is used both as food and as an herbal medicine.

Use: Cranberry juice has a long tradition in American folklore of helping to treat or prevent urinary tract infections (UTIs). Scientific studies have attempted to validate the empiric use of cranberry as a urologic antimicrobial agent and as a potential medicinal herb to help prevent UTIs in susceptible individuals.[1]

Pharmacology: Cranberry juice was originally thought to inhibit urinary bacteria by acidifying the urine or by being excreted as hippuric acid, an antibacterial chemical. More recent investigations have failed to validate these mechanisms.[1] Instead, it is now known that specific proanthocyanidins, condensed tannins from the cranberry fruit (also found in blueberries), can inhibit the adherence of uropathogenic *E. coli* and other bacteria to epithelial cells *in vitro* and *in vivo*.[1-4] A similar constituent has been found to inhibit the co-adhesion of dental plaque bacteria.[5] Cranberry juice has recently been found to have some *in vitro* bactericidal activity as well.[6]

Clinical Trials*: Initial claims that cranberry juice was effective in treating or preventing UTIs were based on case reports or small uncontrolled studies.[1,7] Only three double-blind, placebo-controlled trials have adequately investigated cranberry's clinical effects; two of these trials found clinical benefits. All three studies were conducted in the U.S., but the two positive studies have methodologic weaknesses (e.g., unstated or quasi-randomization procedures, high drop-out rates, no intention-to-treat analysis) that reduce the reliability of the results.[8] Cranberry has not been studied for the treatment of acute symptomatic UTIs.[9]

In one randomized controlled trial (RCT), investigators gave 300 ml/day of cranberry juice cocktail or a placebo beverage to 192 elderly female nursing home residents over a 6-month period.[10] Pyuria with bacteriuria was significantly reduced in the cranberry group (15%) as compared to the placebo group (28.1%) (P = 0.004). Antibiotics for UTIs were prescribed eight times in the cranberry group by subjects' own physicians, and 16 times in the placebo group. Criticisms of this study included important differences in baseline characteristics of the treatment and placebo groups, and a 20% drop-out rate.

In a small RCT using a 6-month crossover-design, investigators gave a daily cranberry extract capsule or placebo to 19 sexually active women (median age 37) with recurrent UTIs; only 10 subjects could be evaluated.[11] Of 21 incidents of UTIs, 6 occurred while taking the cranberry product, and 15 occurred while taking placebo, a statistically significant difference (P < 0.005).

Lastly, no benefits were found in a 6-month crossover study of 15 high-risk children with neurogenic bladder requiring clean intermittent catheterization q.i.d.[12] Subjects drank 2 ounces daily of a cranberry concentrate juice (equivalent to 300 ml of cranberry cocktail) or a placebo, and weekly catheterized urine specimens were obtained at home visits. Cranberry juice, compared to placebo, failed to reduce the frequency of bacteriuria (75% in each group), isolation of *E. coli* (43% vs. 48%, respectively), or symptomatic UTIs (three in each group). No reduction in bacteriuria was found, but the power to detect a difference in the number of clinical UTIs was small due to the low number of UTIs in the children.

Adverse Effects: There are no documented adverse effects with cranberry products.

Interactions: There are no recognized drug interactions.

Cautions: Cranberry juice contains moderately high levels of oxalate, which may increase the risk of kidney stones in susceptible individuals. One man with a distant history of calcium oxalate nephrolithiasis developed recurrent stones following self-administration of cranberry extract tablets for 6 months.[13] A pilot study of an extract taken daily for 1 week in five healthy subjects confirmed an increase in urinary oxalate levels.[13] However, substances known to both induce (e.g., sodium) and inhibit (e.g., magnesium, potassium) stone formation were also increased; the overall effect is still not clear. The large amounts of sugar in many beverage products may be relatively contraindicated for patients with diabetes. Individuals should not rely on cranberry preparations to cure an established, symptomatic UTI, and should not delay in obtaining necessary medical treatment.

Preparations & Doses: Pure cranberry juice is very acidic and sour; the most commonly marketed drink, cranberry juice cocktail, is a mixture of cranberry juice (at least 25% by volume), sweeteners, and vitamin C.[1] Preparations and doses used in the above clinical trials included 300 ml/day (10 oz) of a standard cranberry juice cocktail beverage or 2 oz of concentrate (both supplied by Ocean Spray Cranberries, Inc.) in single or divided doses. A daily dietary supplement capsule containing 400 mg of cranberry extract (Solaray, Inc.) was also used in one trial. There are many other cranberry foods and supplements on the market that would be expected to have similar active constituents, but the optimal preparation and dose is unknown.

Summary Evaluation

Cranberry's anti-infective activity in the urinary tract is well documented. Primarily, it inhibits the adherence of bacteria to urinary epithelial cells. Limited controlled trials suggest that cranberry products may help prevent UTIs in susceptible individuals; however, the available evidence is conflicting, and the studies all have methodologic flaws. Because cranberry is a safe and well-tolerated herbal remedy, it is not unreasonable for individuals with recurrent UTIs to try cranberry products for chronic preventive therapy. However, the potential beneficial effects, if clinically significant, are likely to be small.

---

* **Note added pre-press:** A recent RCT found that 50 ml/day of a cranberry-lingonberry juice concentrate for 6 months reduced recurrences of symptomatic UTIs in 150 women by about 50%.[14] Recurrences were followed for 12 months. This study was not blinded, however, and is therefore not conclusive.

references
1. Lowe FC, Fagelman E: Cranberry juice and urinary tract infections: What is the evidence? Urology 57:407–413, 2001.
2. Ofek I, Goldhar J, Zafriri D, et al: Anti-*Escherichia coli* adhesion activity of cranberry and blueberry juices. New Engl J Med 324:1599, 1991.
3. Howell AB, Vorsa N, Der Marderosian A, Foo LY: Inhibition of the adherence of P-fimbriated *Escherichia coli* to uroepithelial-cell surfaces by proanthocyanidin extracts from cranberries. New Engl J Med 339:1085–1086, 1998.

4. Reid G, Hsiehl J, Potter P, et al: Cranberry juice consumption may reduce biofilms on uroepithelial cells: Pilot study in spinal cord injured patients. Spinal Cord 39:26–30, 2001.

5. Weiss EI, Lev-Dor R, Kashamn Y, et al: Inhibiting interspecies coaggregation of plaque bacteria with a cranberry juice constituent. J Am Dent Assoc 129:1719–1723, 1998.

6. Lee Y-L, Owens J, Thrupp L, Cesario TC: Does cranberry juice have antibacterial activity? JAMA 283:1691, 2000.

7. Siciliano AA: Cranberry. HerbalGram 38:51–54, 1996.

8. Jepson RG, Mihaljevic L, Craig J: Cranberries for preventing urinary tract infections (Cochrane Review). In The Cochrane Library, Issue 4. Oxford, Update Software, 2000.

9. Jepson RG, Mihaljevic L, Craig J: Cranberries for treating urinary tract infections (Cochrane Review). In The Cochrane Library, Issue 4. Oxford, Update Software, 2000.

10. Avorn J, Monane M, Gurwitz JH, et al: Reduction of bacteriuria and pyuria after ingestion of cranberry juice. JAMA 271:751–754, 1994.

11. Walker EB, Barney DB, Mickelsen JN, et al: Cranberry concentrate: UTI prophylaxis. J Fam Pract 45:167–168, 1997.

12. Schlager TA, Anderson S, Trudell J, Hendley JO: Effect of cranberry juice on bacteriuria in children with neurogenic bladder receiving intermittent catheterization. J Pediatr 135:698–702, 1999.

13. Terris MK, Issa MM, Tacker JR: Dietary supplementation with cranberry tablets may increase the risk of nephrolithiasis. Urology 57:26–29, 2001.

14. Kontiokari T, Sundqvist K, Nuutinen M, et al. Randomised trial of cranberry-lingonberry juice and *Lactobacillus* GG drink for the prevention of urinary tract infections in women. BMJ 322:1571–1573, 2001.

Devil's Claw
(*Harpagophytum procumbens*)
rating: 🐾 🐾

> - Used as an anti-inflammatory and analgesic
> - Mild benefits demonstrated by controlled clinical trials, but findings not conclusive
> - Appears safe and well tolerated

The medicinal preparations of devil's claw are made from the dried roots of *Harpagophytum procumbens*, a South African plant. Other common names include grapple plant, and wood or wool spider plant. The fruits have long, branching arms with "claw-like" hooks.

Uses: Since it's introduction to Europe from Africa in the early 20th century, devil's claw has been used most frequently as an analgesic and anti-inflammatory agent for arthritis and other painful musculoskeletal conditions.[1,2] It has also been used for anorexia and dyspepsia, as a bitter tonic, and as an antipyretic. Topical applications include wounds, ulcers, and pain relief.

Pharmacology: The main active constituent is harpagoside, an iridoid glucoside thought to have anti-inflammatory activity; however, it does not adequately account for all of the herb's anti-inflammatory effects.[2] The anti-inflammatory mechanism of devil's claw appears to be different from that of aspirin or NSAIDs. *In vitro*, devil's claw does not affect prostaglandin synthetase activity.[3] In humans, administration of 2 g of powdered devil's claw produced no effect on eicosanoid biosynthesis, either by the cyclo-oxygenase or the 5-lipoxygenase pathways.[4] In animal models, devil's claw extracts demonstrated inconsistent anti-inflammatory activity in experimentally induced inflammation. Extracts administered parenterally were more effective than oral administration, and aqueous extracts consistently demonstrated more anti-inflammatory activity than alcohol extracts or isolated constituents.[1,2,5]

Concern about degradation of active constituents by gastric acid supports the use of enteric coated preparations.[5–7]

Devil's claw extracts have anti-arrhythmic activity in animal models, but this effect has not been tested in humans.[8,9]

Clinical Trials: The effectiveness of devil's claw has been evaluated in a number of controlled clinical trials for osteoarthritis, low back pain, and other rheumatic and musculoskeletal complaints. Several studies are not available in English, and are thus summarized from other sources.[2,5,10] Dosage and preparations varied in the clinical trials, but treatment was generally administered for 4–8 weeks; some involved comparisons with nonsteroidal anti-inflammatory drugs (NSAIDs).

For osteoarthritis, four double-blind, controlled clinical trials have been published. In two placebo-controlled studies (n = 50, 100), treatment with 2.4 g/day of devil's claw dried root or standardized extract produced a statistically significant reduction of pain compared to placebo.[2,5] Another randomized placebo-controlled trial reported improvement in pain and spinal mobility with a dose of 2 g/day in 89 patients with joint pain.[10] The largest study (n = 122) compared the efficacy of devil's claw to diacerhein, a European non-NSAID drug for osteoarthritis. Devil's claw (2.6 g/day root powder) was as effective as standard doses of diacerhein for treatment of hip or knee osteoarthritis, but the reduction of pain and functional disability did not reach statistical significance for either group. There was a statistically significant reduction in the need for analgesic and NSAID medication in the devil's claw group compared to the diacerhein group.[11]

For acute exacerbation of chronic low back pain, two similar, randomized, double-blinded trials conducted by the same research group evaluated a commercial devil's claw extract (WS1532) for 1 month.[12,13] Outcomes were measured by a validated low back pain index. The primary outcome measure chosen was the number of patients who were pain-free without rescue medication (for 5 days out of the last week) at the end of the trial. In the larger trial (n = 197), this outcome measure was reported in 9% and 15% in the 600- and 1200-mg/day treatment groups, respectively, vs. 5% in the placebo group (P = 0.027).[13] However, the decrease in the overall low back pain index was similar among placebo and treatment groups. Similar results were found in the smaller trial (n = 118) with different patients, which compared the 600-mg dose vs. placebo.[12] Although the results appear to be mixed, and the absolute benefits minimal, these two studies were considered to have the best methodologic quality of all of the randomized controlled trials for devil's claw included in a systematic review of herbal anti-inflammatories.[10]

Based on subjective assessment of patients with digestive disorders, a devil's claw decoction was reported to "improve small intestine complaints," normalize constipation and diarrhea, eliminate flatulence, and stimulate appetite.[5] There are no controlled trials of devil's claw for gastrointestinal disorders.

Adverse Effects: Devil's claw appears to be well tolerated. Most clinical trials reported no side effects other than occasional cases of mild gastrointestinal upset.[1,2,10] One patient withdrew from an uncontrolled clinical study reporting a throbbing frontal headache, tinnitus, anorexia, and loss of taste.[14]

Interactions: There are no well-documented drug interactions. A theoretical concern about interactions with warfarin, and NSAIDs and other antiplatelet agents, has been raised in the literature. This is based based on one case report of purpura in a patient receiving warfarin and devil's claw; details of this case are unknown.[15] However, no hematologic problems have been observed in clinical trials or in animal models.[2,3] Anti-arrhythmic effects demonstrated in animal experiments suggest that caution is advisable in using devil's claw with anti-arrhythmics and cardiac glycosides.[5]

Cautions: Herbal authorities advice caution when using devil's claw (considered a "bitter" herb, which is thought to stimulate gastric acid) in the presence of peptic ulcers,[1] although this potential effect has not been reported or evaluated. Devil's claw is best avoided in pregnancy due to oxytoxic effects in animals.[16] Its safety has not been evaluated during pregnancy or lactation.

Preparations & Doses: Traditionally, 3–6 g/day of dried root is taken in three divided doses for analgesic and anti-inflammatory activity. A smaller daily dose of 0.5–1.5 g has been recommended for anorexia.[5] Clinical trials for pain relief have used doses ranging as low as 0.75–2.6 g/day of dried root, but most studies used extracts corresponding to about 3–6 g/day (2–2.4 g/day of a 2.5:1 solid extract, or 0.6–1.2 g/day of a 5:1 powdered extract).[1] Liquid preparations are taken as teas, tinctures, or fluid extracts. Some devil's claw products are standardized to harpagoside.

--------- **Summary Evaluation** ---------

Devil's claw has traditionally been employed to treat joint pain and digestive problems and appears to be relatively well tolerated.

Pharmacologic studies suggest that it has anti-inflammatory and analgesic effects that may occur through mechanisms other than inhibition of arachidonic acid metabolism. Several clinical trials support its use as a mild anti-inflammatory and analgesic herb; however, results are mixed in higher-quality studies. Thus, there is insufficient evidence to validate its effectiveness. Devil's claw has not been adequately evaluated for other indications.

references

1. Mills S, Bone K: Principles and Practice of Phytotherapy: Modern Herbal Medicine. Edinburgh, UK, Churchill Livingstone, 2000.
2. Wegener T: Devil's claw: From African traditional remedy to modern analgesic and anti-inflammatory. HerbalGram 50:47–54, 2000.
3. Whitehouse L, Znamirowska M, Paul C: Devil's claw (*Harpagophytum procumbens*): No evidence for anti-inflammatory activity in the treatment of arthritic disease. Can Med Assoc J 129: 249–251, 1983.
4. Moussard C, Alber D, Toubin MM, et al: A drug used in traditional medicine, *Harpagophytum procumbens:* No evidence for NSAID-like effect on whole blood eicosanoid production in humans. Prostagl Leuk Essent Fatty Acids 46:283–286, 1992.
5. European Scientific Cooperative on Phytotherapy: Harpagophyti Radix: Devil's Claw. Monographs on the Medicinal Uses of Plant Drugs, Exeter, UK, ESCOP, March 1996.
6. Soulimani R, Younos C, Mortier F, Derrieu C: The role of stomachal digestion on the pharmacological activity of plant extracts, using as an example extracts of *Harpagophytum procumbens*. Can J Physiol Pharmacol 72:1532–1536, 1994.
7. Lanhers MC, Fleurentin J, Mortier F, et al: Anti-inflammatory and analgesic effects of an aqueous extract of *Harpagophytum procumbens*. Planta Med 58:117–123, 1992.
8. Circosta C, Occhiuto F, Ragusa S, et al: A drug used in traditional medicine: *Harpagophytum procumbens* DC. II. Cardiovascular activity. J Ethnopharmacol 11:259–274, 1984.
9. Costa De Pasquale R, Busa G, Circosta C, et al: A drug used in traditional medicine: *Harpagophytum procumbens* DC. III. Effects on hyperkinetic ventricular arrhythmias by reperfusion. J Ethnopharmacol 13:193–199, 1985.
10. Ernst E, Chrubasik S: Phyto-anti-inflammatories: A systematic review of randomized, placebo-controlled, double-blind trials. Rheum Dis Clin North Am 26:13–27, 2000.
11. Leblan D, Chantre P, Fournie B: *Harpagophytum procumbens* in the treatment of knee and hip osteoarthritis. Four-month results of a prospective, multicenter, double-blind trial versus diacerhein. Joint Bone Spine 67:462–467, 2000.
12. Chrubasik S, Zimpfer CH, Shutt U, et al: Effectiveness of *Harpagophytum procumbens* in the treatment of acute low back pain. Phytomed 3:1–10, 1996.

13. Chrubasik S, Junck H, Breitschwerdt H, et al: Effectiveness of *Harpagophytum* extract WS 1531 in the treatment of exacerbation of low back pain: A randomized, placebo controlled, double-blind study. Eur J Anaesthesiol 16:118–129, 1999.

14. Grahme R, Robinson BV: Devil's claw (*Harpagophytum procumbens*): Pharmacological and clinical studies. Ann Rheum Dis 40:632, 1981.

15. Shaw D, Leon C, Kolev S, Murray V: Traditional remedies and food supplements: A 5-year toxicological study (1991-1995). Drug Safety 17:342–356, 1997.

16. Newall CA, Anderson LA, Phillipson JD: Herbal Medicine: A Guide for Health-Care Professionals. London, The Pharmaceutical Press, 1996.

Dong Quai (*Angelica sinensis*)

rating: 🐾

> - A traditional Chinese herbal medicine commonly used for women's health
> - Appears to have no estrogenic effects and no benefits for menopausal symptoms
> - Well tolerated with minimal or no side effects

Dong quai is also known as dang gui, tang-kuei, Chinese Angelica, or "female ginseng," and is a member of the carrot and parsley family. A. *sinensis* is the most widely used of the Angelica species, although other species are found in traditional medicines of different cultures. The roots and rhizomes are the most extensively used parts of the plant.

Uses: Dong quai is a popular Chinese medicinal herb, frequently used in formulations for gynecologic disorders. In the U.S., it is often marketed as a general female tonic, labeled simply for "female balance and well being"; it is also used specifically to treat premenstrual syndrome, amenorrhea, irregular menses, dysmenorrhea, and menopausal symptoms.[1,2] In traditional Chinese medicine, dong quai is used for general health promotion, "blood deficiency" conditions, and for many gynecologic and obstetric disorders.[1–5]

Pharmacology: Important chemical constituents reported to be in A. *sinensis* include ligustilide, ferulic acid, polysaccharides, and furanocoumarins (such as psoralen).[3,6] However, a recent analysis failed to find coumarins in commercial dong quai products.[6,7]

The biologic activity of A. *sinensis* extracts has been investigated in a wide range of *in vitro* and animal experiments, primarily in China and Japan. In the 1950s, two different extracts demonstrated opposing uterine muscle activity in animal models.[3,8,9] A volatile oil component of dong quai was found to inhibit spontaneous uterine contractions in isolated uteri (less marked effect was seen after intravenous administration to whole animals). In contrast, a water- or alcohol-based component administered intravenously strengthened and increased uterine contractions *in vivo*. Ferulic acid, a component of A. *sinensis*, was found to have an inhibitory effect on contractions of the rat uterus in oral doses of 300 mg/kg.[10] For Chinese practitioners and herbalists searching to scientifically substantiate traditional Chinese medicine, these studies support the belief that dong quai may help to normalize or "correct imbalances" of uterine muscle contractions in women.

Numerous other *in vitro* and animal studies have been published in the Asian literature documenting the pharmacologic activity of dong quai extracts or isolated chemical components. These include various cardiovascular, hematologic, immunologic, anti-inflammatory, and analgesic effects.[3,6,8,9,11–13] However, because of the widely varying experimental conditions, doses, and animal models, it is difficult to extrapolate these effects to human use.

Dong quai is not considered to be estrogenic in the Chinese literature,[8] but modern western herbalists often ascribe estrogenic activity to this herb. In Chinese pharmacologic studies, no estrogenic effects were seen on vaginal smears of mice, and rodents fed dong quai as 5% of their diet did not develop increased uterine weights.[3,8] This lack of hormonal effect is supported by an *in vitro* U.S. study, in which dong quai did not bind to estrogen receptors (ERs), nor did it stimulate cell proliferation in ER-positive human breast cancer cells.[14] However, contrasting results were found in an unpublished study in which dong quai did bind to estrogen receptors *in vitro*, and adding the herb to the feed of ovariectomized rats reportedly increased uterine weight.[15]

Clinical Trials: A well-designed U.S. clinical trial evaluated dong quai as a single herb for the treatment of menopausal symptoms.[16] This randomized, double-blind, placebo-controlled trial evaluated 71 postmenopausal women with hot flashes. Subjects were randomized to treatment with a placebo or 4.5 g/day of a standardized dong quai root product (500 mg/capsule; 3 capsules t.i.d.) for 24 weeks. Subjects were evaluated for serum hormone concentrations, vaginal cell maturation, endometrial proliferation with transvaginal ultrasonography, and menopausal symptoms with a self-reported diary of hot flashes and a menopausal index score. There were no statistically significant differences between the dong quai group and the placebo group in any parameter that was tested. Participants were unable to distinguish between herb and placebo, and both groups noted similar incidence of side effects (burping, gas, and headache).

One small, randomized, double-blind, and placebo-controlled U.S. study evaluated a combination of dong quai with four other herbs in 13 women with menopausal symptoms over 3 months.[17] The authors reported improvement in menopausal symptoms, but the results were difficult to interpret due to lack of data and the small study size. A Japanese double-blind, placebo-controlled trial found a combination of dong quai with five other herbs to have significant analgesic effects in 40 women with dysmenorrhea.[18] Hormone levels were not affected. A single U.S. case report of a decoction made from dong quai and peony root was associated with improvement of erythropoietin-resistant anemia secondary to chronic renal failure.[19]

Traditional dong quai–containing formulas, in combination with other herbs, have been reported in the Chinese and herbal literature to be effective for dysmenorrhea, amenorrhea, menopausal symptoms, pelvic infections, premenstrual syndrome, hepatitis, chronic obstructive pulmonary disease, chronic glomerulonephritis, and other disorders.[5,8,20] Chinese physicians have also administered dong quai by injection (IV, IM, or into acupuncture sites) to treat conditions such as pain syndromes, thromboangiitis obliterans, chronic pelvic infections, Raynaud's disease, rheumatoid arthritis, stroke, and allergic rhinitis.[3,8,13] However, most of this literature relies partially or completely on traditional Chinese medicine theories of diagnosis and treatment, and these primarily uncontrolled studies and case series are methodologically inadequate to allow scientific evaluation of efficacy.

Adverse Effects: Dong quai is generally thought to have few, if any, adverse effects. Side effects were not different from placebo in the largest controlled trial.[16] One case report of hypertension accompanied by headache, weakness, and vomiting was associated with ingesting two helpings of a traditional dong quai soup in a 32-year-old woman; her 3-week-old son also had mildly elevated blood pressure while breast feeding.[21] A cause and effect relationship with the dong quai component of the soup is unclear. Herbalists often state that dong quai has mild laxative properties, which is most likely based on ancient Chinese writings that it "lubricates the bowel,"[3] but this effect has not otherwise been reported.

Interactions: Two case reports suggest that dong quai may potentiate the anticoagulant effects of warfarin. A 46-year-old woman therapeutically maintained on warfarin experienced a two-fold elevation of the international normalized ratio (INR) after taking 1–2 tablets daily of dong quai (565 mg/tab; Nature's Way), which resolved over several weeks after discontinuation of the herb.[22] Another patient stabilized on warfarin for 10 years presented with widespread bruising and an INR of 10, 1 month after starting dong quai for menopausal symptoms; details of this case are not provided.[23]

Cautions: Based on animal experiments, Chinese scientists have been concerned that dong quai may similarly affect the uterus and blood coagulation of humans, and thus recommend that it be avoided in early pregnancy, bleeding disorders, and menorrhagia.[3] Because dong quai may contain furanocoumarins (e.g., psoralen), some feel that users should be cautioned about potential photosensitization (occasionally seen in persons collecting plants that contain these chemicals), and even about the potential photocarcinogenic or mutagenic effects of psoralens.[24,25] However, to put this in the proper perspective, these chemicals are also found in many edible plants, such as parsnip, celery, and parsley.[25] Ingestion of large amounts may increase the risk of phototoxicity in patients undergoing treatment with psoralen ultraviolet A (PUVA)[26]; however, a recent analysis failed to find furanocoumarins in dong quai products.[6,7]

Preparations & Doses: The daily dose of dong quai prescribed by practitioners of traditional Chinese medicine is usually 4–15 g, administered as the whole root or root slices.[1,4] Dong quai is traditionally used in combination with many other herbs, often prepared in teas, soups, or other dishes, but commercial products are also available in a variety of powdered root or extract formulations. North American consumers can purchase dong quai as a single or combination herbal preparation that contains about 100–500 mg of root or root extract per dosage form, with a wide variety of recommended dosing regimens.[22]

--------- **Summary Evaluation** ---------

Beneficial claims for dong quai are based primarily on theories of traditional Chinese medicine, *in vitro* and animal studies, and uncontrolled clinical trials and case series—all of which suggest beneficial effects but are methodologically inadequate to establish effectiveness. The only well-designed, controlled clinical trial of dong quai used alone did not demonstrate any estrogenic activity or benefits for menopausal symptoms, and thus there is no high-quality evidence to support its use. The use of dong quai in combination with other herbs has been evaluated in few adequately controlled, clinical trials. Based on long historical use and limited clinical studies, dong quai appears safe and well tolerated.

---

references

1. Foster S, Yue C: Herbal Emissaries: Bringing Chinese Herbs to the West. Rochester, VT, Healing Arts Press, 1992.
2. McCaleb RS, Leigh E, Morien K (eds): The Encyclopedia of Popular Herbs. Roseville, CA, Prima Health, 2000.
3. Zhu DPQ: Dong Quai. Am J Chinese Med 15(3–4):117–125, 1987.
4. Bensky D, Gamble A: Chinese Herbal Medicine: Materia Medica. Seattle, Eastland Press, 1993.
5. Belford-Courtney R: Comparison of Chinese and Western uses of *Angelica sinensis*. Aust J Med Herbalism 5:87–91, 1993.
6. Dong quai. The Review of Natural Products. St. Louis, MO, Facts and Comparisons, July 2000.
7. Zschocke S, Liu J-H, Stuppner H, Bauer R: Comparative study of roots of *Angelica sinensis* and related Umbelliferous drugs by thin layer chromatography, high-performance liquid chromatography, and liquid chromatography-mass spectrometry. Phytochem Anal 9:283–290, 1998.
8. Chang H-M, But PP-H: Pharmacology and Applications of Chinese Materia Medica. Vol. 1. Philadelphia, World Scientific, 1986.
9. Qi-bing M, Jing-yi T, Bo C: Advances in the pharmacological studies of radix *Angelica sinensis* (Oliv) diels (Chinese danggui). Chinese Med J 104:776–781, 1991.
10. Ozaki Y, Ma J-P: Inhibitory effects of tetramethylpyrazine and ferulic acid on spontaneous movement of rat uterus in situ. Chem Pharm Bull 38:1620–1623, 1990.
11. Chen JYP: Pharmacologic actions and therapeutic uses of ginseng (*Panax ginseng, Angelica sinensis*). Intl J Chinese Med 1:23–27, 1984.
12. Huang KC: The Pharmacology of Chinese Herbs, 2nd ed. New York, CRC Press, 1999.
13. Noé JE: *Angelica sinensis:* a monograph. J Naturopathic Med (Winter):66–72, 1997.
14. Zava DT, Dollbaum CM, Blen M: Estrogen and progestin bioactivity of foods, herbs, and spices. Proc Soc Exp Biol Med 217:369–378, 1998.
15. Fackelmann K: Medicine for menopause: Researchers study herbal remedies for hot flashes. Science News 153:392–393, 1998.
16. Hirata JD, Swiersz LM, Zell B, et al: Does dong quai have estrogenic effects in postmenopausal women? A double-blind, placebo-controlled trial. Fertility Sterility 68:981–986, 1997.
17. Hudson TS, Standish L, Breed C, et al: Clinical and endocrinological effects of a menopausal botanical formula. J Naturopathic Med 7:73–77, 1998.
18. Kotani N, Oyama T, Sakai I, et al: Analgesic effect of a herbal medicine for treatment of primary dysmenorrhea - A double-blind study. Am J Chin Med 25:205–212, 1997.

19. Bradley RR, Cunniff PJ, Pereira BJG, Jaber BL: Hematopoietic effect of *Radix angelicae sinensis* in a hemodialysis patient. Am J Kidney Dis 34:349–354, 1999.

20. Zhiping H, Dazeng W, Lingyi S, Zuqian W: Treating amenorrhea in vital energy-deficient patients with angelica sinensis-astragalus membranaceus menstruation-regulating decoction. J Trad Chin Med 6(3):187–190, 1986.

21. Nambiar S, Schwartz RH, Constantino A: Hypertension in mother and baby linked to ingestion of Chinese herbal medicine. West J Med 171:152, 1999.

22. Page RL, Lawrence JD: Potentiation of warfarin by dong quai. Pharmacother 19:870–876, 1999.

23. Ellis GR, Stephens MR: Untitled (photograph and brief case report). BMJ 319:650, 1999.

24. Foster S, Tyler VE: Tyler's Honest Herbal, 4th ed. New York, Haworth Herbal Press, 1999.

25. Ivie GW, Holt DL, Ivey MC: Natural toxicants in human foods: Psoralens in raw and cooked parsnip root. Science 213:909–910, 1981.

26. Puig L: Pharmacodynamic interaction with phototoxic plants during PUVA therapy. Br J Dermatol 136:973–974, 1997.

Echinacea (*Echinacea* spp.)

rating: 🐞 🐞 🐞

> - Evidence supports benefits for the treatment of acute viral URI symptoms.
> - Minimal or no effect has been found for prophylaxis of URIs.
> - No well-documented adverse effects or interactions.

Echinacea, or coneflower, is a native North American wildflower that is a member of the Asteraceae family. Of the nine known Echinacea species, three are favored for medicinal purposes: *E. purpurea*, *E. angustifolia*, and *E. pallida*.

Uses: Echinacea is commonly marketed to help treat or prevent colds, flu, and other mild upper respiratory infection (URI)-like illnesses. The plant was traditionally used by Native Americans to treat infections and wounds, and as a general cure-all. Although popular in the 19th and early 20th centuries, echinacea's use declined greatly in the U.S. after the introduction of antibiotics. It was introduced in Germany in the early 1900s, where in recent years it has been avidly researched and promoted as an immune system stimulant to help the body fight infections.[1,2]

Pharmacology: Alkylamides, caffeic acid derivatives (e.g., echinacosides and chicoric acid derivatives), and polysaccharides are the best-studied constituents.[1-3] The polysaccharides may not be in finished products and may not be absorbed orally to a significant extent.[4] Concentrations of individual components vary between different species and plant parts (e.g., roots vs. above-ground portions).[3]

The pharmacologic effects of whole extracts and individual components have been investigated in hundreds of *in vitro* and animal studies. In summary, oral preparations appear to stimulate nonspecific phagocytosis by leukocytes.[1-4] Cellular immune enhancement of T-cells and cytokines (e.g., TNF-alpha, certain interleukins) has been demonstrated, mainly with polysaccharide components administered by injection or evaluated *in vitro*[1-3]; however, these effects may not be observed clinically with oral products.[4] Some studies in humans have demonstrated enhanced phagocytosis or limited cellular immune effects using oral extract preparations,[1,4,5] while other studies have shown mixed or no activity.[6,7] At least part of these apparent discrepancies are due to differences in assays, outcome measures, and products and doses used. Anti-inflammatory effects have been demonstrated in animal studies, and weak anti-viral properties have been reported *in vitro*.[2,8]

Clinical Trials: Two high-quality, systematic reviews of the worldwide literature have evaluated echinacea for preventing or treating the common cold or viral-type URIs.[9–11] Focusing on double-blind, randomized, controlled trials (RCTs), both found 13 published European studies (primarily from Germany) that met criteria for inclusion. Almost identical trials were included in both reviews, and individual trial sizes ranged from 95 to 646 subjects. A variety of different echinacea preparations were studied, including extracts from all three species and different plant parts (roots vs. above-ground portions); seven of the studies utilized echinacea mono-preparations (not combined with other herbs). Although reported to be randomized and double-blind, many trials contain potential biases such as lack of objective validated measures, inadequate descriptions of methods, and lack of intention to treat analysis. The results of both systematic reviews were similar.

• Acute Treatment of URIs—In the eight European trials that evaluated echinacea for acute treatment of URIs (four trials used echinacea mono-preparations), almost every study demonstrated beneficial results for the echinacea product compared to placebo.[9–11] These trials found that echinacea reduced the signs or symptoms or shortened the duration of a viral URI-like illness when initiated in the first few days of symptoms and continued for 8–10 days. Benefits compared to placebo were modest, but were statistically significant in all studies. In addition, a recent U.S. double-blind RCT of an echinacea tea product found similar symptomatic improvements on a simple three-question form given to the 95 subjects 14 days after starting therapy (P < 0.001).[12] One unpublished Canadian trial of an *E. angustifolia* product failed to find any benefits compared to placebo, and other trials with negative results are known to have not been published.[9,11]

• Prevention of URIs—Four large European trials (three using echinacea mono-preparations) conducted over 2–3 months for prevention of illness found positive trends, but no statistically significant benefits compared to placebo.[9–11] A recent experimental prophylaxis trial also found no statistically significant benefits for a U.S. echinacea product.[13] In this double-blind trial, 117 adults were given echinacea or placebo for 2 weeks and then challenged with rhinovirus culture. Again, positive trends were found in the echinacea group, but no statistically significant differences compared to placebo were demonstrated for infection rate (by viral culture and antibody response), development of clinical colds, or individual cold symptoms.

• Other Uses—Many other European clinical trials have reported beneficial effects for other infectious disorders (e.g., pertussis, recurrent candida infections), malignancies, and in the reduction of undesirable effects of anti-neoplastic therapy.[1,2,14] However, most of these studies contain significant methodologic weaknesses,[14] and reported benefits are not convincing. For the prophylaxis of recurrent genital herpes, a recent double-blind RCT of an *E. purpurea* product found no significant benefit compared to placebo.[15]

Adverse Effects: Echinacea preparations are very well tolerated. In the clinical trials, side effects were similar to those seen in the placebo groups. No adverse effects have been reported with oral products other than rare allergic reactions[1,16] and a single case of recurrent erythema nodosum.[17]

Interactions: In an *in vitro* study, echinacea inhibited activity of the 3A4 isozyme of cytochrome P450, a common drug-metabolizing enzyme.[18] This has not been validated *in vivo*, and there are no documented drug interactions reported for echinacea.

Cautions: People with allergies to plants of the Asteraceae family (e.g., daisy, sunflower, chrysanthemum, ragweed) may be allergic to echinacea as well. Echinacea is considered to be a mild immunostimulant; the German Commission E discouraged its use in patients with immune disorders such as AIDS, systemic lupus, and multiple sclerosis, and for chronic use longer than 8 weeks.[19] However, this notion that echinacea may worsen immune-mediated diseases is controversial. Adverse effects in these populations have not been reported, and research does not necessarily support these limitations.[20] In fact, in a 12-week phase 1 study in 14 HIV-positive patients, 1000 mg t.i.d. of *E. angustifolia* was associated with reduction in viral loads by 0.32 log-10 ($p < 0.05$).[21] CD4 counts did not change significantly, and there were no toxic or adverse events.

Based on the evidence to date, it would be prudent to monitor patients with immune disorders or those taking immunosuppressants more closely, and to avoid echinacea in high-risk populations (for example, transplant patients). But note that adverse effects and absolute contraindications remain theoretical.[2]

Although generally best avoided by pregnant and breast-feeding women due to limited data, a prospective cohort study of 207 women using echinacea products during pregnancy found no increased risk for malformations or other adverse pregnancy outcomes.[22]

Preparations & Doses: Dosing recommendations are confounded by a wide variety of preparations using different species, plant parts, and extracts. Unlike other herbal medicines researched in Germany, there are no standardized preparations. Extracts of 1–5 g or more of dried herb per day have been traditionally recommended by herbalists, typically divided t.i.d.[2,8]

Of the European products found effective for acute URI symptoms in clinical trials, three are distributed in the U.S. under the brand names EchinaGuard (by Nature's Way), Echinaforce (by Bioforce), and Esberitox (by Enzymatic Therapy; also contains white cedar and wild indigo). All contain different extracts and have very different dosing regimens. Most of the other preparations used in the European clinical trials are ethanolic extracts of *E. purpurea* or *E. pallida*. They were dosed at 2–4 droppersful (about 2–4 ml) daily, equivalent to about 900 mg/day of the crude herb.

The tea product found effective in the U.S. trial, Echinacea Plus (Traditional Medicinals, Inc.), contains the equivalent of 1275 mg of dried echinacea (from all three species) per tea bag.

─────────── **Summary Evaluation** ───────────

The available evidence supports a modest benefit for the treatment of acute URI symptoms, although publication bias and potential methodologic flaws tempers interpretation of the published trials. Nevertheless, based on the overall evidence, the herb's relative safety, the relatively benign nature of the illness, and lack of other proven therapies, echinacea is a reasonable therapeutic option for the symptomatic treatment of acute viral URIs. Echinacea has minimal or no benefits for prophylaxis of URIs, and other indications have not been adequately evaluated.

references

1. Chavez ML, Chavez PI: Echinacea. Hosp Pharm 33:180–188, 1998.
2. Mills S, Bone K: Principles and Practice of Phytotherapy: Modern Herbal Medicine. Edinburgh, Churchill Livingstone, 2000.
3. Bauer R: Echinacea: Biological effects and active principles. In Lawson LD, Bauer R (eds): Phytomedicines of Europe: Chemistry and Biological Activity. Washington, DC, American Chemical Society, 1998, pp 140–157.
4. Bone K: Echinacea: What makes it work? Altern Med Rev 2:87–93, 1997.
5. Berg A, Northoff H, König D, et al: Influence of Echinacin (EC31) treatment on the exercise-induced immune response in athletes. J Clin Res 1:367–380, 1998.
6. Melchart D, Linde K, Worku F, et al: Results of five randomized studies on the immunomodulatory activity of preparations of echinacea. J Altern Complem Med 1:145–160, 1995.
7. Elsässer-Beile U, Willenbacher W, Bartsch HH, et al: Cytokine production in leukocyte cultures during therapy with echinacea extract. J Clin Lab Analysis 10:441–445, 1996.
8. Boon H, Smith M: The Botanical Pharmacy: The Pharmacology of 47 Common Herbs. Kingston, Ontario, Quarry Press, Inc, 2000.
9. Barrett B, Vohmann M, Calabrese C: Echinacea for upper respiratory infection. J Fam Pract 48:628–635, 1999.
10. Barrett B: Echinacea for upper respiratory infection: An assessment of randomized trials. Healthnotes Rev Complem Integr Med 7:211–218, 2000. [Update of reference 9]
11. Melchart D, Linde K, Fischer P, Kaesmayr J: Echinacea for preventing and treating the common cold (Cochrane Review). In The Cochrane Library, Issue 3. Oxford, Update Software, 2000.
12. Lindenmuth GF, Lindenmuth EB: The efficacy of echinacea compound herbal tea preparation on the severity and duration of upper respiratory and flu symptoms: A randomized, double-blind, placebo-controlled study. J Altern Comlement Med 6:327–334, 2000.
13. Turner RB, Riker DK, Gangemi JD: Ineffectiveness of echinacea for prevention of experimental rhinovirus colds. Antimicrob Agents Chemother 44:1708–1709, 2000.
14. Melchart D, Linde K, Worku F, et al: Immunomodulation with Echinacea-A systematic review of controlled clinical trials. Phytomed 1:245–254, 1994.
15. Vonau B, Chard S, Mandalia S, et al: Does the extract of the plant Echinacea purpurea influence the clinical course of recurrent genital herpes? Int J STD AIDS 12:154–158, 2001.
16. Mullins RJ: Echinacea-associated anaphylaxis. Med J Australia 168:170–171, 1998.
17. Soon SL, Crawford RI: Recurrent erythema nodosum associated with echinacea herbal therapy. J Am Acad Dermatol 44:298–299, 2001.
18. Budzinski JW, Foster BC, Vandenhoek S, Arnason JT: An in vitro evaluation of human cytochrome P450 3A4 inhibition by selected commercial herbal extracts and tinctures. Phytomed 7:273–282, 2000.
19. Blumenthal M, Goldberg A, Brinckmann J (eds): Herbal Medicine: Expanded Commission E Monographs. Newton, MA, Integrative Medicine Communications, 2000.

20. Bone K: Echinacea: When should it be used? Eur J Herbal Med (Phytotherapy) 3(Winter):13–17, 1997–1998.
21. See D, Berman S, Justis J, et al: A phase 1 study on the safety of *Echinacea angustifolia* and its effect on viral load in HIV-infected individuals. J Am Nutraceut Assoc 1:14–17, 1998.
22. Gallo M, Srkar M, Au W, et al: Pregnancy outcome following gestational exposure to echinacea. Arch Intern Med 160:3141–3143, 2000.

Elderberry (*Sambucus nigra*)

rating: 🐿️ 🐿️

> - Popular in European countries for upper respiratory tract illnesses
> - Controlled clinical trials only of combination herbal formulas
> - May be of value in influenza

The tree and its products are quite popular in Europe, where it is known as elder, elderberry tree, or bour tree. Several species of *Sambucus* are well known, especially *S. nigra*, which is native to Europe, and *S. canadensis* from North America. The flowers, or cymes, are the parts that are most favored in herbal therapy; the berries, bark, and leaves are used less frequently.

Uses: In Europe, elder flowers have been popular for treating colds and fevers, and to help expectoration in bronchitis and asthma.[1,2] Elder is commonly described as being a diaphoretic.[2] It is often incorporated in herbal mixtures to treat influenza, sinusitis, and bronchitis. Other recommended uses include neuralgia, nervous conditions, inflammatory diseases, rheumatism, diabetes, and various infections.[3–5] It is also employed as a laxative, a diuretic, for weight loss, and as a topical preparation for skin disorders.[4] The blue or black berries are used as a food, in wine and other drinks, and in jams. Its popularity today relates in large part to its importance in traditional European folklore, where it is credited with legendary properties.

Pharmacology: The flowers are the source of an essential oil that has a buttery consistency because it contains palmitic and other fatty acids, and alkanes.[3,4] The leaves and seeds contain cyanidin glycosides.[3] Over 60 compounds have been extracted from elder, including triterpenes, glycosides (e.g., sambucin, sambucyanin, sambunigrin), various anthocyanins, flavonoids, sterols, and lectins. The lectins have been shown to have antiviral and hemagglutinin properties *in vitro*.[1,3,6,7] Laboratory studies suggest that elder flowers have anti-inflammatory effects,[2] and animal models indicate that elder preparations may protect the liver against toxins.[5] Clinical experience in Germany suggests that elderberry (or elderberry-containing products) may have mucosecretory properties.[1,8]

Clinical Trials: The clinical value of elder flowers and fruits has not been clearly demonstrated, and no individual component has been shown to have specific clinical value. However, elder's use in herbal mixtures has been evaluated in several controlled clinical trials. An elderberry combination product, Sinupret (elder flowers combined with gentian root, primrose flowers, sourdock, and vervain), has been evaluated for upper respiratory infections in several controlled clinical trials in Germany, and some benefit has been demonstrated in sinusitis and bronchitis. Sinupret was compared to placebo in four double-blind clinical trials for sinusitis of 1- to 2-week duration.[2] Two small trials (n = 31 and 39) reported benefits in headache symptoms and sinus x-rays, and a larger study of 177 patients also reported significant improvement in x-rays vs. placebo (87% vs. 70%) and in self-rating of symptoms (96% vs. 75%). However, a separate trial of 139 patients with chronic sinusitis found little symptomatic difference between Sinupret and placebo.

In several studies, Sinupret has been compared to established mucokinetic drugs, including acetylcysteine and ambroxol (derived from the Ayuverdic herb, vasaka) for patients with acute bronchitis. Similar clinical benefits were shown, and there was equivalent improvement in mucociliary clearance.[7] In an observational study involving over 300 centers, 3187 patients with acute bronchitis or exacerbations of chronic bronchitis were evaluated. Similar symptomatic benefits were reported with Sinupret as were seen with the standard mucokinetic drugs.[7]

These studies did not evaluate elderberry separately, and those for bronchitis did not evaluate Sinupret against a placebo. Since the beneficial effects of allopathic expectorants and mucolytics have not been adequately demonstrated, Sinupret and elder flowers cannot be regarded as having objectively proved their value.

Using a standardized black elderberry extract (Sambucol), a double-blind, placebo-controlled trial of 40 Israeli subjects was carried out during an influenza outbreak.[9] Symptoms and fever improved significantly within 2 days in 93.3% of subjects in the treatment group, whereas the same degree of improvement was achieved by 91.7% of the controls at 6 days (P < 0.001). The preparation was also reported to increase hemagglutination inhibition titers to infuenza B, and to inhibit replication of strains of influenza A and B. Although this surprisingly successful outcome has led to the promotion of Sambucol for influenza, the study has yet to be replicated.

Adverse Effects: There are no recognized adverse effects, although data is limited. It is suggested that a diuretic effect may result in hypokalemia,[3] but this has not been objectively reported or studied.[5]

Interactions: There are no recognized drug interactions.

Cautions: The stems, roots, unripe berries, and seeds may contain cyanide, and could cause vomiting and severe diarrhea if chewed or eaten uncooked.[5,10] Ripe berries are safe when prepared for use in foods.

Preparations & Doses: The flower preparations are usually administered as teas and alcoholic extracts, and are often found in composite herbal remedies. The traditional dose is 3–5 g of the flower, and this is typically administered 2–3 times a day. Topical cosmetic preparations are used for the skin and eyes.[5] Sinupret contains 18 mg of powdered elder flower extract per dose in combination with other herbs, and Sambucol (a standardized elderberry extract) is marketed in the U.S. by both J.B. Harris and Nature's Way.

Summary Evaluation

Elder products including the flower and berry are pleasant traditional preparations, especially for use in mild sinus and bronchial infections. There is some evidence in support of using elder flower in combination with other herbs for these indications, but there aren't enough well-designed clinical trials to determine its individual or synergistic value. Its potential value in influenza needs to be confirmed.

---

references

1. Blumenthal M, Goldberg A, Brinckmann J: Herbal Medicine: Expanded Commission E Monographs. Newton, MA, Integrative Medicine Communications, 2000.
2. Schulz V, Hänsel R, Tyler VE: Rational Phytotherapy. A Physicians' Guide to Herbal Medicine, 4th ed. Berlin, Springer, 2001.
3. Newall CA, Anderson LA, Phillipson JD: Herbal Medicines: A Guide for Health-Care Professionals. London, The Pharmaceutical Press, 1996.
4. Bisset NG, Wichtl M (eds): Herbal Drugs and Phytopharmaceuticals. Boca Raton, CRC Press, 1994.

5. Bruneton J: Pharmacognosy, Phytochemistry, Medicinal Plants. Secaucus, NY, Lavoisier Publishing Inc, 1995.
6. Elderberry. The Review of Natural Products. St. Louis, MO, Facts and Comparisons, July 1992.
7. März RW, Matthys H: Phytomedicines in the treatment of the lower respiratory tract. What is proven? In Loew D, Rietbrock N (eds): Phytopharmaka III. Forschung und klinische Anwendung. Darmstadt, Germany, Steinkopff Verlag, 1997, pp 161–178.
8. März RW, Ismail C, Popp MA: Action profile and efficacy of a herbal combination preparation for the treatment of sinusitis. Wien Med Wschr 149:202–208, 1999.
9. Azkay-Rones Z, Varsano N, Zlotnek M, et al: Inhibition of several strains of influenza virus in vitro and reduction of symptoms by an elderberry extract (*Sambucus nigra* L.) during an outbreak of influenza B Panama. J Altern Complem Med 1:361–369, 1995.
10. McGuffin M, Hobbs C, Upton R, Goldberg A (eds): American Herbal Products Association's Botanical Safety Handbook. Boca Raton, FL, CRC Press, 1997.

Ephedra, or Ma Huang
(*Ephedra sinica*)
rating: 🐾🐾 –

- Ephedra, or ma huang, is the herbal source of ephedrine and pseudoephedrine.
- These drugs are of value in asthma and for nasal and sinus congestion.
- The use of ephedra as an energizer and as a weight loss agent has potential toxicity, and lacks adequate proof of value.

The best known ma huang comes from the stems of the Chinese ephedra bush, *Ephedra sinica*, although some may be derived from *E. equisetum* species; similar plants are used in India and in the Near East. The ephedra species found in the U.S. are used to produce Mormon tea, which has none of the major properties of Chinese ephedra.

Uses: The ephedra plant has been used in Chinese medicine for thousands of years, probably as an astringent, diuretic, and antipyretic, and for treating cough.[1] It was found to contain ephedrine, and this agent was introduced in the U.S. as an oral drug for asthma in 1924. The ephedra plant also contains pseudo-ephedrine. These sympathomimetic agents are still useful drugs for treating respiratory disorders and nasal congestion. Ephedrine is also used intravenously as a vasopressor. Ma huang remains an important constituent of Chinese herbal medicines, and is incorporated in many multi-herb formulations. In the U.S., it is a controversial dietary supplement for mood elevation and weight loss, and is advertised as an appetite suppressant, energizer, performance enhancer, and psychic stimulant. Other uses have included motion sickness, bradycardia, spastic or hypermotile bowel, diabetic neuropathic edema, and myasthenia gravis.[2]

Pharmacology: The important components in ephedra are the alkaloids found in the stems.[3–5] The most abundant is d-pseudo-ephedrine, but the most active is l-ephedrine. Additional constituents include l-methylephedrine, n-methyl-ephedrine, l-norephedrine, and other isomers. Tannins, glycans (ephedrans), flavonoids, and other active compounds are usually present. The total alkaloid content of any product can vary considerably, but is usually around 1.3%.[6] The constituents of the roots of ephedra plants (e.g., ephedranines, makonine, feruloylhistamine, ephedrannin and mahuannins) differ chemically from those of the stems.[3] Their effects also differ; the root components may cause less sweating and can produce hypotension.[4] The nodes of the stems have been reported to contain more toxic constituents, and these can cause convulsions.[5]

It has been well established that ephedrine and pseudoephedrine have potent sympathomimetic effects, with alpha-, beta$_1$-, and beta$_2$-agonist therapeutic uses. The physiologic action of ephedrine is to release norepinephrine from ganglia; after repeated use, the availability of norepinephrine in adrenergic nerves is depleted, and ephedrine loses its effect. This is the phenomenon of tachyphylaxis, which makes ephedrine an unreliable drug in chronic therapy.[7]

Ephedra alkaloids have anorexiant and thermogenic, or ergogenic, effects that result in increased metabolism in animals and in humans.[8,9] These qualities provide a basis for using ma huang as a weight-reducing supplement. It is known that alpha$_1$-adrenergic stimulation of the paraventricular nuclei in the brain leads to a reduction in appetite, and the peripheral effects on muscles and fat may result in increased fat oxidation and weight loss.[8]

Clinical Trials: The clinical benefits of ephedrine and pseudoephedrine are long established.[7] Ephedrine and other ephedra constituents are moderately effective bronchodilators, vasoconstrictors, and decongestants. Evidence has been published showing its benefits in cough when used in a multi-herb formulation.[7] Moreover, in a randomized, double-blind, placebo-controlled trial of 20 women, ephedrine sulfate was shown to facilitate sexual arousal. However, the drug was not assessed in women with impaired function.[10] The specific effectiveness of ma huang has not been adequately demonstrated for these indications.

Ephedra alkaloids and ma huang have gained considerable popularity as anorexiants and stimulants. Animal models suggest that these effects may be potentiated by caffeine and by catechol-polyphenols in green tea.[11] However, in eight human clinical trials of ephedra or ephedrine-caffeine combinations, with or without other drugs, results have been inconsistent. Six of these trials studied

14–42 obese subjects, while the two others studied 103 and 180 subjects; no study lasted more than 6 months, and dropout rates were high.[12] Weight loss was not dramatic in any study. No significant differences from placebo were found in five of the trials, while one showed benefit that was apparently significant, and two (each using ephedrine combined with caffeine) found significant benefits of the combination when compared to either drug alone or to placebo. Moreover, there were significant, but usually tolerable, side effects, particularly when ephedra was combined with caffeine.

Another proposed use of ephedra is as an ergogenic drug to improve oxygen consumption and exercise efficiency. In a study of 12 healthy, untrained men, the combination of caffeine (4 mg/kg) and ephedrine (0.8 mg/kg) had a significant ergogenic effect during exercise that was similar to that of higher doses of caffeine (5 mg/kg) and of ephedrine (1 mg/kg), but with fewer side effects.[13] However, this effect has not been adequately evaluated in well-designed, randomized, controlled trials.

Adverse Effects: Numerous adverse effects of ephedrine alkaloids are recognized, including hypertension, tachycardia, dangerous arrhythmias, nervousness, tremor, insomnia, and anorexia.[7] Ephedra/ma huang is said to be less likely to cause hypertension than ephedrine. Nevertheless, a sufficient number of reports have been submitted to the FDA to suggest that ma huang can cause hypertensive events, strokes, and heart attacks. In addition, psychoses and deaths have been attributed to this herb.[14] However, the reliability of many of these reports is questionable. A recent review of 140 reports of alleged adverse effects from the use of dietary supplements containing ephedra alkaloids concluded that 31% were related to the herb.[15]

Although the association has been questioned,[16,17] it is apparent that overuse of ma huang can be harmful and can cause severe impairment or death. Prolonged use has been reported to lead to dependency and to be associated with eating disorders in female athletes.[18] Individual susceptibility, unreliability of marketed products, variations in daily dosing, and taking ephedra with other sympathomimetic agents appear to be relevant. Renal stones resulting from ephedrine and ephedra use has been described; excessive doses of pseudoephedrine could possibly produce the same complication.[19]

Interactions: Combining ephedrine and monoamine oxidase inhibitors can result in severe toxicity.[20] Combinations with other sympathomimetic drugs or stimulants may result in additive cardiovascular or nervous system effects.

Cautions: Ephedra, like other sympathomimetic agonists, is relatively contraindicated in diseases such as hypertension, heart disease, thyroid disease, diabetes mellitus, prostatic hypertrophy, narrow angle glaucoma, and anxiety. Overuse of ephedra alkaloids can cause mild to serious disturbances in sleep and appetite, as well as tremor and nervousness. The more serious outcomes are particularly likely to occur in those who use larger doses in combination with other stimulants. Some patients who abuse ephedrine have developed an "addiction" with apparent dependency, and athletes have tolerated doses as high as 750 mg per day.[18] In such cases, withdrawal symptoms can occur upon abstinence. Patients should be warned not to escalate the dosage with chronic use since unexpected adverse effects may ensue.

Ephedrine, pseudoephedrine, and related drugs (including ma huang) are banned from use in Olympic sport competitions.[21] Ephedrine and ma huang are considered to be relatively safe for the management of mild asthma in pregnancy, since they have long been given to pregnant women. Their use by children, adolescents, and breast-feeding mothers should be discouraged.

Preparations & Doses: Ma huang and ephedra are available in numerous Chinese herbal preparations, mostly in mixtures with several other plant extracts and sometimes with animal constituents and minerals.[22] Ma huang is also marketed in many U.S. products as a diet and performance aid. The amounts of active drugs in these preparations vary enormously, and excess dosage is readily experienced.[12,23] A typical adult dose of the herb is 2 g, and this may contain about 13 mg of total alkaloids. Proprietary products have been shown to contain 0 to 18.5 mg of alkaloids per dose.[23] The FDA has proposed that labeling of dietary supplement products be required to stipulate that dosages should not exceed 8 mg t.i.d. to be taken for not more than 1 week, but this recommendation has proved to be both inappropriate and unenforceable. The German Commission E and other herbal authorities recommend that ma huang and ephedra alkaloid dosages should be limited to 300 mg/day.[6] A U.S. panel of experts claim that adverse events have not been shown to be related to ephedrine alkaloids when single doses are limited to 25 mg with not more than a total of 100 mg/day.[17]

Summary Evaluation

Ephedrine, ephedra, and ma huang have sympathomimetic effects that have long been recognized as effective in the treatment of mild asthma, nasal congestion, and sinusitis. Loss of effectiveness usually occurs with continued use (tachyphylaxis). The common side effects of low doses are annoying, but may be acceptable. The anorexiant, anti-obesity, and ergogenic properties that are exploited in over-the-counter dietary supplements have not been adequately established, and ingesting high dosages of ephedra constituents could cause serious cardiac and cerebral damage. Because of its effects on the sympathetic nervous system, ephedra is one of the most potent and dangerous herbal medications in common use. Daily use of ephedra for more than a week or two or any dose in excessive amounts should be discouraged, since the herb's risk:benefit ratio is so high.

references

1. Hsu H-Y, Chen Y-P, Lu C-F, Ying L: A study of the methods of processing Ma huang (Ephedrae Herba). Bull Orient Heal Arts Inst 7(3):28–40, 1982.
2. Reynolds JEF (ed): Martindale. The Extra Pharmacopoeia, 31st ed. London, Royal Pharmaceutical Society, 1996.
3. Karch SB: Ma huang and the Ephedra alkaloids. In Cupp MJ (ed): Toxicology and Clinical Pharmacology of Herbal Products. Towata, NJ, Humana Press, 2000, pp 11–30.
4. Hikino H: The constituents of ma huang (Ephedra). Bull Orient Heal Arts Inst 8(6):1–10, 1983.
5. Masatoshi H: A pharmacological study of ma huang. Bull Orient Heal Arts Inst 8(2):15–20, 1983.
6. Blumenthal M, Goldberg A, Brinckmann J (eds): Herbal Medicine. Expanded Commission E Monographs. Newton, MA, Integrative Medicine Communications, 2000.
7. Ziment I: Respiratory Pharmacology and Therapeutics. Philadelphia, WB Saunders Company, 1978.
8. Astrup A, Breum L, Toubro S: Pharmacological and clinical studies of ephedrine and other thermogenic agonists. Obes Res 3 (Suppl. 4):537S–540S, 1995.
9. Greenway FL, Raum WJ, DeLany JP. The effect of an herbal dietary supplement containing ephedrine and caffeine on oxygen consumption in humans. J Altern Complement Med 6:553–555, 2000.
10. Meston CM, Heiman JR: Ephedrine-activated physiological sexual arousal in women. Arch Gen Psychiatry 55:652–656, 1998.
11. Dulloo AG, Seydoux J, Girardier L, et al: Green tea and thermogenesis: Interactions between catechin-polyphenols, caffeine, and sympathetic activity. Int J Obes Relat Metab Disord 24:252–258, 2000.

12. Fugh-Berman A, Allina A: Ephedra for weight loss. Atlanta, GA, American Health Consultants newsletter, Alternative Therapies in Women's Health 2(11):81–84, 2000.

13. Bell DG, Jacobs I, McLellan TM, Zamecnik J: Reducing the dose of combined caffeine and ephedrine preserves the ergogenic effect. Aviat Space Environ Med 71:415–419, 2000.

14. Adverse events associated with ephedrine-containing products-Texas, December 1993-September 1995. MMWR 45:689–693, 1996.

15. Haller CA, Benowitz NL: Adverse cardiovascular and central nervous system events associated with dietary supplements containing ephedra alkaloids. N Engl J Med 343:1833–1838, 2000.

16. Fleming GA: The FDA, regulation, and the risk of stroke. N Engl J Med 343:1886–1887, 2000.

17. Editorial. No association between reported adverse events and Ephedra when consumed as directed. Accessed November 25, 2000 at www.medscape.com/MedscapeWire/ 2000/0800/medwire.0816.No.htm

18. Gruber AJ, Pope HG Jr: Ephedrine abuse among 36 female weightlifters. Am J Addict 7:256–261, 1998.

19. Powell T, Hsu FF, Turk J, Hruska K: Ma-huang strikes again: Ephedrine nephrolithiasis. Am J Kidney Dis 32:153–159, 1998.

20. Dawson JK, Earnshaw SM, Graham CS: Dangerous monoamine oxidase inhibitor interactions are still occurring in the 1990s. J Accid Emerg Med 12:49–51, 1995.

21. Catlin D, Murray TH: Performance-enhancing drugs, fair competition, and Olympic sport. JAMA 276:231–237, 1996.

22. Hsu H-Y, Easer DH: A Practical Introduction to Major Chinese Herbal Formulas. Los Angeles, Oriental Healing Arts Institute, 1980.

23. Gurley BJ, Gardner SF, Hubbard MA: Content versus label claims in ephedra-containing dietary supplements. Am J Health Syst Pharm 57:963–969, 2000.

Evening Primrose Oil
(*Oenothera biennis*)
rating: 🦃🦃

> - Rich source of gamma-linolenic acid (GLA)
> - Used for the treatment of eczema, breast pain associated with premenstrual syndrome, and other inflammatory conditions
> - Evidence in controlled trials mixed; benefits not proven
> - Well tolerated without significant side effects, but practical limitations include large dose (number of capsules) needed daily

Evening primrose is a member of the fuchsia and willow herb family. The common name of the plant is derived from the flower, which opens and releases its scent during the evening. The seeds contain oils that are used therapeutically.

Uses: Evening primrose oil (EPO), along with borage and black currant oils, are rich sources of gamma-linolenic acid (GLA). These plant oils are used for premenstrual syndrome and associated breast pain, eczema, and arthritis. EPO has also been recommended for diabetic peripheral neuropathy, chronic fatigue syndrome, hyperlipidemia, inflammatory bowel disease, schizophrenia, menopausal hot flushes, and many other ailments.[1-4] Patients with these disorders are thought to be unable to sufficiently convert their dietary essential fatty acids to GLA, a precursor of anti-inflammatory eicosanoids[5-7]; thus, supplementation with GLA-rich plant oils is considered beneficial.

Pharmacology: The key constituents of the seeds are fixed oils containing essential omega-6 fatty acids such as linoleic acid (LA), and especially its derivative gamma-linolenic acid (GLA). EPO contains 7–10% GLA, while borage seed oil contains 23%, and black currant oil contains 15–20%.[1,5]

The metabolic pathway of GLA is well established in humans and other animals.[4,5,8] Dietary linoleic acid, an essential fatty acid, is converted to GLA by a rate-limiting enzymatic step. GLA is then rapidly converted to dihomo-gammalinolenic acid (DGLA), which is further metabolized to 1-series prostaglandins (PGs, such as PGE_1) and 3-series leukotrienes (LTs), which have anti-inflammatory properties. DGLA is also metabolized to arachidonic acid (AA) in limited amounts, which is converted by cyclo-oxygenases and lipoxygenases to proinflammatory mediators such as the 2-series prostaglandins (e.g., PGE_2), the 4-series leukotrienes (e.g., LTB_4), and platelet activating factor.

LA → GLA → DGLA → 1-series PGs, 3-series LTs (anti-inflammatory)
  \
    → AA → 2-series PGs, 4-series LTs (pro-inflammatory)

GLA supplementation has been shown to attenuate the *in vitro* inflammatory response by enriching cells with DGLA, the immediate precursor of PGE1, without increasing corresponding amounts of AA.[4,5] DGLA or another metabolite, 15-hydroxy-DGLA, appear to inhibit the AA pathway to its inflammatory byproducts, further inhibiting inflammation, and have direct immune modulating effects on T-lymphocytes. A variety of anti-inflammatory effects from GLA supplementation have been demonstrated.

Based on an increase in anti-inflammatory eicosanoids that affect platelet function, GLA should be expected to reduce platelet aggregation. Controlled studies in humans have reported varying results, however, with most studies reporting an increase or no change in aggregation.[1] Bleeding time data has not been evaluated.

Clinical Trials: Numerous clinical trials have evaluated the use of EPO. Problems with several studies include inadequate controls (some used olive oil or other potentially active substances as the placebo) and trials that did not run long enough (based on some studies, it may take many months to ameliorate disease).

• Atopic Dermatitis/Eczema—Dozens of trials have evaluated EPO for the treatment of eczema and related skin disorders.[2,7,9] An early meta-analysis of nine mostly small trials that were randomized, double-blind, and placebo-controlled found a modest but significant benefit of EPO for the treatment of eczema in a total of 311 patients taking 2–6 g/day (160–480 mg/day GLA) for several months.[10] Improvement was found in itching, scaling, inflammation, dryness, and erythema.

However, several more recent double-blind, randomized, controlled trials (RCTs) failed to find beneficial effects. One RCT of 39 patients with chronic hand dermatitis evaluated 6 g/day EPO

(600 mg/day GLA) for 24 weeks; no benefit of EPO over placebo was shown.[11] An RCT of 102 patients with atopic dermatitis evaluated EPO, with and without fish oil, for 16 weeks and found no improvement in either group compared to placebo.[12] Similarly, an RCT in 60 children with atopic dermatitis for 16 weeks found no benefit for EPO supplementation vs. placebo.[13]

• Cyclical Mastalgia and Premenstrual Syndrome—EPO is a commonly used therapy for women with premenstrual syndrome and cyclical mastalgia. In non-blinded studies from two mastalgia clinics (n = 170 and 117), women given 2–3 g/day of EPO had a complete response rate of 26% in one study,[14] and at least a partial response of 58% and 38% (cyclical and noncyclical mastalgia, respectively) in the other.[15,16] EPO was as effective as bromocriptine in one study, but less effective than danazol in both studies. In a systematic review of controlled trials of EPO for premenstrual syndrome symptoms, only two high-quality, double-blind RCTs were identified.[17] In contrast to other studies, these controlled trials failed to demonstrate statistically significant benefits for EPO compared to placebo.[18,19]

• Rheumatoid Arthritis and Related Disorders—The results of EPO in clinical trials for rheumatoid arthritis have been mixed.[8] One double-blind RCT of 49 patients found positive results over one-year. EPO at a dose of 6 g/day (540 mg/day GLA) was significantly better than placebo in reducing subjective symptoms and the need for nonsteroidal anti-inflammatory medication, although objective clinical assessments and biochemical indicators of disease were not decreased. Improvements were demonstrated at 6–12 months, but not at 3 months.[20]

In contrast, a double-blind RCT of 40 patients that compared 6 g/day of EPO to placebo for 6 months showed there was no improvement with EPO compared to the placebo group.[21] Larger doses of GLA (1.4–2.8 g/day), using borage or black currant oils, have demonstrated more consistent benefits for rheumatoid arthritis. Mixed results in small placebo-controlled clinical trials (n = 21–38) have been found for other rheumatic disorders such as Raynaud's disease (positive results), psoriatic arthritis (negative results), and Sjögren's syndrome (mixed results).[8]

• Diabetic Peripheral Neuropathy—Positive animal and human experimental data initiated the clinical study of EPO for peripheral nerve damage related to diabetes.[3] In one high-quality, double-blind RCT in 111 diabetic patients, 6 g/day EPO (480 mg/day

GLA) caused improvement in peripheral neuropathy over a 1-year period, although pain was not assessed.[22] Another RCT of 22 patients treated with 4 g/day EPO (360 mg/day GLA) for 6 months also showed improvement in peripheral neuropathy based on symptoms and nerve conduction testing.[23] A third RCT found EPO (480 mg/day GLA), given over 1 year, to have no benefits over placebo in peripheral and autonomic neuropathy.[24]

• Miscellaneous—EPO has been evaluated in controlled trials for many other disorders.[1-4] Beneficial effects on lipid levels have been found in several trials in hyperlipidemic patients, although other studies found no effects.[1] Uremic pruritis was evaluated in two small, double-blind, placebo-controlled trials; statistically insignificant trends were observed.[25,26] For post-viral fatigue syndrome, one double-blind RCT of 63 adults over a 3-month period reported significant symptomatic improvement in the EPO group compared with the placebo group,[27] although a more recent double-blind RCT in chronic fatigue syndrome found no benefit.[28] In a 6-month RCT for ulcerative colitis, modest improvements were found for stool consistency, but not for stool frequency or rectal bleeding.[29] Negative results were reported in double-blind controlled trials for recurrence of breast cysts,[30] menopausal symptoms,[31] psoriasis,[32] chronic hepatitis B,[33] and asthma.[3,13,34]

Adverse Effects: EPO and other GLA-containing plant oils are well tolerated in clinical trials lasting up to 1 year. A few cases of diarrhea or soft stools, belching, abdominal bloating, and headache have been reported.[3,5]

Interactions: There are no documented drug interactions.

Cautions: In early studies of chronic schizophrenia, EPO was reported to worsen the psychosis of three patients, who on electroencephalography evaluation were subsequently found to have temporal lobe epilepsy.[35] Based on this single report, EPO has since been considered to be able to "lower the seizure threshold" in patients with epilepsy. This effect has not been corroborated. There has been one additional report of seizures in a patient taking a combination herbal regimen that included EPO, black cohosh, and chaste tree.[36] Although a cause-and-effect relationship is unlikely, caution is nonetheless warranted in patients with seizure disorders. There are no data on the use of EPO during pregnancy or lactation.

Preparations & Doses: EPO contains about 8–9% GLA. Almost all the clinical trials have used brands such as Efamol,

Epogam, and Efamast.[9] Efamol (available in the U.S.) contains 500 mg of oil and 45 mg of GLA/capsule; Epogram (available in Europe) contains 40 mg GLA. Some products contain a combination of EPO with eicosapentanoic acid, also found in fish oils. The typical dosage of EPO used in most clinical trials is 6 g/day (12 capsules containing about 480–560 mg GLA) in adults, and half that dose in children, in divided doses. For some indications (e.g., cyclical mastalgia) 2–4 g/day of EPO has been used. Because these doses require large numbers of capsules, many patients cannot tolerate this amount or prefer using borage oil or black currant oil, which contain higher concentrations of GLA.

Summary Evaluation

EPO is a well-tolerated source of GLA, an omega-6 fatty acid that has shown promise in many experimental studies and has been used for a variety of clinical disorders. Positive results from well-designed controlled clinical trials have been documented for diabetic peripheral neuropathy, rheumatoid arthritis, and eczema; however, efficacy is not well established due to mixed or limited trial results. Practical drawbacks to the use of EPO are the large number of capsules required daily, and the onset of action that may take many months.

references

1. Barre DE. Potential of evening primrose, borage, black currant, and fungal oils in human health. Ann Nutr Metab 2001;45:47–57.
2. Mills S, Bone K. Principles and Practice of Phytotherapy. Edinburgh, UK, Churchill Livingstone, 2000.
3. Boon H, Smith M. The Botanical Pharmacy: The Pharmacology of 47 Common Herbs. Kingston, Ontario, Quarry Press Inc, 1999.
4. Newall CA, Anderson LA, Phillipson JD. Herbal Medicines: A Guide for Healthcare Professionals. London, Pharmaceutical Press, 1996.
5. Fan Y-Y, Chapkin RS. Importance of dietary gamma-linolenic acid in human health and nutrition. J Nutr 1998;128:1411–1414.
6. Brush MG, Watson SJ, Horrobin DR, Manku MS. Abnormal fatty acid levels in plasma of patients with premenstrual syndrome. Am J Gynecol 1984;150: 363–366.
7. Horrobin DF. Essential fatty acid metabolism and its modification in atopic eczema. Am J Clin Nutr 2000; 71(suppl):367S–372S.
8. Belch JF, Hill A. Evening primrose oil and borage oil in rheumatologic conditions. Am J Clin Nutr 2000; 71(suppl):352S–356S.
9. Kemper K. Evening Primrose Oil. Longwood Herbal Taskforce. Accessed June 2001 at http://www.mcp.edu/herbal/default.htm

10. Morse PF, Horrobin DF, Manku MS, et al. Meta-analysis of placebo-controlled studies of the efficacy of Epogam in the treatment of atopic dermatitis. Relationship between plasma essential fatty acid changes and clinical response. Br J Dermatol 1989;121:75–90.

11. Whitaker DK, Cilliers J, de Beer C. Evening primrose oil (Epogam) in the treatment of chronic hand dermatitis: Disappointing therapeutic results. Dermatol 1996;193:115–120.

12. Berth-Jones J, Graham-Brown RAC. Placebo-controlled trial of essential fatty acid supplementation in atopic dermatitis. Lancet 1993;341:1557–1560.

13. Hederos C-A, Berg A. Epogam evening primrose oil treatment in atopic dermatitis and asthma. Arch Dis Child 1996;75:494–497.

14. Wetzig NR. Mastalgia: A 3-year Australian study. Aust NZ J Surg 1994;64: 329–331.

15. Pye JK, Mansel RE, Hughes LE. Clinical experience of drug treatments for mastalgia. Lancet,1985;2:373–377.

16. Gateley CA, Miers M, Mansel RE, Hughes LE. Drug treatments for mastalgia: 17 years experience in the Cardiff mastalgia clinic. J Roy Soc Med. 1992;85:12–15.

17. Budeiri D, Li Wan Po A, Dornan JC. Is evening primrose oil of value in the treatment of premenstrual syndrome? Controlled Clinical Trials 1996;17:60–68.

18. Khoo SK, Munro C, Battistutta D. Evening primrose oil and treatment of premenstrual syndrome. Med J Australia 1990;153:189–192.

19. Collins A, Cerin Å, Coleman G, Landgren B-M. Essential fatty acids in the treatment of premenstrual syndrome. Obstet Gynecol 1993;81:93–98.

20. Belch JJF, Ansell D, Madhok R, et al. Effects of altered dietary essential fatty acids on requirements for non-steroidal anti-inflammatory drugs in patients with rheumatoid arthritis: A double-blind, placebo-controlled study. Ann Rheum Dis 1988;47:96–104.

21. Brzeski M, Madhok R, Capell HA. Evening primrose oil in patients with rheumatoid arthritis and side effects of nonsteroidal anti-inflammatory drugs. Br J Rheumatol 1991;30:370–372.

22. Keen H, Payan J, Allawi J, et al. Treatment of diabetic neuropathy with gamma-linolenic acid. Diabetes Care 1993;16:8–15.

23. Jamal JA, Carmichael H. The effects of gamma-linolenic acid on human diabetic peripheral neuropathy: A double-blind placebo-controlled trial. Diabetic Med 1990;7:319–323.

24. Purewal TS, Evans PMS, Harvard F, O'Hare JP. Lack of effect of evening primrose oil on autonomic function tests after 12 months of treatment. Diabetologia 1997;40 (Suppl 1):A556 [Abstract].

25. Yoshimoto-Furuie K, Yoshimoto K, Tanaka T, et al. Effects of oral supplementation with evening primrose oil for six weeks on plasma essential fatty acids and uremic skin symptoms in hemodialysis patients. Nephron 1999;81: 151–159.

26. Tamimi NAM, Mikhail AI, Stevens PE. Role of gamma-linolenic acid in uraemic pruritus. Nephron 1999;83:170–171.

27. Behan PO, Behan WMH. Effect of high doses of essential fatty acids on postviral fatigue syndrome. Acta Neurologic Scand 1990;82:209–216.

28. Warren G, McKendricki M, Peet M. The role of essential fatty acids in chronic fatigue syndrome. Acta Neurol Scand 1999; 99:112–116.

29. Greenfield SM, Green AT, Teare JP, et al. A randomized controlled study of evening primrose oil and fish oil in ulcerative colitis. Aliment Pharmacol Ther 1993;7:159–166.

30. Mansel RE, Harrison J, Melhuish J, et al. A randomized trial of dietary intervention with essential fatty acids in patients with categorized cysts. Ann NY Acad Sci. 1990;586:288–294.

31. Chenoy R, Hussain S, Tayob Y, et al. Effect of oral gamolenic acid from evening primrose oil on menopausal flushing. BMJ 1994;308:501–503.

32. Oliwiecki S, Burton JL. Evening primrose oil and marine oil in the treatment of psoriasis. Clin Exp Dermatol 1994;19:127–129.

33. Jenkins AP, Green AT, Thompson RPH. Essential fatty acid supplementation in chronic hepatitis B. Aliment Pharmacol Ther 1996;10:665–668.

34. Ebden P, Bevan C, Banks J, et al. A study of evening primrose seed oil in atopic asthma. Prostagl Leukotr Essent Fatty Acids 1989;35:69–72.

35. Vaddadi KS. The use of gamma-linolenic acid and linoleic acid to differentiate between temporal lobe epilepsy and schizophrenia. Prostagl Med. 1981; 6:375–379.

36. Shuster J. Black cohosh root? Chaste tree? Seizures! Hospital Pharmacy 1996;31:1553–1554.

Fenugreek (*Trigonella foenum-graecum*)

rating: 🐾🐾 +

> - Currently used for lowering blood glucose
> - Beneficial effects reported, but only in poorly controlled studies
> - Safe and well tolerated in usual doses

Fenugreek bears hard, irregularly shaped seeds, which are used both as a spice and as an herbal medicine. The seeds have a characteristic odor and a somewhat bitter taste. Fenugreek is native to Asia and southeastern Europe.

Uses: Fenugreek came from the herbal medicine traditions of the Middle East, India, and Egypt, and later in China and Europe, and was favored as a digestive aid for dyspepsia, intestinal gas, anorexia, and diarrhea. It was also used to treat chronic cough, bronchitis, fever, sore throat, and mouth ulcers. Poultices and other external formulations have been used for wounds and skin irritations. Fenugreek's most common modern indications include diabetes and hyperlipidemia.[1,2]

Pharmacology: Fenugreek seeds contain 45–60% carbohydrates (mainly mucilaginous fiber), proteins high in lysine and tryptophan, 5–10% fixed oils, flavonoids, alkaloids such as trigonelline, saponins such as fenugreekine, and coumarins.[2,3]

Lipid-lowering activity has been reported in animal studies.[4,5] The steroidal saponins were thought to account for many of the pharmacologic effects of fenugreek, particularly the inhibition of cholesterol absorption and synthesis.[4,6] However, debitterized fenugreek (the bitter tasting lipid fraction and saponins were removed) was reported to lower serum lipids in one clinical trial.[7] Alternatively, the high fiber content has been hypothesized to account for the hypocholesterolemic activity,[5] but fenugreek does not affect HDL cholesterol, which is usually lowered by other sources of dietary fiber.[8]

Similarly, various hypotheses about the mechanism of the hypoglycemic activity of fenugreek have been postulated, including delayed gastric emptying and an agonist effect on insulin receptors.[9,10]

Both the coumarins and the fenugreek alkaloid, trigonelline, caused hypoglycemia or inhibited experimentally-induced hyperglycemia in different animal models.[11,12]

Clinical Trials: The hypoglycemic and lipid-lowering effects of fenugreek seed have been studied in many clinical trials, almost all from India. Although all of these studies reported positive effects, most of the trials were small, and study methodology and reporting of data were generally of poor quality. Most of the trials were uncontrolled, and none of the controlled studies were blinded.

• Hypoglycemic Activity—In an initial uncontrolled trial of type II diabetics, decreased post-prandial blood sugar (PPBS) and serum insulin levels were reported with a single dose of 15 g of fenugreek seeds soaked in water.[13] In an uncontrolled study of six diabetic and healthy subjects over 3 weeks, the hypoglycemic effects were highest for whole seeds, followed by gum isolate, extracted seeds, and cooked seeds (degummed seeds and leaves had no effect).[14]

Several controlled trials also reported beneficial effects, although none were randomized or blinded. In two crossover trials of type II diabetics, each with only 10 patients over 10–14 days, fenugreek liberally added to the diet was found to decrease serum glucose levels (and cholesterol levels in one trial), compared to control diets.[10,15] One trial used 100 g/day of debitterized fenugreek powder and the other used 15 g/day of fenugreek seeds. In a larger trial over 6 months, 60 type II diabetics were given a daily diet with 25 g of fenugreek in two divided doses, and compared to 10 control patients. There was a significant decrease in fasting blood sugar (FBS), an improvement in the glucose tolerance test, and decreases in glycosylated hemoglobin in the fenugreek group, but not in the control group.[16] In a comparative trial of 111 type II diabetics, 51 patients were given 3 g b.i.d. of fenugreek seed, and 60 patients were given other Indian herbal preparations, for 6 weeks. The patients in the fenugreek arm showed significant decreases in FBS, PPBS, and serum cholesterol compared to the other groups.[17]

In the only placebo-controlled trial, 2.5 g b.i.d. of encapsulated fenugreek seed administered to 20 type II diabetics resulted in reductions in glucose (about 15–20%) in patients with mild diabetes (FBS averaging 175 mg/dl) after 1 month. There was no benefit in patients with more severe diabetes (FBS averaging 220 mg/dl).

This trial was not randomized; there was no mention of blinding; and the data were poorly reported.[18]

• Hypolipidemic Activity—Lipid-lowering effects have been reported in several uncontrolled trials. Two such studies in type II diabetics reported reductions in total cholesterol, LDL, VLDL, and/or triglycerides. One study gave 25 g b.i.d. of fenugreek in a soup for 6 months; the other gave 9 g/day of encapsulated fenugreek seed powder for 3 months.[19,20] In an uncontrolled trial of 20 patients with hypercholesterolemia given either 12.5 g or 18 g of fenugreek seed powder daily for 30 days, both groups had a significant decrease in total and LDL cholesterol, but no change in HDL, VLDL, or triglycerides.[21]

In a placebo-controlled trial of 2.5 g b.i.d. of encapsulated fenugreek seed, no effect was seen on cholesterol in healthy subjects, and platelet aggregation, fibrinolytic activity, and fibrinogen levels also were not affected.[18] However, in a subgroup of 30 patients with type II diabetes and coronary artery disease, reductions in total cholesterol (about 6%) and triglycerides (about 16%) were reported by the end of 3 months. However, this trial was not randomized; there was no mention of blinding; and the data were poorly reported—thus casting doubts on the reported beneficial results.[18] In a recent RCT with 18 type II diabetics, 25- and 50-g doses of defatted fenugreek were compared to placebo for 20 days. There were significant decreases in total cholesterol, triglycerides, and VLDL.[7] Characteristics of blinding were not mentioned in the study.

Adverse Effects: No significant adverse effects were reported in any of the clinical trials, apart from occasional flatulence and diarrhea.[15] Rare allergic symptoms, including numbness, swelling, and wheezing, have been reported with fenugreek applied topically.[22] An interesting side effect is the peculiar odor of maple syrup that fenugreek has been reported to impart to urine when ingested in large amounts.[23]

Interactions: The absorption of drugs taken concomitantly with fenugreek may be delayed or impaired because of the herb's high mucilaginous fiber content.[3] This effect has not been studied. In a patient previously stabilized on warfarin, oral consumption of one fenugreek capsule and 10 drops of a boldo (*Peumus boldus*) extract, both with meals, was associated with an elevation of the INR (from 2.3 to 3.4).[24] The effect was confirmed with rechallenge, but the cause and effect relationship with fenugreek is not known.

Cautions: Occupational exposure to fenugreek has been reported to cause asthma, and inhalation of seed powder may cause allergic symptoms such as rhinorrhea and wheezing.[25] Because of reported oxytocic and isolated uterine stimulant activity in animals,[3] fenugreek in doses larger than those encountered in foods is not recommended during pregnancy.[26]

Preparations & Doses: Common oral preparations include pulverized seeds, capsules with seed powder, and teas. Pulverized seeds have been mixed with water to make a paste and used as a poultice. Typically, the recommended dose for oral use is 1–6 g three times a day.[2,3] Doses as high as 50–100 g/day have been used in clinical trials.

──────────── **Summary Evaluation** ────────────

Animal studies and inadequately controlled clinical trials suggest that fenugreek lowers serum cholesterol and glucose levels. However, high-quality controlled trials are lacking, and thus efficacy has not been adequately demonstrated. Because the herb appears safe and well tolerated, and may be a good source of fiber, it is not unreasonable for diabetic or hypercholesterolemic patients to try fenugreek supplements, as long as clinical effects are monitored. None of the other claimed uses or indications for fenugreek have been evaluated clinically.

references

1. Peirce A. The American Pharmaceutical Association's Practical Guide to Natural Medicines. New York, William Morrow and Co, 1999.
2. Blumenthal M, Goldberg A, Brinckmann J (eds). Herbal Medicine: Expanded Commission E Monographs. Newton, MA, Integrative Medicine Communications, 2000.
3. Newall CA, Anderson LA, Philipson DJ. Herbal Medicines. A Guide for Healthcare Professionals. London, The Pharmaceutical Press, 1996.
4. Sharma RD. An evaluation of hypocholesterolemic factor of fenugreek seeds in rats. Nutr Rep Int 33:669–677, 1986.
5. Valette G, Sauvaire Y, Baccou JC, Ribes G. Hypocholesterolaemic effect of fenugreek seeds in dogs. Atherosclerosis 50:105–111, 1984.
6. Sauvaire Y, Ribes G, Baccou JC, et al. Implication of steroid saponins and sapogenins in the hypocholesterolemic effects of fenugreek. Lipids 26: 191–197, 1991.
7. Prasanna M. Hypolipidemic effect of fenugreek: A clinical study. Indian J Pharmacol 32:34–36, 2000.
8. Rodriguez-Moran M, Guerrero-Romero F, Lazcano-Burciaga G. Lipid- and glucose-lowering efficacy of plantago psyllium in type II diabetics. J Diabetes Complicat 12:273–278, 1998.

9. Mazdar Z. New sources of dietary fibre. Int J Obes 11(suppl 1):57–65, 1987.

10. Raghuram TC, Sharma RD, Sivakumar B. Effect of fenugreek seeds on intravenous glucose disposition in noninsulin-dependent diabetic patients. Phytother Res 8:83–86, 1994.

11. Mishkinsky JS, Goldschmied A, Joseph B, et al. Hypoglycemic effect of *Trigonella foenum-graecum* and *Lupinus termis* (Leguminosae) seeds and their major alkaloids in alloxan-diabetic and normal rats. Arch Int Pharmacodyn Ther 210:27–37, 1974.

12. Mishkinsky J, Joseph B, Sulman FG. Hypoglycemic effect of trigonelline. Lancet 2:1311–1312, 1967.

13. Mazdar Z, Abel R, Samish S, Arad J. Glucose-lowering effect of fenugreek in noninsulin-dependent diabetics. Eur J Clin Nutr 42:51–54, 1988.

14. Sharma RD. Effect of fenugreek seeds and leaves on blood glucose and serum insulin responses in human subjects. Nutr Res 6:1353–1364, 1986.

15. Sharma RD, Raghuram TC, Rao SN. Effect of fenugreek seeds on blood glucose and serum lipids in type I diabetes. Europ J Clin Nutr 44: 301–306, 1990.

16. Sharma RD, Sarkar A, Hazra DK, et al. Use of fenugreek seed powder in the management of noninsulin-dependent diabetes mellitus. Nutr Res 16: 1331–1339, 1996.

17. Kumar N, Kumar A, Sharma ML. Clinical evaluation of single and herbo-mineral compound drugs in the management of Madhumeha (diabetes). J Res Ayurveda Siddha 20(1–2):1–9, 1999.

18. Bordia A, Verma SK, Srivastava KC. Effect of ginger and fenugreek on blood lipids, blood sugar and platelet aggregation in patients with coronary artery disease. Prostagl Leukotr Essent Fatty Acids 56:379–384, 1997.

19. Sharma RD, Sarkar A, Hazra DK, et al. Hypolipidemic effect of fenugreek seeds: A chronic study in noninsulin-dependent diabetic patients. Phytother Res 10:332–334, 1996.

20. Kuppurajan K, Srivatsa A, Krishnaswami CV, et al. Hypoglycemic and hypotriglyceridemic effects of methica churna (fenugreek). The Antiseptic (3):78–79, 1995.

21. Sowmya A, Rajyalakshmi P. Hypocholesterolemic effect of germinated fenugreek seeds in human subjects. Plant Food Human Nutr 53:359–365, 1999.

22. Patil SP, Niphadkar PV, Bapat MM. Allergy to fenugreek. Ann Allergy Asthma Immunol 78:297–300, 1997.

23. Bartley GB, Hilty MD, Andreson BD, et al. "Maple syrup" urine odor due to fenugreek ingestion. New Engl J Med 305:467, 1981.

24. Lambert J-P, Cormier J. Potential interaction between warfarin and boldofenugreek. Pharmacother 21:509–512, 2001

25. Dugue P, Bel J, Figueredo M. Fenugreek causing a new type of occupational asthma. Presse Med 22:922, 1999.

26. McGuffin M, Hobbs C, Upton A, Goldberg A (eds). American Herbal Products Association's Botanical Safety Handbook. Boca Raton, CRC Press, 1997.

Feverfew (*Tanacetum parthenium*)

rating: 🐜🐜

> - May be effective for migraine headache prophylaxis; benefits not clearly established
> - No other clinical value demonstrated

Feverfew, *Tanacetum parthenium*, is a member of the Asteraceae family. Other common names of feverfew include featherfew, febrifuge plant, and wild chamomile. The leaves of the plant are most commonly used in herbal preparations.

Uses: Feverfew has been used traditionally by herbalists for headaches, arthritis, menstrual irregularity, difficulties in labor, psoriasis, stomach ache, asthma, and fever.[1–3] It gained popularity in Great Britain in the 1980s as a headache remedy and is now commonly used for migraine prophylaxis as well as for other painful disorders such as arthritis.

Pharmacology: The numerous constituents of feverfew include sesquiterpene lactones, monoterpenes, flavonoids, polyacetylenes, and an essential oil.[1,2] The sesquiterpene lactones, of which parthenolide is the major constituent, were initially thought to be most important. Parthenolide is found in many other plants, and the concentrations vary widely among different chemotypes of *T. parthenium* species grown in different geographic areas.[3]

Feverfew extracts, with parthenolide causing most of the activity, have been found to inhibit release from platelets of storage granules containing serotonin, which at one time was thought to play a role in migraine headaches.[3,4] Extracts also inhibit pro-inflammatory prostaglandin (arachidonic acid and thromboxane) production, by interfering with phospholipase A2 in some studies, and by inhibiting cyclo-oxygenase and lipoxygenase enzymes in others.[3,4] Parthenolide can inhibit expression of inducible COX-2 and pro-inflammatory cytokines (TNF-alpha and IL-1) in macrophages, and can also interfere with contractile and relaxant mechanisms in blood vessel.[2,3] In limited animal studies, injectable feverfew extracts were reported to have anti-inflammatory activity, and to inhibit experimentally induced bronchoconstriction.[2,4]

Feverfew extracts and parthenolide can prevent platelet aggregation in vitro[3,4]; however, hematologic effects have not been observed in vivo. In 10 patients taking feverfew for several years, platelet aggregation induced by adenosine diphosphate or thrombin was indistinguishable from that of four control patients.[6] In a blinded crossover study with 20 patients taking feverfew for 2 months, no effect was found on platelet serotonin uptake and activity.[7] All of the in vitro effects described above have proved difficult to detect in vivo, and have not been correlated with clinical benefits.

Clinical Trials: In an initial uncontrolled survey of 270 migraine patients in Great Britain, over 70% of patients reported improvements when eating an average of 2–3 fresh leaves of feverfew daily over several months to years.[2] Subsequently, six double-blind randomized controlled trials from outside the U.S. have evaluated feverfew for the prophylaxis of migraine headaches[8,9]; four studies found beneficial results.

In the initial investigation, 17 patients were evaluated who chronically ate feverfew leaves for self-prophylaxis of migraines. Switching patients to a placebo caused a significant increase in migraine symptoms, compared to those who were placed on a feverfew capsule preparation (50 mg daily).[10] The second positive trial, using a crossover study design of two 4-month treatment periods, evaluated 76 migraine patients. Feverfew capsules, 70–114 mg daily, significantly decreased the number of attacks by 24% (3.6 vs. 4.7 attacks per 2-month period; $P < 0.005$), and decreased symptoms of nausea and vomiting compared to a placebo ($P < 0.02$).[11] A similar crossover trial of 57 migraine patients also demonstrated beneficial effects for feverfew capsules at a dose of 100 mg daily, which significantly decreased pain, vomiting, and sensitivity to light and noise compared to a placebo ($P < 0.01$).[12] One 3-month study, reported only in abstract form at a symposium, evaluated three different doses (2.08 mg, 6.25 mg, and 18.75 mg) of a specific feverfew extract given t.i.d. to 147 migraine patients.[9] The feverfew group had significantly fewer migraine attacks than the placebo group, and the optimal effective dose was 6.25 mg of the extract t.i.d.

In contrast, a Dutch crossover study found that feverfew, in a dose of 143 mg/day, was no better than a placebo for migraine prophylaxis. Fifty migraine patients took an ethanolic feverfew extract standardized for parthenolide content, as opposed to powdered dry leaf products used in most of the previous studies.[13] The negative findings of this study might have been the result of degradation of active ingredients during processing, or standardization to the wrong chemical entity. Because of these results, there is now doubt that parthenolide is the major active constituent.[14] In addition, a randomized, double-blind, crossover study of 20 migraine patients reported that 100 mg/day of feverfew for 2 months was ineffective in the prophylaxis of migraine.[7] This study was published only as an abstract, and few details were described.

Although the overall results suggest that feverfew may be beneficial for migraine headaches, methodologic quality of these studies was questioned in a critical systematic review.[8,9] None of the crossover-design trials contained adequate washout periods; intention-to-treat analyses were not performed in two positive studies; and one negative trial was considered to have the highest methodologic quality. The reviewers emphasized that while feverfew may have beneficial effects for migraine prophylaxis, firm conclusions cannot be drawn from the literature.

Feverfew was found to be ineffective for the treatment of rheumatoid arthritis in a double-blind, placebo-controlled study using an encapsulated dried leaf product at a dose of 70–86 mg/day.[15] Compared to placebo, there was no clinical or laboratory evidence of improvement in 40 rheumatoid arthritis patients over 6 weeks.

Adverse Effects: In an uncontrolled survey of feverfew leaf users, adverse effects occurred in 18% of 270 patients. The main side effects included oral disturbances (e.g., mouth ulceration, sore tongue, unpleasant taste, swollen lips and mouth) and mild gastrointestinal disturbances, in 9.8% and 4.3% of patients, respectively.[2] Oral side effects appear to be more common when chewing the fresh leaves. Reported side effects from the clinical trials using encapsulated products were similar to placebo (actually less than placebo in two trials).[8] Results of hematologic and biochemical safety tests were also not affected by feverfew products.

The term "post-feverfew syndrome" was coined by one investigator, who reported rebound headache, anxiety, insomnia, and joint and muscle stiffness or pain in about 10% of chronic feverfew users who discontinued the herb.[10] Other studies have not reported this effect.

Interactions & Cautions: Feverfew affects platelet activity *in vitro*, but this has not been demonstrated *in vivo*,[3,6,7] and there have been no reported clinical cases of untoward laboratory abnormalities, unexpected bleeding, or other interactions in patients who were also taking anticoagulant or antiplatelet drugs. Adverse effects on coagulation are thus doubtful, but caution and monitoring is advised for patients at high risk of bleeding. Contact allergy to feverfew is well documented with occupational exposures, and there is cross-allergenicity between similar plants containing sesquiterpene lactones (e.g., chrysanthemums, ragweed, daisies).[5,16] The feverfew plant can cause abortions in cattle, and is therefore contraindicated during pregnancy.[16]

Preparations & Doses: Commercial products usually consist of the leaves or other above-ground parts of the plant, often powdered and freeze-dried; these preparations are presumably safer than chewing the fresh leaves. The daily dose used in successful controlled trials was approximately 50–100 mg of encapsulated dried leaf preparations (roughly equivalent to 2–4 fresh leaves), but daily doses of up to 200–600 mg have been recommended by some herbal authorities.[1,2,17] Preparations are typically standardized to contain at least 0.2% parthenolide. However, while standardization can be useful to ensure the correct identity of the *T. parthenium* chemotype, it may not provide an index of effectiveness.[14]

Summary Evaluation

Feverfew has been shown to be beneficial for migraine headache prophylaxis in the majority of randomized controlled trials conducted; however, efficacy has not been adequately established beyond a reasonable doubt. Feverfew appears to be safe and well tolerated, and thus it is not unreasonable for chronic migraine sufferers to try this herbal medicine. Feverfew has not been investigated for treatment of acute migraine attacks or for other types of headaches. It has been found to be ineffective in one trial for rheumatoid arthritis, and none of its other purported clinical uses have been investigated.

---

references
1. Newall CA, Anderson LA, Phillipson JD: Herbal Medicines: A Guide for Health-Care Professionals. London, The Pharmaceutical Press, 1996.

2. Mills S, Bone K: Principles and Practice of Phytotherapy: Modern Herbal Medicine. Edinburgh, Churchill Livingstone, 2000.

3. Heptinstall S, Awang DVC: Feverfew: A review of its history, its biological and medicinal properties, and the status of commercial preparations of the herb. In Lawson LD, Bauer R (eds): Phytomedicines of Europe: Chemistry and Biological Activity. ACS Symposium Series 691. Washington DC, American Chemical Society, 1998, pp 158–175.

4. Groenewegen WA, Knight DW, Heptinstall S: Progress in the medicinal chemistry of the herb feverfew. Prog Med Chem 29:217–238,1992.

5. Kemper KJ: The Longwood Herbal Task Force. Feverfew (Tanacetum parthenium), revised Nov. 9, 1999. Accessed Dec. 24, 2000 at http://www.mcp.edu/herbal/default.htm

6. Biggs MJ, Johnson ES, Persaud NP, Ratcliffe DM: Platelet aggregation in patients using feverfew for migraine. Lancet 2:776, 1982.

7. Kuritzky A, Elhacham Y, Yerushalmi Z, Hering R: Feverfew in the treatment of migraine: Its effect on serotonin uptake and platelet activity. Neurology 44(Suppl 2):A201(293P), 1994.

8. Pittler MH, Vogler BK, Ernst E: Feverfew for preventing migraine (Cochrane Review). In The Cochrane Library, Issue 4. Oxford, Update Software, 2000.

9. Ernst E, Pittler MH: The efficacy and safety of feverfew (Tanacetum parthenium L.): An update of a systematic review. Public Health Nutr 3(4A):509–514, 2000.

10. Johnson ES, Kadam NP, Hylands DM, Hylands PJ: Efficacy of feverfew as prophylactic treatment of migraine. BMJ 291:569–573, 1985.

11. Murphy JJ, Heptinstall S, Mitchell JRA: Randomised double-blind placebo-controlled trial of feverfew in migraine prevention. Lancet ii:189–192, 1988.

12. Palevitch D, Earon G, Carasso R: Feverfew (Tanacetum parthenium) as a prophylactic treatment for migraine: A double-blind placebo-controlled study. Phytotherapy Res 11:508–511, 1997.

13. De Weerdt CJ, Bootsma HPR, Hendriks H: Herbal medicines in migraine prevention. Phytomedicine 3:225–230, 1996.

14. Awang DVC: Prescribing therapeutic feverfew (Tanacetum parthenium) and Chrysanthemum parthenium. Integrative Med 1:11–13, 1998.

15. Pattrick M, Heptinstall S, Doherty M: Feverfew in rheumatoid arthritis: A double-blind, placebo-controlled study. Ann Rheum Dis 48:547–549, 1989.

16. Hausen BM: Sesquiterpene lactones-Tanacetum parthenium. In De Smet PAGM (ed): Adverse Effects of Herbal Drugs. Vol 1. Berlin, Springer, 1992, pp 255–260.

17. Tanaceti Parthenii Herba/Folium: Feverfew. European Scientific Cooperative on Phytotherapy. Monographs on the Medicinal Uses of Plant Drugs. Exeter, UK, ESCOP, March 1996.

Garlic (*Allium sativum*)
rating: 🐾 🐾

> - Commonly used to help prevent cardiovascular disease and cancer
> - Mixed study results regarding benefits for cardiovascular disease
> - Well tolerated with few adverse effects

Garlic has many varieties, such as ramson (wild garlic, A. ursinum), garlic chives, and elephant garlic. The name *Allium* is derived from the Celtic word for pungent, hot, or burning; the species name, *sativum*, means cultivated or planted. The cloves in the garlic bulb are used medicinally and as a food component.

Uses: Garlic is one of the oldest herbal remedies; it was a favored food in the Old Testament and has been accorded almost magical properties in various cultures. It was considered a cure-all and aphrodisiac. Garlic has been employed to treat infections, wounds, respiratory conditions, diarrhea, rheumatism, heart disease, diabetes, and many other disorders. Currently, it is most often used as an antithrombotic and antioxidant herb to help prevent heart disease, atherosclerosis, and cancer. It is widely promoted to reduce abnormal cholesterol and blood pressure levels.[1–3]

Pharmacology: There is an enormous body of literature on garlic, and the following is a simplification of the controversial reports on its constituents and properties.[4–8] Garlic contains pharmacologically active, organic sulfur compounds; the main ones are S-alkylcysteine sulfoxides and their precursors, derivatives of the amino acid cysteine such as alliin (S-allyl-L-cysteine sulfoxide). The active constituent is thought to be allicin (diallyldisulfide-S-oxide) or a variety of allicin byproducts, which are formed only when the garlic bulb is cut, chewed, or crushed. This releases the enzyme alliinase from cells, which converts alliin into the unstable allicin. Allicin and related diallyl sulfide dimerization products provide the characteristic garlic odor, and are considered to be the most important pharmacologic and medicinal compounds—many commercial products are standardized to their allicin yield.

Another compound in garlic is ajoene, which is a condensation product of allicin, found mainly in garlic oil macerates. Ajoene and similar compounds are much more stable than allicin, although it is uncertain if they are formed or have any function in the body after a garlic preparation is eaten. Less odorous allicin degradation products such as S-allylcysteine (SAC) are also reported to have biologic activity.

There is no consensus regarding exactly which constituents are primarily responsible for the proposed effects *in vivo*. Allicin and its breakdown products are believed to be the major ingredient responsible for antilipidemic effects, based on animal studies.[2,9]

Garlic components stimulate fibrinolysis, inhibit arachidonic acid conversion into prostaglandins, and can reduce platelet aggregation *in vitro* and in animal studies.[4] Note that cooking garlic significantly reduces this activity.[9] A systematic review of human studies revealed that four of five controlled trials found modest but significant decreases in platelet aggregation with garlic treatment compared with placebo; the other trial found mixed effects.[10] Mixed results were observed on fibrinolytic activity, while effects on serum fibrinogen and homocysteine levels were insignificant.

Garlic has antioxidant properties that can activate endogenous protective mechanisms against free-radical formation.[4] Hypotensive effects of aqueous garlic extracts have been reported in animal models.[9] Garlic has antimicrobial effects against various bacteria, protozoa, and fungi.[4] Allicin, ajoene, diallyl sulfide, and other thiosulfinate constituents have antifungal and other antimicrobial properties.[11,12] Garlic also has been shown to have antimutagenic and anticarcinogenic effects in animal and *in vitro* studies.[4,9,12] It has been suggested that the most effective anticancer components worthy of study are the allyl sulfides.[4] Other attributes include reducing inflammation and improving immune responses, detoxifying chemical carcinogens, and stimulating antitumor cytokine production.[4,12]

Clinical Trials: Numerous controlled clinical trials have been published.[1,2] The most comprehensive critical evaluation of this literature, commissioned by the U.S. Agency for Heathcare Research & Quality (AHRQ), has recently been published as a systematic review and meta-analysis.[10,13] Many trials were found to have methodologic weaknesses, such as unclear randomization procedures, difficulty in adequately blinding for garlic's smell or odor, and lack of intention-to-treat analysis.

• Lipid-Lowering Effects—Epidemiologic studies have suggested that people who habitually eat garlic and onions have lower lipid and cholesterol levels.[14] This was initially supported by two meta-analyses published in 1993 and 1994, which analyzed 16 randomized controlled trials (RCTs), and found that garlic preparations lowered cholesterol levels by 8–15%.[15,16] In the recent AHRQ meta-analysis of 45 RCTs lasting at least 4 weeks, garlic was similarly associated with an average reduced total cholesterol at 1 and 3 months of 7.2 and 17.1 mg/dl, respectively. Comparable results were found with triglycerides and LDL-cholesterol, while HDL-cholesterol was not significantly affected. However, nine trials reporting outcomes at 6 months did not show persistence of significant cholesterol reductions. Results of trials limited to subjects with hyperlipidemia or using double-blind methods did not vary significantly from the overall results. The Agency review asserted that garlic does not appear to offer long-term reduction of cholesterol.[10]

A separate meta-analysis of 13 randomized, double-blind, placebo-controlled trials found similar results in patients with elevated total cholesterol levels (> 200 mg/dl). Garlic preparations were found to reduce total cholesterol levels more than placebo ($P < 0.01$), with a weighted mean difference of 15.7 mg/dl (a 4–6% reduction). However, the six diet-controlled trials with the best methodologic quality revealed a nonsignificant difference between garlic and placebo groups.[17]

Of the more recent well-designed, double-blind RCTs evaluating hypercholesterolemia, both positive and negative results have been published,[18–24] inspiring vigorous debate. Some claim that the negative results are due to specific trials that used inferior products or brands.[25–27] Others assert that most of the negative studies are simply better diet-controlled than the positive ones, and that the trials with better methodology more accurately reflect the true lack of antilipidemic effects. Firm conclusions have not been reached.

• Hypertension—A 1994 meta-analysis of eight RCTs on blood pressure found mild blood pressure–lowering effects (about 6%), but many of these trials had methodologic shortcomings.[16] Of the 23 placebo-controlled trials that evaluated blood pressure included in the AHRQ analysis, four demonstrated small but statistically significant reductions (2–7%), while the rest found no significant benefit.[10] Of six recent, well-designed RCTs, two found mild reductions of blood pressure,[20,28] and four found no difference compared to placebo.[21,23,29,30]

• Cardiovascular Disease—In clinical trials evaluating garlic's effect on cardiovascular morbidity or mortality, significant reductions in established disease have not been proven. An unpublished 3-year RCT in 432 patients with evidence of prior myocardial infarctions initially reported a significant reduction of reinfarction in the garlic extract group vs. the placebo group, but a reanalysis of the statistics revealed no statistically significant differences.[10] Garlic pills allegedly slowed carotid or femoral artery plaque formation in a 4-year randomized, double-blind study;[31] however, reanalysis showed statistical benefits in women, but not in men, and there were several methodologic inadequacies.[10,32] A double-blind RCT in 80 patients with claudication from peripheral arterial disease reported a statistically significant improvement in pain-free walking distance, but the absolute measure of improvement (a difference of 15 meters between the garlic and placebo group) was not clinically significant.[33]

• Anti-Cancer Effects—Over 20 case-control or cohort studies have evaluated the association of garlic with the incidence of cancers in different cultures.[34] In multiple studies, dietary garlic consumption is correlated with a decreased incidence of gastric and colorectal cancer, and limited studies have also shown promising inverse relationships with head and neck, prostate, and breast cancer. A few studies of garlic supplements, however, have failed to find a protective association with cancer incidence.[13,34] An indication of publication bias was found upon evaluation of all the studies,[34] and thus adequate evidence of a beneficial effect is lacking.

• Other Uses—Statistically significant reductions in serum glucose (in nondiabetics) were found in only one of 12 trials that assessed the effect of garlic on glucose levels.[10] A topical 1% ajoene cream was found to be effective for superficial tinea infections.[35] In a RCT of 20 Helicobacter pylori-positive, dyspeptic patients, garlic oil capsules had no affect on symptoms, histologic gastritis grade, or H. pylori density.[36]

Adverse Effects: Garlic can cause malodorous breath or body odor.[10] Less commonly, dyspepsia, flatulence, anorexia, rhinitis, asthma, dermatitis, and other allergic reactions can also occur.[37] Of more concern are two case reports of prolonged bleeding during surgical procedures, and one report of a spontaneous spinal epidural hematoma associated with heavy garlic use in an

87-year-old man.[38–40] The cause and effect relationship between garlic and bleeding is not well established in these cases; however, since garlic may affect fibrinolysis and platelet aggregation, garlic supplementation should be considered a possible risk factor for bleeding.

Interactions: In two patients taking warfarin, increased (roughly doubled) international normalized ratios (INRs) were attributed to the use of garlic products. However, these case reports lacked sufficient details to adequately assess causality.[41] Theoretically, excessive garlic may potentiate bleeding if patients are taking anticoagulant drugs or otherwise have compromised hemostasis.

Cautions: Sensitive patients can develop dermatitis, asthma, rhinitis, or even anaphylaxis with oral, topical, or respiratory exposure to garlic products. Such reactions are usually seen upon prolonged contact with raw garlic or after massive occupational exposure.[37,42,43]

Preparations & Doses: Garlic cloves can be used in several forms: whole or chopped, powdered and dried, or oil extracts. Freeze-dried garlic powder, in which alliinase is inactivated, is the prepared form that is most representative of the true composition of the fresh clove. To preserve the allicin constituents, most products are manufactured to protect alliinase from degradation by the stomach acids with a protective enteric-coating. Alternatively, oil extracts are manufactured (by maceration, steam distillation, or soaking in ethanol) that contain little allicin, but are instead composed mainly of products such as ajoene, disulfides, and SAC.

The choice of popular commercial preparations is confusing. Supporters of major products (such as powdered, freeze-dried garlic[4,27] or a garlic oil called Aged Garlic Extract (marketed under the name Kyolic)[26] cite large bodies of convincing scientific literature to support their individual claims.

The majority of the clinical trials used 600–900 mg/day of a concentrated freeze-dried garlic powder (Kwai tablets, by Lichtwer Pharma) standardized to 1.3% alliin or 0.6% allicin yield, containing 3.6–5.4 mg allicin/day. This dose is roughly equivalent to one small clove or about 2–3 g of fresh garlic. There are many different powder products on the market that vary widely in their allicin yield. A few controlled trials used Kyolic (600 mg/day) or other garlic oil products (oil macerates, steam-distilled, etc.) that contain primarily SAC and other allicin degradation products; these are mostly devoid of alliin and allicin.

Summary Evaluation

Garlic is one of the most popular herbal medicines, and a large variety of different types of products are available. Despite common claims and advertising, the evidence for garlic's beneficial effects on cholesterol and blood pressure is inconsistent and controversial; effects are likely to be small or clinically insignificant. Garlic supplementation appears safe for most patients who desire to use an herbal product for cardiovascular health, but the extent of any long-term beneficial effect is not well established.

references

1. Blumenthal M, Goldberg A, Brinckmann J (eds). Herbal Medicine: Expanded Commission E Monographs. Newton, MA, Integrative Medicine Communications, 2000.
2. Schulz V, Hänsel R, Tyler VE. Rational Phytotherapy: A Physicians' Guide to Herbal Medicine, 4th ed. New York, Springer, 2001.
3. Boon H, Smith M. The Botanical Pharmacy: The Pharmacology of 47 Common Herbs. Kingston, Ontario, Quarry Press, 1999.
4. Koch HP, Lawson LD (eds). Garlic. The Science and Therapeutic Applications of *Allium sativum L.* and Related Species. Baltimore, Williams and Wilkins, 1996.
5. Bruneton J. Pharmacognosy, Phytochemistry, Medicinal Plants. Secaucus, New York, Lavoisier Publishing, Inc., 1999.
6. Block E. The organosulfur chemistry of the genus *Allium:* Implications for the organic chemistry of sulfur. Angew Chem Int Ed Engl 31:1135–1178, 1992.
7. Block E. The chemistry of garlic and onions. Sci Am 252:114–119, 1985.
8. Leung A, Foster S. Encyclopedia of Common Natural Ingredients Used in Food, Drugs and Cosmetics, 2nd ed. New York, John Wiley & Sons, 1996.
9. Ali M, Thomson M, Afzal M. Garlic and onions: Their effect on eicosanoid metabolism and its clinical relevance. Prostaglandins Leuk Essent Fatty Acids 62:55–73, 2000.
10. Ackermann RT, Mulrow CD, Ramirez G. Garlic shows promise for improving some cardiovascular risk factors. Arch Intern Med 161:813–824, 2001.
11. Dietz V. Garlic for the treatment of topical infections: does it help? Atlanta, GA, American Health Consultants, Alternative Medicine Alert 2(3):28–31, 1999.
12. Nagourney RA. Garlic: Medicinal food or nutritious medicine? J Medicinal Food 1:13–28, 1998.
13. Anon. Garlic: Effects on cardiovascular risks and disease, protective effects against cancer, and clinical adverse effects. Summary. Agency for Healthcare Research and Quality Evidence Report/Technology Assessment (AHRQ Pub. No. 01-E022), Oct. 2000.
14. Kleijnen J, Knipschild P, Ter Riet G. Garlic, onions and cardiovascular risk factors. A review of the evidence from human experiments with emphasis on commercially available preparations. Br J Clin Pharmac 28:535–544, 1989.

15. Warshafsky S, Kamer RS, Sivak SL. Effect of garlic on total serum cholesterol: A meta-analysis. Ann Intern Med 119:599–605, 1993.

16. Silagy C, Neil A. Garlic as a lipid lowering agent: A meta-analysis. J R Coll Phys London 28:39–45, 1994.

17. Stevinson C, Pittler MH, Ernst E. Garlic for treating hypercholesterolemia: A meta-analysis of randomized clinical trials. Ann Intern Med 133:420–429, 2000.

18. Rahman K. Historical perspective on garlic and cardiovascular disease. J Nutr 131:977S–979S, 2001.

19. Lash JP, Cardoso LR, Mesler PM,et al. The effect of garlic on hypercholesterolemia in renal transplant patients. Transplant Proc 30:189–191, 1998.

20. Adler AJ, Holub BJ. Effect of garlic and fish-oil supplementation on serum lipid and lipoprotein concentrations in hypercholesterolemic men. Am J Clin Nutr 65:445–450, 1997.

21. McCrindle BW, Helden E, Conner WT. Garlic extract therapy in children with hypercholesterolemia. Arch Pediatr Adolesc Med 152:1089–1094, 1998.

22. Superko HR, Krauss RM. Garlic powder, effect on plasma lipids, postprandial lipemia, low-density lipoprotein particle size, high-density lipoprotein subclass distribution and lipoprotein(a). J Am Coll Cardiol 35:321–326, 2000.

23. Zhang X-H, Lowe D, Giles P, et al. A randomized trial of the effects of garlic oil upon coronary heart disease risk factors in trained male runners. Blood Coagul Fibrinolysis 11:67–74, 2000.

24. Gardner CD, Chatterjee LM, Carlson JJ. The effect of garlic preparation on plasma lipid levels in moderately hypercholesterolemic adults. Atherosclerosis 154:213–220, 2001.

25. Lawson LD. Effect of garlic on serum lipids. JAMA 280:1568, 1998.

26. Amagase H, Petesch BL, Matsuura H, et al. Intake of garlic and its bioactive components. J Nutr 131:955S–962S, 2001.

27. Lawson LD, Wang ZJ, Papadimitriou D. Allicin release under simulated gastrointestinal conditions from garlic powder tablets employed in clinical trials on serum cholesterol. Planta Med 67:13–18, 2001.

28. Steiner M, Khan AH, Holbert D, Lin RIS. A double-blind crossover study in moderately hypercholesterolemic men that compared the effect of aged garlic extract and placebo administration on blood lipids. Am J Clin Nutr 64:866–870, 1996.

29. Simons LA, Balasubramaniam S, von Konigsmark M, et al. On the effect of garlic on plasma lipids and lipoproteins in mild hypercholesterolaemia. Atherosclerosis 113:219–225, 1995.

30. Saradeth T, Seidl S, Resch KL, Ernst E. Does garlic alter the lipid pattern in normal volunteers? Phytomedicine 1:183–185, 1994.

31. Koscielny J, Klüssendorf D, Latza R, et al. The antiatherosclerotic effect of Allium sativum. Atherosclerosis 144:237–249, 1999.

32. Siegel G, Klüssendorf D. The anti-atherosclerotic effect of Allium sativum: statistics re-evaluated. Atherosclerosis 150:437–438, 2000.

33. Kieswetter H, Jung F, Jung EM, et al. Effects of garlic coated tablets in peripheral arterial occlusive disease. Clin Investig 71:383–386, 1993.

34. Fleischauer AT, Poole C, Arab L. Garlic consumption and cancer prevention: meta-analyses of colorectal and stomach cancers. Am J Clin Nutr 72:1047–1052, 2000.

35. Ledezma E, Marcano K, Jorquera A, et al. Efficacy of ajoene in the treatment of tinea pedis: A double-blind and comparative study with terbinafine. J Am Acad Dermatol 43:829–832, 2000.

36. Aydin A, Ersöz G, Tekesin O, Akçiçek E. Garlic oil and *Helicobacter pylori* infection. Am J Gastroenterol 95:563–564, 2000.

37. Morbidoni L, Arterburn JM, Young V, et al. Garlic: Its history and adverse effects. J Herbal Pharmacother 1:63–83, 2001.

38. German K, Kumar U, Blackford HN. Garlic and the risk of TURP bleeding. Br J Urol 76:518, 1995.

39. Burnham BE. Garlic as a possible risk for postoperative bleeding. Plastic Reconstr Surg 95:213, 1995.

40. Rose KD, Croissant PD, Parliament CF, Levin MB. Spontaneous spinal epidural hematoma with associated platelet dysfunction from excessive garlic ingestion: A case report. Neurosurgery 26:880–882, 1990.

41. Sunter W. Warfarin and garlic. Pharmaceut J 246:722, 1991.

42. Perez-Pimiento AJ, Moneo I, Santaolalla M, de Paz S, et al. Anaphylactic reaction to young garlic. Allergy 54:626–629, 1999.

43. Sieger C-P. *Allium sativum.* In De Smet PAGM, Keller K, Hänsel R, Chandler RF (eds): Adverse Effects of Herbal Drugs. Vol 1. New York, Springer-Verlag, 1992, pp 73–77.

Ginger (*Zingiber officinale*)

rating: 🐜🐜🐜 +

> - Beneficial for treatment of nausea and motion sickness
> - Anti-inflammatory and other clinical claims not well substantiated
> - Safe and well tolerated in usual doses

Ginger is noted for its aroma and pungent flavor. The fresh or dried rhizome (usually referred to as the root) is a valuable spice and condiment, as well as a traditional herbal medicine.

Uses: Ginger root is widely used as a digestive aid for mild dyspepsia, and is commonly promoted to help treat or prevent nausea or motion sickness. Known since ancient times (especially in Asian, Indian, and Arabic herbal traditions), ginger has also been used for arthritis, colic, diarrhea, heart disease, and as a general "warming" herb.[1–3]

Pharmacology: Important chemical constituents are thought to be the phenolic compounds (e.g., gingerols, shogaols) and essential oils (primarily the sesquiterpenes such as zingiberene, zingiberol, and curcumene). Ginger and isolated constituents, primarily gingerols, have been studied in many animal and *in vitro* experiments; the details of these studies have been extensively reviewed.[2–4] In summary, ginger was found to enhance gastrointestinal motility in some (but not all) animal studies, and to decrease chemotherapy-induced vomiting. It reduces experimentally induced gastric lesions, and enhances bile excretion. *In vitro*, ginger is an antioxidant; inhibits formation of inflammatory prostaglandins and leukotrienes; and inhibits platelet aggregation.

In human pharmacologic studies, oral administration of dried or fresh ginger root has produced variable results. Enhanced gastrointestinal motility was found in one investigation,[5] but not in others.[6,7] An indirect antivertigo effect on the vestibular system was also demonstrated; this is thought to be similar to the effect of anticholinergic agents.[8] Platelet aggregation inhibition (demonstrated *in vitro*) appears to be dose dependent *in vivo*, and may not be clinically significant at usual therapeutic doses. In placebo-controlled trials, typical doses of up to 4 g daily had no effect on bleeding time or platelet aggregation,[9,10] while larger doses of 5 and 10 g reduced aggregation.[10,11] In contrasting studies, a reduction in thromboxane production was found with doses of 5 g, but not with 15 g.[12,13] In spite of some claims to the contrary, no changes in lipid or glucose levels have been found with 4 g/day of dried ginger compared to placebo.[10]

Clinical Trials: Ginger root, primarily in doses of 0.5–1 g, has been well-studied for motion sickness and as an antiemetic; results of controlled trials are generally positive, but are not all consistent. Ginger was more effective than placebo and dimenhydrinate (Dramamine) in an initial single-blind experiment for motion sickness, measuring the tolerance of 36 students in a rotating chair.[14] Although one small, placebo-controlled study also reported an anti-vertigo effect to caloric stimulation of the vestibular apparatus,[8] three subsequent controlled studies of experimental motion sickness (using a rotating chair or turntable) found ginger to be no more effective than placebo.[7,15,16]

Better results were found in "real-life" clinical studies of motion sickness. Ginger was reported to help prevent or reduce sea-sickness on ocean vessels in three double-blind, randomized controlled trials (RCTs). In 79 naval cadets, a single dose of ginger reduced vomiting and cold sweats more effectively than placebo.[17] In 60 cruise passengers, ginger had equivalent effects to standard doses of antiemetic antihistamines when given every 4 hours, and in 1741 tourists on whale safaris when given in two doses shortly before and after departure.[18,19] In a separate RCT of 28 children (ages 4–8) prone to travel sickness, 0.25 g every 4 hours reduced symptoms of travel sickness more effectively, and with less side effects, than dimenhydrinate.[20]

To treat nausea and vomiting during pregnancy, two double-blind RCTs (n = 27, 70) found ginger root, in doses of 0.2 and 0.25 g q.i.d. for 4 days, to reduce symptoms more effectively than placebo.[21,22] Results were both statistically and clinically significant.

Mixed results were found for postsurgical nausea following laparoscopic gynecologic procedures in four large double-blind RCTs; results were positive in two studies and negative in the other two. In the positive studies, 1 g of a ginger root product before surgery reduced the incidence of nausea as effectively as a standard dose of metoclopramide, and decreased the need for post-operative medications.[23,24] In the other two studies, there was a nonsignificant trend for benefit with ginger in one, but ginger caused more vomiting than placebo in the other.[25,26] The pooled absolute risk reduction, using both positive and only one negative trial, indicated a non-significant difference between the ginger and the placebo groups.[27]

Ginger's potential anti-inflammatory effects have been reported in uncontrolled case series of patients with arthritis and related musculoskeletal disorders[28]; these findings have not been substantiated in controlled clinical trials. In a crossover double-blind RCT (without washout periods) in 56 patients with osteoarthritis, a statistically significant benefit of a ginger extract was found prior to the first crossover period with a placebo, but not when the results of all study periods were evaluated.[29] Ginger was less effective than 1200 mg of ibuprofen daily during all periods of the study.

Adverse Effects: Ginger has no known clinical adverse effects other then rare heartburn.[27,30]

Interactions: Drug interactions have not been studied or reported in humans. In a rat model, ginger did not interact with warfarin's activity on blood coagulation.[31]

Cautions: Although ginger has antiprostaglandin and antiplatelet effects *in vitro*, increased risk of bleeding has not been demonstrated with oral doses up to 4 g daily, and there have been no case reports of bleeding.[9,10,30] Because doses greater than 4 g/day may affect platelet function, it would be prudent to recommend lower doses for patients who are taking anticoagulant drugs or are otherwise at high bleeding risk.

Despite its widespread use in foods, ingestion of ginger during pregnancy is controversial. Ginger extract and isolated ginger constituents have mutagenic and antimutagenic properties, depending on the *in vitro* experimental test.[1,2,30] Embryotoxic effects have been described in pregnant rats.[32] In the two controlled clinical trials of pregnant women (totaling 59 women who received ginger), there were no significant adverse effects detected on pregnancy outcome.[26,27] Based on the experience of its widespread use in foods, it is unlikely that ginger has detrimental effects during pregnancy; nevertheless, it would be prudent to be cautious and to avoid higher doses (> 2 g daily).[4]

Preparations & Doses: Common preparations include powdered ginger capsules, liquid extracts, tinctures, and candies. The doses examined in various clinical trials range from 0.2 to 1 g of dried ginger root, usually administered in capsules, as a single dose or repeated every 4 hours or q.i.d. depending on the study. Doses recommended by herbal authorities are similar, usually 0.5–1 g two to four times a day, up to 4 g daily.[1,2,4] Larger daily doses of up to 9 g of fresh or dried ginger are often used in traditional Chinese medicine.[1] Substantial ginger content is found in highly spiced meals or strong ginger ales and teas.

Summary Evaluation

Although the results of controlled trials are not consistently positive, the evidence demonstrates that ginger root has some clinical benefits for the prevention or treatment of nausea and motion sickness, and may have effects similar to standard antiemetic antihistamine-type drugs. Unlike most antiemetic agents, however, ginger is nonsedating and has no other significant adverse effects. It is not unreasonable for patients to try ginger as a mild herbal antiemetic or for motion sickness. Anti-inflammatory and other purported clinical claims are not well substantiated.

references

1. Blumenthal M, Goldberg A, Brinckmann J: Herbal Medicine: Expanded Commission E Monographs. Newton, MA, Integrative Medicine Communications, 2000.
2. World Health Organization: WHO Monographs on Selected Medicinal Plants. Vol. 1. Geneva, WHO, 1999.
3. Kemper KJ: The Longwood Herbal Task Force. Ginger (*Zingiber officinale*), revised Nov. 3, 1999. Accessed December 11, 2000 at http://www.mcp.edu/herbal/default.htm
4. Mills S, Bone K: Principles and Practice of Phytotherapy: Modern Herbal Medicine. Edinburgh, Churchill Livingstone, 2000.
5. Micklefield GH, Redeker Y, Meister V, et al: Effects of ginger on gastroduodenal motility. Int J Clin Pharmacol Ther 37:341–346, 1999.
6. Phillips S, Hutchinson S, Ruggier R: *Zingiber officinale* does not affect gastric emptying rate. Anaesthesia 48:393–395, 1993.
7. Stewart JJ, Wood MJ, Wood CD, Mims ME: Effects of ginger on motion sickness susceptibility and gastric function. Pharmacol 42:111–120, 1991.
8. Grøntved A, Hentzer E: Vertigo-reducing effect of ginger root. ORL 48:282–286,1986.
9. Lumb AB: Effect of dried ginger on human platelet function. Thromb Haemost 71:110–111, 1994.
10. Bordia A, Verma SK, Srivastava KC: Effect of ginger (*Zingiber officinale* Rosc.) and fenugreek (*Trigonella foenumgraecum* L.) on blood lipids, blood sugar and platelet aggregation in patients with coronary artery disease. Prostag Leukot Essent Fatty Acids 56:379–384, 1997.

11. Verma SK, Singh J, Khamesra R, Bordia A: Effect of ginger on platelet aggregation in man. Indian J Med Res 98:240–242, 1993.

12. Srivastava KC: Effect of onion and ginger consumption on platelet thromboxane production in humans. Prostag Leukot Essent Fatty Acids 35:183–185, 1989.

13. Janssen PLTMK, Meyboom S, van Staveren WA, et al: Consumption of ginger (*Zingiber officinale* Roscoe) does not affect ex vivo platelet thromboxane production in humans. Eur J Clin Nutr 50:772–774, 1996.

14. Mowrey DB, Clayson DE: Motion sickness, ginger, and psychophysics. Lancet 1(8273):655–657, 1982.

15. Stott JRR, Hubble MP, Spencer MB: A double-blind comparative trial of powdered ginger root, hyosine hydrobromide, and cinnarizine in the prophylaxis of motion sickness induced by cross-coupled stimulation. NATO Advisory Group for Aerospace Research and Development, Conference Proceedings no. 372, Nov. 1984, Reference 39, pp 1–6.

16. Wood CD, Manno JE, Wood MJ, et al: Comparison of efficacy of ginger with various antimotion sickness drugs. Clin Res Pract Drug Reg Affairs 6:129–136, 1988.

17. Grøntved A, Brask T, Kambskard J: Ginger root against seasickness. Acta Otolaryngol (Stockh) 105:45–49, 1988.

18. Riebenfeld D, Borzone L: Randomized double-blind study comparing ginger (Zintona) and dimenhydrinate in motion sickness. Reviewed by Fulder S, Brown D in Healthnotes Complem Integr Med 6:98–101, 1999.

19. Schmid R, Schick T, Steffen R, et al: Comparison of seven commonly used agents for prophylaxis of seasickness. J Travel Med 1:203–206, 1994.

20. Careddu P: Motion sickness in children: Results of a double-blind study with ginger (Zintona) and dimenhydrinate. Reviewed by Fulder S, Brown D in Healthnotes Complem Integr Med 6:102–107, 1999.

21. Bone ME, Wilkinson DJ, Young JR, et al: Ginger root—A new antiemetic: The effect of ginger root on postoperative nausea and vomiting after major gynaecological surgery. Anaesthesia 45:669–671, 1990.

22. Phillips S, Ruggier R, Hutchinson SE: *Zingiber officinale* (ginger)—An antiemetic for day case surgery. Anaesthesia 48:715–717, 1993.

23. Arfeen Z, Owen H, Plummer JL, et al: A double-blind randomized controlled trial of ginger for the prevention of postoperative nausea and vomiting. Anaesth Intens Care 23:449–452, 1995.

24. Visalyaputra S, Petchpaisit N, Somcharoen K, Choavaratana R: The efficacy of ginger root in the prevention of postoperative nausea and vomiting after outpatient gynaecological laparoscopy. Anaesthesia 53:506–510, 1998.

25. Ernst E, Pittler MH: Efficacy of ginger for nausea and vomiting: A systematic review of randomized clinical trials. Br J Anaesthesia 84:367–371, 2000.

26. Fischer-Rasmussen W, Kjaer SK, Dahl C, Asping U: Ginger treatment of hyperemesis gravidarum. Eur J Obstet Gynecol Reprod Biol 38:19–24, 1990.

27. Vutyavanich T, Kraisarin T, Ruangsri R-A: Ginger for nausea and vomiting in pregancy: Randomized, double-blind, placebo-controlled trial. Obstet Gynecol 97:577–582, 2001.

28. Srivastava KC, Mustafa T: Ginger (*Zingiber officinale*) in rheumatism and musculoskeletal disorders. Med Hypotheses 39:342–348, 1992.

29. Bliddal H, Rosetzsky A, Schlichting P, et al: A randomized, placebo-controlled, cross-over study of ginger extracts and ibuprofen in osteoarthritis. Osteoarth Cartilage 8:9-12, 2000.
30. Corrigan D: *Zingiber officinale*. In De Smet PAGM (Ed): Adverse Effects of Herbal Drugs. Vol. 3. Berlin, Springer, 1997, pp 215–228.
31. Weidner MS, Sigwart K: The safety of a ginger extract in the rat. J Ethnopharmacol 73:513–520, 2000.
32. Wilkinson JM: Effect of ginger tea on the fetal development of Sprague-Dawley rats. Reprod Toxicol 14:507–512, 2000.

Ginkgo (*Ginkgo biloba*)
rating: 🐿️🐿️

> - Mild benefits for the treatment of dementia and intermittent claudication
> - Other indications (e.g., memory enhancement and treatment of vertigo and tinnitus) not well established
> - Generally well tolerated; small increased risk of bleeding

Ginkgo biloba is one of the oldest living tree species. Almost extinct following the Ice Age, the ginkgo tree survived only in Asia, and was imported to Europe and America in the 18th century as an ornamental street tree. An extract is prepared from the dried green leaves.

Uses: A standardized *Ginkgo biloba* extract (GBE) first became popular in Germany in the 1960s when a group of scientists found it to be particularly active while investigating the effects of exotic herbs on circulation.[1] This extract was extensively researched and used for cognitive defects and peripheral vascular disorders in European countries, and is now commonly promoted for similar uses in the U.S., particularly for the treatment of dementia and the enhancement of memory. GBE is used to treat circulatory impairment (cerebrovascular and peripheral arterial insufficiency), vertigo, tinnitus, impotence, asthma, allergies, premenstrual syndrome, depression, and many other disorders.[1–3]

Pharmacology: More than 40 components of *Ginkgo biloba* have been identified. Two of the most important groups of active chemicals are the flavonoids (e.g., quercetin, kaempferol, isorhamnetin) and the terpene lactones or terpenoids, which include bilobalide and several ginkgolides (A, B, C, J, and M).[2,4] GBE, standardized to 24% flavonoids and 6% terpenoids, and the individual constituents have been studied in hundreds of *in vitro*, animal, and human pharmacologic experiments.[1,2,4,5]

In summary, GBE improves cerebral and peripheral bloodflow in animal and human experiments, at least in part via nitric oxide–induced vasodilation. The flavonoid components have antioxidant activity that can also prevent cellular damage. One or both of these effects result in protection against neuronal, myocardial, and retinal damage in laboratory experiments and animal models, especially resulting from hypoxia or ischemia. *In vitro*, the ginkgolides (especially ginkgolide B) inhibit binding of platelet-activating factor (PAF), which is normally a potent mediator of inflammatory and allergic responses. Additionally, activation of various cerebral neurotransmitter systems (especially the cholinergic system) may contribute to ginkgo's cerebral properties. GBE causes behavioral changes in animals that include increased task performance and behavior adaptation, and produces enhanced alpha-wave activity on human EEG profiles that are similar to other cognitive-activator drugs such as tacrine.[5,6]

While multiple biologic mechanisms have been well characterized, doses and routes of administration used in these experiments do not always correspond with oral doses in humans.

Clinical Trials:

• Dementia and Cerebral Insufficiency—GBE has been used and studied in Europe for many years for the treatment of "cerebral insufficiency," an ill-defined syndrome consisting of dementia or cognitive defects and a group of related physical and affective symptoms (e.g., tinnitus, vertigo, fatigue, headache, depression, anxiety). A 1992 critical review evaluated 40 controlled trials of GBE for the treatment of this syndrome. All but one trial reported positive results, but only eight trials were of acceptable quality or were well performed.[7] Recent research has concentrated on defined diagnoses with more stringent inclusion criteria for dementia of the Alzheimer's type (DAT) and vascular or multi-infarct dementia (MID). In a recent systematic review, nine of 18 double-blind, randomized, controlled trials met inclusion criteria for the treatment of mild-moderate DAT or MID.[8] Statistically significant benefits were found in eight of nine trials. While some of these studies had methodologic faults, the overall results demonstrated that ginkgo appeared efficacious in delaying the clinical deterioration of patients with dementia or in bringing about symptomatic improvement.

In a meta-analysis of ginkgo for mild-moderate DAT, four double-blind RCTs met strict inclusion criteria.[9] A small but significant effect was calculated after 6 months of treatment (mean effect size 0.41; 95% CI 0.22–0.61). These reviews also include one well-designed, year-long U.S. trial that found modest beneficial results in two of three primary outcome measurements for DAT and MID.[10] In general, the benefit of 120–240 mg/day GBE for Alzheimer's disease is comparable to that shown for acetylcholinesterase inhibitors such as donepezil and tacrine.[9,11] Nevertheless, a recent rigorous, 6-month, double-blind RCT of 160 or 240 mg/day GBE failed to demonstrate any benefit (in intention-to-treat and per-protocol analyses) in a subset of 63 elderly patients with mild-moderate dementia.[12]

• Memory/Cognition—Several double-blind RCTs have evaluated GBE's role in improving memory or cognitive functioning in healthy adults without dementia or cerebral insufficiency, but results are mixed and inconclusive. In young healthy volunteers, one small, single-dose trial (n = 8) found benefits on a test for short-term memory reaction time, but only with a very large dose, 600 mg of GBE.[13] These results were *not* confirmed in another small trial (n = 12) using the same memory test and GBE dosage.[14] In two subacute trials in normal volunteers (n = 36, 20) taking 120 to 360 mg/day GBE for 2–4 days, large batteries of tests showed faster short-term memory performance compared to placebo,[15] and improvements in tests of speed of reaction time that assessed attention.[16] However, there were many inconsistencies (e.g., other tests did not demonstrate benefits; and one study found better results at lower doses of 120 mg/day,[15] while the other found better results at higher doses of 240 and 360 mg/day[16]). In the only chronic study of normal healthy adults without a history of memory impairment, 180 mg/day of GBE given for 6 weeks improved four out of five tests evaluating speed of information processing, but only one test reached statistical significance; objective tests for memory and recall were not affected.[17]

Several double-blind RCTs have evaluated GBE in middle-age to elderly subjects with mild memory impairment without dementia (Folstein mini-mental status exam generally > 24). A small trial in 18 subjects using large, single doses of 320 and 600 mg GBE found no difference in absolute recall, but reported subtle improvement in the speed of information processing.[18] A 3-month trial (n = 60) of a Swiss "GB8" ginkgo product showed significant improvement in attention, concentration, and short-term memory testing; results were statistically significant with 120 mg/day, but not with 240 mg/day.[19] Two 6-month trials (n = 27, 241) found beneficial results for a few tests of memory reaction time, but most other test results were not affected.[20,21] One of the largest and most rigorous RCTs, in 151 patients in old-age homes taking 160 or 240 mg/day of GBE for 6 months, found no affect on cognitive testing in either the intention-to-treat or per-protocol analyses.[12]

• Peripheral Arterial Insufficiency—Many European studies on patients with intermittent claudication due to peripheral vascular disease suggest that GBE decreases symptoms and increases walking distance by as much as 50%. In a recent meta-analysis of double-blind RCTs in which eight studies met inclusion criteria, seven studies favored ginkgo, and four reached statistical significance.[22] The meta-analysis found an overall positive statistical benefit for GBE. The difference in pain-free walking between the ginkgo and placebo group was 26–43 meters, and for maximal walking distance was 36–189 meters. The effect was considered modest, but not dissimilar to that found with pentoxifylline in separate studies. A separate dose-response study found 240 mg/day to be superior to 120 mg/day.[23]

• Tinnitus—Studies on the use of GBE for chronic tinnitus have yielded inconsistent results. A systematic review found five heterogeneous RCTs using four different ginkgo products for several months. Although four trials found positive outcomes, the only one with acceptable methodologic quality showed only mild reduction (42 dB to 39 dB) in the loudness of tinnitus by audiometry.[24] Since this review, a randomized, double-blind, placebo-controlled trial of 489 matched pairs of patients with chronic tinnitus failed to find beneficial effects from 150 mg/day of GBE administered for 12 weeks.[25] This large study demonstrated that there is unlikely to be a practical benefit of ginkgo for chronic tinnitus.

• Other—Other single- or double-blind, placebo-controlled trials have reported benefits for: mountain sickness, vertigo, diabetic retinopathy, macular degeneration, premenstrual syndrome, depression, and airway hyperactivity in asthmatics. Benefits have also been reported in open or uncontrolled trials.[1,3,26] In negative double-blind, placebo-controlled trials, ginkgo was *not* beneficial for the treatment of winter depression,[27] for acute ischemic strokes,[28] or for acute multiple sclerosis.[1]

Adverse Effects: GBE is well tolerated. Less than 2% of patients develop side effects, which include mild gastrointestinal symptoms, headache, and dermal hypersensitivity.[3,26,29,30] In most controlled clinical trials, the incidence of side effects is similar to that of placebo.

To date, seven case reports in the U.S. literature highlight the potential for bleeding complications, believed to be due to ginkgolide's inhibitory effects on PAF. Two cases were of spontaneous subdural hematoma, two were of intracerebral hemorrhage (one in a 78-year-old man who was also taking warfarin), and there was one case each of subarachnoid hemorrhage, spontaneous eye hyphema (in an elderly man also taking aspirin), and postoperative bleeding.[31-37] The causality of the relationships is not firmly established, and there have been no reports of bleeding from any of the controlled clinical trials or the millions of patients who have been treated in European countries.[30] Thus, any risk of bleeding appears to be extremely small. Similarly, seven cases of seizures associated with ginkgo use have been recently reported to the FDA, and several other anecdotal cases have been noted.[38] Although causality is uncertain, these reports highlight the potential toxicity of an herb with potent pharmacologic properties.

Interactions: Ginkgo extract given with trazodone was associated with acute CNS depression in an 80-year-old woman, which appeared to be reversed with flumazenil.[39] In light of the *in vitro* action of ginkgo on PAF and the case reports of bleeding, ginkgo should be used cautiously with other medications that inhibit clotting or enhance the risk of bleeding.

Cautions: Data from animal studies indicates no teratogenic or embryotoxic effects with ginkgo; however, there is no human data for use in pregnancy or lactation.[29,30] Excessive ingestion of ginkgo seeds (not the leaves) can result in an illness known in Japan as gin-nan poisoning, which includes seizures.

Preparations & Doses: The usual dose of GBE demonstrated to be beneficial in the controlled clinical trials is 120–240 mg/day administered in 2–3 divided doses (i.e., 40–80 mg taken two to three times a day). For chronic conditions, a 6- to 8-week trial of use has been typically recommended to evaluate efficacy. The GBE formulation is a concentrated 35–67:1 (mean 50:1) extract consisting of dried ginkgo leaves, which is standardized to contain 22–27% flavonoid glycosides and 5–7% terpenoids.[3] This extraction technique also removes polyphenolic compounds including the potentially toxic and allergenic ginkgolic acids (to < 5 ppm).

Two European preparations, EGb 761 (Tebonin, by Schwabe; Tanakan, by Ipsen) and LI 1370 (Kaveri, by Lichtwer), were used in almost all of the controlled clinical trials, and are marketed in the U.S as Ginkgold (Nature's Way), Ginkoba (Pharmaton), and

Ginkai (Lichtwer).[3] Many different preparations are available on the market, but the standardized GBE products are considered safer and more reliable.

Summary Evaluation

Ginkgo biloba contains many pharmacologically active constituents and is widely used for cognitive impairment, circulatory disorders, and many other indications. The best evidence for ginkgo's clinical efficacy is for mild-moderate dementia and for intermittent claudication. However, benefits are likely to be small and have not been proven beyond a reasonable doubt. As a general memory-enhancer in the healthy adult, there is some evidence that GBE can improve selected cognitive testing such as speed of information processing. However, the optimal dose is unknown, and many studies failed to demonstrate beneficial effects; thus, the actual clinical and cognitive implications are unclear and inconclusive. Ginkgo's role as a potential therapy for many other indications is not well established. Standardized ginkgo extracts are generally well tolerated, although there may be a very small increased risk of bleeding.

references

1. Mills S, Bone K. Principles and Practice of Phytotherapy: Modern Herbal Medicine. Edinburgh, UK, Churchill Livingstone, 2000.
2. Chavez ML, Chavez PI. Ginkgo (Part 1): History, use, and pharmacologic properties. Hosp Pharm 33:658–672, 1998.
3. Blumenthal M, Goldberg A, Brinckmann J (eds). Herbal Medicine: Expanded Commission E Monographs. Newton, MA, Integrative Medicine Communications, 2000.
4. van Beek TA, Bombardelli E, Morazzoni P, Peterlongo F. *Ginkgo biloba* L. Fitoterapia 69:195–244, 1998.
5. Diamond BJ, Shiflett SC, Feiwel N, et al. *Ginkgo biloba* extract: Mechanisms and clinical indications. Arch Phys Med Rehabil 81:668–678, 2000.
6. Itil TM, Eralp E, Ahmed I, et al. The pharmacological effects of *Ginkgo biloba*, a plant extract, on the brain of dementia patients in comparison with tacrine. Psychopharmacol Bull 34:391–397, 1998.
7. Kleijnen J, Knipschild P. *Ginkgo biloba* for cerebral insufficiency. Br J Clin Pharmacol 34:352–358, 1992.
8. Ernst E, Pittler MH. *Ginkgo biloba* for dementia: A systematic review of double-blind, placebo-controlled trials. Clin Drug Invest 17:301–308, 1999.
9. Oken BS, Storzbach DM, Kaye JA. The efficacy of *Ginkgo biloba* on cognitive function in Alzheimer's disease. Arch Neurol 55:1409-1415, 1998.

10. Le Bars PL, Katz MM, Berman N, et al (North American EGb Study Group). A placebo-controlled, double-blind, randomized trial of an extract of Ginkgo biloba for dementia. JAMA 278:1327–1332, 1997.

11. Wettstein A. Cholinesterase inhibitors and Ginkgo extracts: Are they comparable in the treatment of dementia? Phytomed 6:393–401, 2000.

12. van Dongen MCJM, van Rossum E, Kessels AGH, et al. The efficacy of Ginkgo for elderly people with dementia and age-associated memory impairment: New results of a randomized clinical trial. J Am Geriatr Soc 48:1183–1194, 2000.

13. Subhan Z, Hindmarch I. The psychopharmacological effects of Ginkgo biloba extract in normal healthy volunteers. Int J Clin Pharm Res 4:89–93, 1984.

14. Warot D, Lacomblez L, Danjou Ph, et al. Comparaison des effets d'extraits de Ginkgo biloba sur les performances psychomotrices et la mémoire chez le sujet sain [Comparative effects of Ginkgo biloba extracts on psychomotor performances and memory in healthy volunteers]. Therapie 46:33–36, 1991.

15. Rigney U, Kimber S, Hindmarch I. The effects of acute doses of standardized Ginkgo biloba extract on memory and psychomotor performance in volunteers. Phytother Res 13:408–415, 1999.

16. Kennedy DO, Scholey AB, Wesnes KA. The dose-dependent cognitive effects of acute administration of Ginkgo biloba to healthy young volunteers. Psychopharmacol 151:416–423, 2000.

17. Mix JA, Crews WD. An examination of the efficacy of Ginkgo biloba extract EGb 761 on the neuropsychologic functioning of cognitively intact older adults. J Altern Complement Med 6:219–229, 2000.

18. Allain H, Raoul P, Lieury A, et al. Effect of two doses of Ginkgo biloba extract (EGb 761) on the dual-coding test in elderly subjects. Clin Therapeut 15:549–558, 1993.

19. Winther K, Randløv C, Rein E, Mehlsen J. Effects of Ginkgo biloba extract on cognitive function and blood pressure in elderly subjects. Curr Ther Res 59:881–888, 1998.

20. Rai GS, Shovlin C, Wesnes KA. A double-blind, placebo controlled study of Ginkgo biloba extract (Tanakan) in elderly outpatients with mild to moderate memory impairment. Curr Med Res Opin 12:350–355, 1991.

21. Brautigam MRH, Blommaert FA, Verleye G, et al. Treatment of age-related memory complaints with Ginkgo biloba extract: A randomized double blind placebo-controlled study. Phytomed 5:425–434, 1998.

22. Pittler MH, Ernst E. Ginkgo biloba extract for the treatment of intermittent claudication: A meta-analysis of randomized trials. Am J Med 108:276–281, 2000.

23. Schweizer J, Hautmann C. Comparison of two dosages of Ginkgo biloba extract EGb 761 in patients with peripheral arterial occlusive disease Fontaine's stage IIb. Arzneim-Forsch/Drug Res 49:900–904, 1999.

24. Ernst E, Stevinson C. Ginkgo biloba for tinnitus: A review. Clin Otolaryngol 24:164–167, 1999

25. Drew S, Davies E. Effectiveness of Ginkgo biloba in treating tinnitus: Double-blind, placebo-controlled trial. BMJ 322:1-6, 2001.

26. Chavez ML, Chavez PI. Ginkgo (Part 2): Clinical efficacy, dosage, and adverse effects. Hosp Pharm 33:1076–1095, 1998.

27. Lingjærde O, Føreland AR, Magnusson A. Can winter depression be prevented by Ginkgo biloba extract? A placebo-controlled trial. Acta Psychiatr Scand 100:62-66, 1999.

28. Garg RK, Nag D, Agrawal A. A double-blind placebo-controlled trial of Ginkgo biloba extract in acute cerebral ischaemia. J Assoc Physicians India 43:760–763, 1995.
29. Woerdenbag HJ, Van Beek TA. *Ginkgo biloba*. In De Smet PAGM (ed): Adverse Effects of Herbal Drugs. Vol 3. Berlin, Springer, 1997, pp 51–66.
30. DeFeudis FV. *Ginkgo Biloba* Extract (Egb 761): From Chemistry to Clinic. Wiesbaden, Germany, Ullstein Medical, 1998.
31. Rowin J, Lewis SL. Spontaneous bilateral subdural hematomas associated with chronic *Ginkgo biloba* ingestion. Neurology 46:1775–1776, 1996.
32. Gilbert GJ. Ginkgo biloba. Neurology 48:1137, 1997.
33. Matthews MK. Association of *Ginkgo biloba* with intracerebral hemorrhage. Neurology 50:1933–1934, 1998.
34. Benjamin J, Muir T, Briggs K, Pentland B. A case of cerebral haemorrhage—Can *Ginkgo biloba* be implicated? Postgrad Med J 77:112–113, 2001.
35. Vale S. Subarachnoid haemorrhage associated with *Ginkgo biloba*. Lancet 352:36, 1998.
36. Rosenblatt M, Mindel J. Spontaneous hyphema associated with ingestion of *Ginkgo biloba* extract. N Engl J Med 336:1108, 1997.
37. Fessenden JM, Wittenborn W, Clarke L. *Gingko biloba:* A case report of herbal medicine and bleeding postoperatively from a laparoscopic cholecystectomy. Am Surg 67:33–35, 2001.
38. Gregory PJ. Seizure associated with *Ginkgo biloba?* Ann Intern Med 134:344, 2001.
39. Galluzzi S, Zanetti O, Binetti G, et al. Coma in a patient with Alzheimer's disease taking low-dose trazodone and *Ginkgo biloba*. J Neurol Neurosurg Psychiat 68:679–680, 2000.

Glucosamine*

rating: 🐝 🐝 🐝 +

> - Clinical trial results support benefits for osteoarthritis
> - Symptom reduction similar to that achieved with low- to moderate-dose NSAIDs
> - Well tolerated, with only mild gastrointestinal side effects

Glucosamine (2-amino-2-deoxy beta-D-glucopyranose) is a substrate for the production of articular cartilage and is present in most human tissue. Commercial products are prepared from the shells of crabs and other crustaceans.

Uses: Glucosamine is commonly employed for musculoskeletal and other types of chronic pain. It has been studied primarily for pain due to osteoarthritis.

Pharmacology: Endogenous glucosamine is used to produce glycosaminoglycans and other proteoglycans within articular cartilage. In osteoarthritis, the rate of production of new cartilage is exceeded by the rate of degradation of existing cartilage, resulting in a net loss.[1] Administration of exogenous glucosamine provides a greater supply of "building blocks," and stimulates production of glycosaminoglycans,[2,3] resulting in an increase in, or maintenance of, existing cartilage.[4] Animal and human studies of glucosamine given orally or by injection into affected large joints have demonstrated increases in thickness and histological normalization of damaged cartilage.[2,5,6] In addition, some mild anti-inflammatory action by non-prostaglandin–related mechanisms has been observed in both *in vitro* and animal studies.[7,8] Oral glucosamine is 90% absorbed, but undergoes a significant hepatic first-pass effect of up to 70%.[9]

Clinical Trials: See Chondroitin, page 129, for discussion of combined glucosamine and chondroitin trials.

---

* *Editor's Note:* Although not an herb, glucosamine is a dietary supplement that is included here because of its current popularity.

• Osteoarthritis (OA)—Early European and Asian trials in patients with OA found some benefits with intra-articular, intravenous, and intramuscular glucosamine, as well as combinations of injectable and oral doses.[10] More recent, controlled trials using oral doses relied on objective comparison scales that provide reliable measures of clinical benefits. For example, a high-quality, randomized, placebo-controlled trial that met statistical power used glucosamine sulfate (GS) 500 mg or placebo three times daily for 4 weeks, in 252 patients with knee OA. Significant differences were found in favor of GS in the change in Lequesne index (a validated disability scale used in OA trials) as well as outcomes as defined by physician assessment of global efficacy.[11]

A number of controlled clinical studies of glucosamine have reported similar benefits for pain or disability due to knee OA. A meta-analysis of randomized, double-blind, placebo-controlled trials found six (five oral and one intra-articular dosing) that lasted at least 4 weeks; study size varied from 20 to 329 patients. The treatment effect size of glucosamine was calculated to be 0.44, a moderate effect. However, methodological limitations common to most of the trials (e.g., inadequate allocation concealment, absence of intent-to-treat analysis) tended to overestimate effects, and therefore the actual treatment effect size is likely to be smaller than the calculated value.[10] A Cochrane Review identified 16 double-blind, randomized, controlled trials (13 vs. placebo, 12 using oral glucosamine), mostly in patients with knee OA but also one trial each with spine and multiple OA sites. Glucosamine was found to be superior to placebo in all but one study; a moderate effect size was also calculated.[12]

In contrast to the positive findings of almost all of the previous studies, a recent U.S. randomized, double-blind, placebo-controlled 2-month trial of 98 patients with knee arthropathy found no significant difference between treatment groups in reduction of pain at rest and pain while walking. Investigators believed the greater average severity and duration of disease in these patients, as opposed to those in other trials, might have accounted in part for the negative results.[13]

A recent, randomized, double-blind, placebo-controlled trial was the first long-term study to specifically evaluate joint structural changes radiographically.[6] This trial randomized 212 patients with knee OA to 1500 mg oral GS or placebo once daily. At 3 years, joint-space width was increased in the GS group compared to placebo, implying an increase in cartilage formation or other structural benefit. Small but statistically significant differences between the GS and placebo groups, respectively, were seen for primary outcomes of both mean joint space width (+0.07 mm vs. −0.031 mm; P = 0.038) and minimum joint space width (+0.11 mm vs. −0.40 mm; P = 0.002). Symptoms decreased by 24.3% for GS patients and increased 9.8% for placebo patients. There was no significant difference in use of concomitant analgesics between groups. Analysis by both per protocol and intent-to-treat approaches resulted in similar beneficial findings for glucosamine, and the trial met statistical power. Investigators noted that correlation between symptom outcomes and joint structure changes was poor, i.e., many GS patients who evidenced disease progression by radiographic changes tended to have improvements in symptoms.[6]

In studies comparing oral GS with NSAIDs, 1500 mg/day of GS or ibuprofen 1200 mg/day was given in two randomized, double-blind studies of 4-week duration and similar design (n = 178, 40).[14,15] Results at week 4 were similar between GS and ibuprofen groups and reflected > 50% decreases in pain scores. GS treatment effects remained evident in terms of lower pain scores during a 2-week period after stopping therapy. Another randomized, double-blind study included 200 inpatients with knee OA on the same GS and ibuprofen dosage regimens as the preceding studies.[16] At 2 weeks, scores reflected greater decreases in pain for ibuprofen patients, while at 4 weeks there was no significant difference. This delay in onset of symptom relief (with results equivalent to the NSAID group by the end of the treatment period) was also apparent in a randomized, double-blinded trial using piroxicam 20 mg daily, alone and in conjunction with GS for 60 days.[17]

The HCl salt of oral glucosamine has been examined in only one trial. A double-blind, randomized, Canadian trial (n = 98) of 8-week duration compared 1500 mg/day glucosamine HCl to placebo.[18] No significant differences between groups were found at week 8 for the primary outcome measure of change in pain scores, or for as-needed acetaminophen use.

Although efficacy evidence is not definitive for glucosamine, the authors of the Cochrane Review noted that the flaws in the existing clinical trials are, as a group, no worse than the flaws in OA trials for NSAIDs.[12]

• Other Uses—Another oral form, N-acetyl-D-glucosamine, was evaluated in a recent pilot study of 12 children with chronic inflammatory bowel disease. A reduction in symptoms was reported in eight patients. Nine additional children received rectal doses: improvement was noted in three, and remission occurred in two. Biopsies (not done in all cases) showed histological improvement. However, this pilot study was not controlled.[19]

Adverse Effects: Glucosamine is well tolerated.[12] Mild nausea and diarrhea are most commonly reported; frequency is similar to placebo in some controlled trials.[6,12] One trial (n = 1200) noted that gastrointestinal side effects occurred at a higher rate in patients with pre-existing gastroduodenal illnesses or those taking diuretics.[20] There is one case report each of an immediate hypersensitivity reaction and of photosensitivity recurring on rechallenge.[21,22]

Interactions: There are no known drug interactions with glucosamine.

Cautions: A common caution based on animal studies is that glucosamine may increase blood glucose. One human study using intravenous glucosamine did find slight (5.4–9.0 mg/dl) increases in plasma fasting glucose levels.[23] However, clinical effects of oral glucosamine on blood glucose have not been reported, and one study found no changes in fasting glucose over a 3-year period.[6] Safety during pregnancy and lactation has not been determined.

Preparations & Doses: The recommended dose, used in almost all of the clinical trials, is 500 mg three times daily. Theoretically, all salt forms should dissolve and allow glucosamine absorption, but there is some evidence that the sulfate moiety is necessary for clinical efficacy. Animal and human studies have shown a decrease in glycosaminoglycan synthesis in sulfate depletion conditions.[24] No trials comparing the different salt forms have been conducted; however, results of the one clinical trial of glucosamine HCl did not show benefits.[18] Another form, N-acetyl-D-glucosamine, has been shown to increase serum glucosamine levels, but has not been adequately tested clinically.[25] Until more data is available, the recommended form is glucosamine sulfate.

--- **Summary Evaluation** ---

The clinical evidence is sufficient to support the use of oral glucosamine sulfate for symptoms of mild to moderate osteoarthritis.

Symptom reduction appears to be similar to that of analgesic doses of NSAIDs. Glucosamine has a longer onset of action than NSAIDs, but fewer adverse effects. Evidence of positive effects on joint structure is promising. There is no evidence at this time that glucosamine is beneficial for disorders other than osteoarthritis.

---

references

1. Delafuente JC: Glucosamine in the treatment of osteoarthritis. Rheum Dis Clin North Am 26:1–11, 2000.
2. Vidal Y, Plana RR, Karzel K: Glucosamine: Its importance for the metabolism of articular cartilage. Studies on articular cartilage. Fortschr Med 98:801–806, 1980.
3. Bassleer C, Rovati L, Franchimont P: Stimulation of proteoglycan production by glucosamine sulfate in chondrocytes isolated from human osteoarthritic articular cartilage in vitro. Osteoarth Cartilage 6:427–434, 1998.
4. Pavelka K, Gatterova J, Olejarova M, et al: Glucosamine sulfate decreases progression of knee osteoarthritis in a long-term, randomized, placebo-controlled, independent, confirmatory trial. [Abstract]. Philadelphia, PA, American College of Rheumatology, November 1999. Accessed December, 2000 at www.abstracts-on-line.com/rh
5. Drovanti A, Bignamini AA, Rovati AL: Therapeutic activity of oral glucosamine sulfate in osteoarthrosis: A placebo-controlled, double-blind investigation. Clin Therap 3:260–272, 1980.
6. Reginster JY, Deroisy R, Rovati LC, et al: Long-term effects of glucosamine sulphate on osteoarthritis progression: A randomized, placebo-controlled clinical trial. Lancet 357:251–256, 2001.
7. Setnikar I, Pacini MA, Revel L: Antiarthritic effects of glucosamine sulfate studied in animal models. Arzneim-Forsch/Drug Res 41:542–545, 1991.
8. Setnikar I, Cereda R, Pacini, MA, Revel L: Antireactive properties of glucosamine sulfate. Arzneim-Forsch/Drug Res 41:157–161, 1991.
9. Setnikar I, Cereda R, Pacini, MA, Revel L: Pharmacokinetics of glucosamine in man. Arzneim-Forsch/Drug Res 43:1109–1113, 1993.
10. McAlindon TE, LaValley MP, Gulin JP, Felson DT: Glucosamine and chondroitin for treatment of osteoarthritis. A systematic quality assessment and meta-analysis. JAMA 283:1469–1475, 2000.
11. Noack W, Fischer M, Förster KK, et al: Glucosamine sulfate in osteoarthritis of the knee. Osteoarth Cartilage 2:51–59, 1994.
12. Towheed TE, Anastassiades TP, Shea B, et al: Glucosamine therapy for treating osteoarthritis (Cochrane Review). In The Cochrane Library, Issue 2. Oxford, Update Software, 2001.
13. Rindone JP, Hiller D, Collacott E, et al: Randomized, controlled trial of glucosamine for treating osteoarthritis of the knee. West J Med 172:91–94, 2000.
14. Qui G, Gao SN, Giacovelli G, et al: Efficacy and safety of glucosamine sulfate versus ibuprofen in patients with knee osteoarthritis. Arzneim-Forsch/Drug Res 48:469–474, 1998.
15. Lopez Vaz A: Double-blind clinical evaluation of the relative efficacy of ibuprofen and glucosamine sulfate in the management of the knee in outpatients. Curr Med Res Opin 8(3):145–149, 1982.

16. Müller-Fassbender H, Bach GL, Haase W, et al: Glucosamine sulfate compared to ibuprofen in osteoarthritis of the knee. Osteoarth Cartilage 2:61–69, 1994.

17. Rovati LC, Giacovelli G, Annefeld N, et al: A large, randomized, placebo-controlled, double-blind study of glucosamine sulfate vs piroxicam and vs their association on the kinetics of the symptomatic effect in knee osteoarthritis (abstract). Osteoarth Cartilage 2(suppl 1):56, 1994.

18. Houpt JB, McMillan R, Wein C, Paget-Dellio SD: Effect of glucosamine hydrochloride in the treatment of pain of osteoarthritis of the knee. J Rheum 26:2423–2430, 1999.

19. Salvatore S, Heuschkel R, Tomlin S, et al: A pilot study of N-acetyl glucosamine, a nutritional substance for glycosaminoglycan synthesis, in paediatric chronic inflammatory bowel disease. Aliment Pharmacol Therapeut 14:1567–1579, 2000.

20. Tapadinhas MJ, Rivera IC, Bignamini AA: Oral glucosamine sulphate in the management of arthrosis: Report on a multi-centre open investigation in Portugal. Pharmatherapeutica 3:157–168, 1982.

21. Matheu V, Gracia Bara MT, Pelta R, et al: Immediate-hypersensitivity reaction to glucosamine sulfate. Allergy 54:643, 1999.

22. Danao-Camara T: Potential side effects of treatment with glucosamine and chondroitin. Arthritis Rheum 43:2853, 2000.

23. Monauni T, Grazia Zenti M, Cretti A, et al: Effects of glucosamine infusion on insulin secretion and insulin action in humans. Diabetes 49:926–935, 2000.

24. Kelly GS: The role of glucosamine sulfate and chondroitin sulfates in the treatment of degenerative joint disease. Alt Med Rev 3:27–39, 1998.

25. Talent JM, Gracy RW: Pilot study of oral polymeric N-acetyl-D-glucosamine as a potential treatment for patients with osteoarthritis. Clin Therapeut 18:1184–1190, 1996.

Goldenseal (*Hydrastis canadensis*)
rating: 🦫

- A berberine-containing herb commonly used as a tonic and antibiotic
- No clinical trials published
- Topical use possibly justified by antimicrobial and other properties of berberine
- Appears safe and well tolerated in usual doses, based on limited data

---

Goldenseal, also called yellowroot or eyeroot, is a member of the buttercup family and is native to North America. It produces a golden-yellow dye. Goldenseal's popularity in the 1990s led to severe over-harvesting, causing concerns that it was becoming an endangered species in the U.S.; this has stimulated increased cultivation.

Uses: Goldenseal is marketed as a tonic and natural antibiotic, and it is often combined with echinacea to help "strengthen the immune system." As a popular American folk medicine, goldenseal has been used as an antiseptic, astringent, or hemostatic to treat a wide variety of skin, eye, and mucous membrane inflammatory and infectious conditions. Thus, it has been employed as a mouthwash, for canker sores, and as a topical agent for dermatologic disorders. In tonic form, it has been ingested as a "bitter" to aid digestion and treat dyspepsia. Some herbalists also view goldenseal as a mucous membrane "alterative"—increasing and decreasing mucus secretion depending on the body's needs.[1,2]

Pharmacology: Goldenseal contains several active isoquinoline alkaloids such as berberine (0.5–6%), hydrastine (1.5–4%), and canadine.[3,4] Berberine provides the bitter taste and yellow color to the herb, and most of the scientific explanations for goldenseal's use have been attributed to the effects of berberine and related alkaloids. Berberine is very poorly absorbed orally (probably < 1%), although blood levels are measurable after large doses.[5,6]

Extracts of the crude herb, and berberine in particular, have broad *in vitro* antimicrobial activity against gram-positive and gram-negative bacteria, fungi, and protozoa and other parasites.[3,7–10]

Immunologic activity, such as enhanced macrophage, cytokine, and antibody response, has been demonstrated in rodent and *in vitro* studies.[10-12] In contrast, anti-inflammatory and immunosuppressive effects also have been demonstrated.[10,13] High doses of oral berberine reduced the colonic inflammation of drug-induced colitis in rats.[14] Berberine's use as an antidiarrheal agent may be partly explained by inhibition of ion transport secretory activity in intestinal epithelial cells.[15]

Berberine and related alkaloids affect *in vivo* cardiovascular activity and cause contraction or relaxation of isolated smooth muscles; results vary depending on the alkaloid and the animal model studied.[3,4,9,10,16] In humans, very large intravenous doses of berberine (0.2 mg/kg/min for 30 min) to patients with severe congestive heart failure caused significant hemodynamic changes consistent with decreased vascular resistance and increased cardiac output, as well as ventricular tachycardia in some patients.[17]

Clinical Trials: There are no clinical trials in the medical or herbal literature using goldenseal or crude herbal extracts. The only clinical research has been with pure berberine, often isolated from other berberine-containing plants such as *Berberis aristata*. Berberine has been studied in countries such as India for acute diarrhea in children or adults, and for trachoma. It appears to have antimicrobial and clinical activity similar to other antibiotics in unblinded, controlled trials for diarrhea due to enterotoxigenic *Escherichia coli* and giardia, with fewer benefits found for cholera.[18,19] One randomized, double-blind, placebo-controlled trial found only minimal anti-secretory or antibacterial effects for cholera and non-cholera diarrhea.[20] Berberine oral doses usually ranged from 100 mg/day for children to 400 mg/day for adults. For trachoma, a 0.2% berberine eyedrop was found to be similar in efficacy to other standard ophthalmic antibiotics[21,22]; these old studies have not been replicated.

In the Russian literature, very small doses of berberine have been reported to be beneficial in the treatment of cholecystitis or hepatitis (10–60 mg/day), and for thrombocytopenia (15 mg/day).[23,24] However, it is doubtful that enough berberine is absorbed at these doses to have a substantial systemic effect. In uncontrolled Chinese studies, large doses of oral berberine have been found beneficial in patients with severe CHF (1200 mg/day) and diabetes (900–1500 mg/day).[6,10] In other Chinese literature, berbamine (a related alkaloid derived from a variety of berberine-containing plants) is used clinically to treat leukopenia.[25] It is not known if berbamine is a constituent of *H. canadensis*. None of these indications have been evaluated in adequately controlled trials.

Adverse Effects: The herb appears safe and well tolerated based on traditional and common usage; there are no well-documented adverse effects with usual doses. A number of serious reactions have been previously described (e.g., gastrointestinal toxicity, nephritis, ulcerations, convulsions, fatalities from cardiovascular collapse), but these appear to be inappropriately extrapolated from reports of toxicologic studies of berberine administered to animals, or from 19th century literature on homeopathic "provings."[26,27]

Interactions: Goldenseal can inhibit the hepatic cytochrome P450-3A4 drug-metabolizing system *in vitro*, but this has not been verified *in vivo* or clinically.[28] Goldenseal is erroneously believed by drug users to act as a natural substance to mask the detection of illegal drugs in urine tests.[29,30] This myth was originally based on an antiquated chemical reaction described in a novel by the herbalist John Lloyd, published in 1900.

Cautions: Berberine-containing plants have been used as ingredients in abortifacient products and should be avoided during pregnancy.[26] Similarly, use has been associated with cases of kernicterus in the newborn and should be avoided during breastfeeding of the very young.[31] Because goldenseal is at risk of becoming an endangered species, some herbalists advocate the use of alternative berberine-containing plants in its place (e.g., barberry, Oregon grape, Chinese and American goldthread).[1]

Preparations & Doses: The usual oral dose of goldenseal is about 250–500 mg of solid extracts, or 500–1000 mg of dried root and rhizome, usually given t.i.d.[2,3] Various tinctures and fluid extracts are also available. To provide 400 mg of berberine (the adult dose used in many clinical studies), one would have to ingest roughly 20–30 capsules containing 500 mg of goldenseal, an unreasonably large amount.

--- **Summary Evaluation** ---

Clinical trials have not been performed with goldenseal, and there is no evidence that this herb is effective for any clinical indication. There appears to be no rationale for favoring its combination with echinacea. Although the isolated alkaloid berberine is pharmacologically active, the small amount contained in usual oral doses of goldenseal is unlikely to be absorbed to a sufficient degree to provide systemic effects. Herbal extracts do have antimicrobial and other pharmacologic activity; these properties may support some of the herb's traditional uses when applied topically to the skin or mucous membranes, or when used locally in the gastrointestinal tract. These indications, however, have yet to be clinically evaluated.

references

1. McCaleb R, Leigh E, Morien K: The Encyclopedia of Popular Herbs. Roseville, CA, Prima Health, 2000.
2. Boon H, Smith M: The Botanical Pharmacy: The Pharmacology of 47 Common Herbs. Kingston, Ontario, Quarry Health Books, 1999.
3. Newall CA, Anderson LA, Phillipson JD: Herbal Medicines: A Guide for Health-Care Professionals. London, Pharmaceutical Press, 1996
4. Goldenseal. The Review of Natural Products, St. Louis, MO, Facts and Comparisons, February 2000.
5. Miyazaki H, Shirai E, Ishibashi M, Niizima K: Quantitative analysis of berberine in urine samples by chemical ionization mass fragmentography. J Chromatogr 152:79–86, 1978.
6. Zeng X, Zeng X: Relationship between the clinical effects of berberine on severe congestive heart failure and its concentration in plasma studied by HPLC. Biomed Chromatogr 13:442–444, 1999.
7. Gentry EJ, Jampani HB, Keshavarz-Shokri A, et al: Antitubercular natural products: Berberine from the roots of commercial *Hydrastis canadensis* powder. Isolation of inactive 8-oxotetrahydrothalifendine, canadine, β-hydrastine, and two new quinic acid esters, hycandinic acid esters-1 and -2. J Nat Prod 61:1187–1193, 1998.
8. Scazzocchio F, Cometa MF, Palmery M: Antimicrobial activity of *Hydrastis canadensis* extract and its major isolated alkaloids. Fitoterapia 69 (Suppl. 5):58–59, 1998.
9. Birdsall TC, Kelly GS: Berberine: therapeutic potential of an alkaloid found in several medicinal plants. Alternat Med Rev 2:94–103, 1997.
10. Mills S, Bone K: Principles and Practice of Phytotherapy: Modern Herbal Medicine. Edinburgh, UK, Churchill Livingstone, 2000.
11. Kumazawa Y, Itagaki A, Fukumoto M, et al: Activation of peritoneal macrophages by berberine-type alkaloids in terms of induction of cytostatic activity. Int J Immunopharmacol 6:587–592, 1984.
12. Rehman J, Dillow JM, Carter SM, et al: Increased production of antigen-specific immunoglobulins G and M following in vivo treatment with the medicinal plants *Echinacea angustifolia* and *Hydrastis canadensis*. Immunol Letters 68:391-395, 1999.
13. Marinova EK, Nikolova DB, Popova DN, et al: Suppression of experimental autoimmune tubulointerstitial nephritis in BALB/c mice by berberine. Immunopharmacol 48:9–16, 2000.

14. Zhou H, Mineshita S: The effect of berberine chloride on experimental colitis in rats in vivo and in vitro. J Pharmacol Exp Therap 294:822–829, 2000.
15. Taylor CT, Winter DC, Skelly MM, et al: Berberine inhibits ion transport in human colonic epithelia. Eur J Pharmacol 368:111–118, 1999.
16. Sabir M, Bhide NK: Study of some pharmacological actions of berberine. Indian J Physiol Pharmacol 15:111–132, 1971.
17. Marin-Neto JA, Maciel BC, Secches AL, Gallo L: Cardiovascular effects of berberine in patients with severe congestive heart failure. Clin Cardiol 11:253–260, 1988.
18. Sharda DC: Berberine in the treatment of diarrhea of infancy and childhood. J Indian Med Assoc 54:22–24, 1970.
19. Rabbani GH: Mechanism and treatment of diarrhea due to Vibrio cholerae and *Escherichia coli:* Roles of drugs and prostaglandins. Dan Med Bull 43:173–185, 1996.
20. Khin-Maung-U, Myo-Khin, Nyunt-Nyunt-Wai, et al: Clinical trial of berberine in acute watery diarrhea. Br Med J 291:1601–1605, 1985.
21. Babbar OP, Chhatwal VK, Ray IB, Mehra MK: Effect of berberine chloride eye drops on clinically positive trachoma patients. Indian J Med Res 76(Suppl):83–88, 1982.
22. Mohan M, Pant CR, Angra SK, Mahajan VM: Berberine in trachoma (a clinical trial). Indian J Ophthalmol 30:69–75, 1982.
23. Turova AD, Konovalov MN, Leskov AI: [Berberine-An effective cholagoque]. Meditsinskaia Promyshlennost [Medical Industry] 18(6):59–60, 1964. [English Translation]
24. Chekalina SI, Umurzakova RZ, Saliev KK, Abdurakhmanov TR: [The effect of berberin bisulfate on platelet hemostatis in thrombocytopenia patients.] Gematologiya Transfuziologiya [Hematology Transfusiology] 39(5):33–35, 1994.[Abstract]
25. Liu C-X, Xiao P-G, Liu G-S: Studies on plant resources, pharmacology and clinical treatment with berbamine. Phytotherapy Res 5:228–230, 1991.
26. Lampe KF: Berberine. In De Smet PAGM (ed): Adverse Effects of Herbal Drugs. Vol. 1. Berlin, Springer, 1992, pp 97–104.
27. Foster S: Goldenseal: *Hydrastis canadensis.* Botanical series #309. Austin, TX, American Botanical Council, 1996.
28. Budzinski JW, Foster BC, Vandenhoek S, Arnason JT: An *in vitro* evaluation of human cytochrome P450-3A4 inhibition by selected commercial herbal extracts and tinctures. Phytomed 7:273–282, 2000.
29. Foster S: Goldenseal masking of drug tests. HerbalGram Fall 21:7 and 35, 1989.
30. Cone EJ, Lange R, Darwin WD: In vivo adulteration: excess fluid ingestion causes false-negative marijuana and cocaine urine test results. J Analytic Tox 22:460–473, 1998.
31. Chan E: Displacement of bilirubin from albumin by berberine. Biol Neonate 63:201–208, 1993.

Gotu Kola (*Centella asiatica*)

rating: 🐾 🐾

> - Used for mental support, wound healing, and venous disorders
> - Limited evidence, from old studies, of benefits for venous insufficiency
> - Appears safe and well tolerated based on limited data

Gotu kola, also known as hydrocotyle and Indian pennywort, is a thin, creeping perennial that has been used in Asia and India since ancient times. Gotu kola should not be confused with the kola plant (*Cola nitidia*), which is often used as a stimulant.

Uses: Currently, gotu kola is promoted for venous disorders and for "mental support"—to improve mental functioning and memory retention, and for treating anxiety.[1-3] It is used topically to treat skin diseases and promote wound healing. Historical uses included the treatment of high blood pressure, rheumatism, fever, nervous disorders, and a number of dermatologic diseases such as psoriasis, leprosy, abscesses, and other skin eruptions. It has also been touted as an aphrodisiac and to promote long life.[1,4]

Pharmacology: The primary active constituents of gotu kola are thought to be several triterpenoid saponins: asiaticoside, madecassoside, asiatic acid, and madecassic acid.[4] Wound-healing properties have been ascribed to asiaticoside, which induces antioxidants and reticuloendothelial growth and increases angiogenesis. Along with asiaticoside, asiatic and madecassic acid have been reported to promote collagen synthesis.[5] Glycosaminoglycan catabolism, measured by glycuronic and hyduronic acids, has been used to assess these effects.[6] Gotu kola's vascular activity has been measured by the lysosomal enzymes β-glucuronidase, β-N-acetylglucosaminidase, and arylsulfatase, which serve as markers for connective tissue metabolism in the vascular walls.[6]. A screening program by the National Institute of Mental Health demonstrated gotu kola's affinity for gamma aminobutyric acid ($GABA_B$) and cholecystokinin receptors; these effects have been related to the herb's potential ability to affect psychotropic responses.[7]

Clinical Trials: Many uncontrolled, unblinded, and otherwise potentially biased studies with gotu kola have found beneficial effects. Few controlled trials or other relevant studies have been published.

• Psychotropic Uses—A randomized, double-blind, placebo-controlled study was conducted with 40 healthy subjects. A large dose of gotu kola (12 g of crude powder) significantly attenuated the acoustic startle response 30 and 60 minutes after administration compared to placebo,[2] suggesting that the herb could have anxiolytic activity. Two studies investigating improvement in IQ scores in retarded children have been performed with gotu kola. The first was a randomized, double-blind, placebo-controlled trial which examined a dose of 0.5 g daily for six months in 30 severely mentally retarded children. The mean IQ of the active and control groups at baseline were 32.3 and 37.7, respectively. A mild positive effect was observed after 3 months, with an increase of 7.5 points for gotu kola, compared to 3.2 points for placebo; however, this difference was probably not statistically or clinically significant.[8] The second trial, which was uncontrolled, used a dose of 100 mg/kg b.i.d. for 6 months in 12 retarded children with a mean IQ of 60.4. Improvement in IQ (to 94.8) was reported in 8 of the 12 children.[9] These studies have not been replicated, and the unprecedented benefits described in the second (uncontrolled) trial remain unsubstantiated.

• Venous Disorders—Several trials have been conducted using the titrated (or standardized) extract of *C. asiatica* (TECA) and the total titrated fraction of *C. asiatica* (TTFCA). The first was a randomized, double-blind, placebo-controlled trial with 94 patients suffering from venous insufficiency who received TECA, 120 or 60 mg per day, or placebo. Symptomatic improvement was seen in both TECA groups versus placebo, measured subjectively (limb heaviness and an overall evaluation by the patient) and objectively (degree of edema and venous distensibility measured by plethysmography).[10]

Two other studies examined TTFCA for venous insufficiency. The first was a placebo-controlled trial of 62 patients receiving doses of 60 mg, 30 mg, or placebo three times daily. Additionally, 10 normal subjects were treated with 60 mg t.i.d. in an open study. A dose-dependent benefit compared to placebo was seen in both objective parameters (plethysmography and ankle edema) and subjective symptoms.[11] No significant changes in either the placebo group or the normal subjects were reported.

In the second study, the same investigators evaluated three groups: severe venous hypertension (n = 12), moderate venous hypertension (n = 22), and normal subjects (n = 10). All three groups received 60 mg t.i.d., and the two groups with venous hypertension demonstrated symptomatic improvement and improvement in local capillary permeability and microcirculation (based upon the reduction of a wheal induced by a vacuum suction chamber).[12] The different methods of evaluating objective responses points to the difficulty in assessing the effectiveness of these products on the therapy of venous insufficiency.

• Wound Healing—Benefits of topical gotu kola application for a variety of skin disorders (e.g., psoriasis, leprosy) and for wound healing have been reported.[1,4] There are no well-designed controlled clinical trials.

Adverse Effects: The only adverse effects reported with the oral forms are mild gastrointestinal distress and pruritis.[1,4] Contact dermatitis is the most commonly reported side effect associated with topical use.[13,14] Gotu kola has been reported to cause hyperglycemia and hypercholesterolemia in a single trial from 1969[15]; these effects have not been reported in other studies.

Interactions: There are no recognized drug interactions. Caution is advised in patients who are already taking drugs or supplements that have sedative properties to avoid any possible additive effect.

Cautions: Although data is limited, gotu kola has been suggested as an antifertility agent and is thus contraindicated during or prior to pregnancy.[16,17] Reports of gotu kola having carcinogenic properties are largely based on a study in which asiaticoside had a possible carcinogenic effect in hairless mice with topical applications twice weekly for up to 2 years.[18]

Preparations & Doses: Usual or appropriate doses are poorly established. Recommended dosages, from 435 mg of an extract daily to 600 mg of dried leaves t.i.d.,[1,4] differ considerably from those used in clinical trials (30–60 mg t.i.d. of a standardized extract for venous insufficiency, to up to 12 g/day of crude powder for psychotropic effects).

Summary Evaluation

Although few well-designed clinical trials have been published, they do suggest a possible role for gotu kola extracts for venous insufficiency. The evidence for its use in wound healing and for mental support has not been established in controlled studies. Gotu kola appears to be safe and well tolerated based on limited evidence.

references

1. Brinkhaus B, Lindner M, Schuppan D, Hahn EG: Chemical, pharmacological, and clinical profile of the east Asian plant *Centella asiatica*. Phytomed 7:427–448, 2000.

2. Bradwejn J, Zhou Y, Koszycki D, Shlik J: A double-blind, placebo-controlled study on the effects of Gotu Kola (*Centella asiatica*) on acoustic startle response in healthy subjects. J Clin Psychopharmacol 20:680–684, 2000.

3. Chittaranjan A, Sudha S, Venkataraman BV: Herbal treatments for ECS-induced memory deficits: A review of research and a discussion on animal models. J ECT 16:145–156, 2000.

4. Kartnig T: Clinical applications of *Centella asiatica*. Herbs Spices Med Plants 3:146–173, 1988.

5. Shukla A, Rasik AM, Jain GK, et al: *In vitro* and *in vivo* wound healing activity of asiaticoside isolated from *Centella asiatica*. J Ethnopharmacol 65:1–11, 1999.

6. Arpaia MR, Ferrone R, Amitrano M, et al: Effects of *Centella asiatica* extract on mucopolysaccaride metabolism in subjects with varicose veins. Int J Clin Pharm Res 10:229–233, 1990.

7. Cott J: Medicinal plants and dietary supplements: Sources for innovative treatments or adjuncts? Psychopharm Bull 31:131–137, 1995.

8. Appa Rao MVR, Srinivasan K, Koteswara RTL: The effect of *Centella asiatica* on the general ability of mentally retarded children. Ind J Psych 19:54–59, 1977.

9. Sharma R, Jaiswal AN, Kumar S, et al: Role of bhrami (*Centella asiatica*) in educable mentally retarded children. J Res Educ Ind Med 4:55–57, 1985.

10. Pointel JP, Boccalon H, Cloarec M, et al: Titrated extract of *Centella asiatica* (TECA) in the treatment of venous insufficiency of the lower limbs. Angiology 38:46–50, 1987.

11. Belcaro GV, Rulo A, Grimaldi R: Capillary filtration and ankle edema in patients with venous hypertension treated with TTFCA. Angiology 41:8–12, 1990.

12. Belcaro GV, Grimaldi R, Guidi G: Improvement of capillary permeability in patients with venous hypertension after treatment with TTFCA. Angiology 41:533–540, 1990.

13. Izu R, Aguirre A, Gil N, Diaz-Perez JL: Allergic contact dermatitis from a cream containing *Centella asiatica* extract. Contact Dermatitis 26:192–193, 1992.

14. Danese P, Carnevali C, Bertazzoni MG: Allergic contact dermatitis due to *Centella asiatica* extract. Contact Dermatitis 31:201, 1994.
15. Oliver-Bever B: Medicinal plants in tropical West Africa. Cambridge, MA, Cambridge University Press, 1986.
16. Dutta T, Basu UP: Crude extract of *Centella asiatica* and products derived from its glycosides as oral antifertility agents. Indian J Exp Biol 6:181–182, 1968.
17. Brinker F: The Toxicology of Botanical Medicines, 3rd ed. Sandy, Oregon, Eclectic Medical Publications, 2000.
18. Lacrum OH, Iversen OH: Reticuloses and epidermal tumors in hairless mice after topical skin applications of cantharidin and asiaticoside. Cancer Res 32:1463–1469, 1972.

Hawthorn (*Crataegus* species)
rating: 🐝 🐝 🐝

- Typically used for CHF and related cardiovascular conditions
- Promising results for mild CHF in several short-term controlled trials; benefits not verified for chronic therapy
- Well tolerated with few reported side effects

Hawthorn is a member of the rose family and the genus Crataegus. The most commonly employed species of hawthorn are *C. laevigata* (also known as *C. oxyacantha*) and *C. monogyna*. Herbal formulations may contain a mixture of these species.

Uses: In modern herbal medicine, hawthorn is primarily used to treat congestive heart failure (CHF). Other clinical applications have included therapy for angina and coronary artery disease, hypertension, and cardiac arrhythmias. Traditionally, hawthorn has been considered a "cardiotonic" herb.[1-3]

Pharmacology: Hawthorn differs from foxglove in that it does not produce cardioactive glycosides. Some of the chemical constituents in hawthorn include oligomeric and polymeric procyanidins, flavonoids (e.g., hyperoside, vitexin- and acetyl-vitexin-2"-O-rhamnoside), catechins, triterpene saponins, and amines.[3] Of these, the oligomeric procyanidins (OPCs) and flavonoids are most likely to contribute pharmacologic activity [3]. In animal and *in vitro* studies, flavonoids inhibit phosphodiesterase (PDE) activity.[4] As a result, they may promote vasodilation and coronary blood flow, decrease vascular resistance, and increase heart rate and contractility.[4] The vasodilation may be due to PDE inhibition or the release of endothelium-derived vasoactive factors, such as nitric oxide.[4,5] The inotropic effects, however, appear to be unrelated to PDE or beta-sympathomimetic effects. *In vitro*, Crataegus inhibits the Na^+/K^+ ATPase in human myocardial cells, similar to the digitalis glycosides, leading to a rise in intracellular calcium and enhanced force of contraction.[6,7]

In contrast to other inotropic drugs (e.g., digoxin, amrinone, milrinone, epinephrine), hawthorn increases cardiac refractoriness by prolonging the action potential duration (similar to a Class III antiarrhythmic) and delaying sodium channel recovery (similar to a Class I antiarrhythmic).[8–10] Other inotropes shorten the refractory period, and thus can induce arrhythmias.[9,10] Standardized hawthorn extracts reduce ischemia-induced arrhythmias and markers of ischemic injury in most animal models.[11–13] One recent study, however, demonstrated a pro-arrhythmic effect of hawthorn.[14]

Although unlikely to be related to its inotropic activity, flavonoid-rich preparations exhibit antioxidant properties and reduce parameters of lipid peroxidation in animal models of atherosclerosis.[15] The OPC fraction also has antioxidant effects.[16]. *In vitro*, various constituents in hawthorn have been shown to inhibit platelet aggregation by blocking thromboxane A2 synthesis, and to stimulate platelet aggregation by enhancing prostacyclin synthesis.[17]

Clinical Trials: Hawthorn has been primarily studied in patients with mild CHF (mostly New York Heart Association Class II) in at least 10 clinical trials from European countries. Only one study was published in the English language,[18] but all the studies have been reviewed and summarized.[3,19] Seven of these clinical trials were controlled and had similar outcome measurements; five were randomized and all were double-blinded. Six of the seven were placebo-controlled, and one compared hawthorn extract to captopril, an angiotensin-converting enzyme inhibitor. These controlled trials contained 30–136 patients each, lasted 4–8 weeks, and used doses of standardized hawthorn extract products ranging from 160 to 900 mg/day. Primary study outcomes were the pressure rate product (PRP)—the product of heart rate multiplied by systolic blood pressure divided by 100; exercise tolerance as measured by a bicycle ergometer; and subjective symptoms (e.g., shortness of breath, fatigability).

Of the six placebo-controlled trials, four of five noted statistically significant improvements in the PRP, three of four in exercise tolerance, and five of six in subjective symptoms. One placebo-controlled trial that did not observe any benefit in PRP, work tolerance, or symptoms had a study duration of 4 weeks, compared to 8 weeks for most of the others. This study, however, did note a significant improvement in ejection fraction in the hawthorn group. The trial that compared hawthorn extract (900 mg/day) to low doses of captopril (37.5 mg/day) for 8 weeks noted significant and equivalent improvements in work tolerance and severity of symptoms.

Adverse Effects: Hawthorn is very well tolerated. Mild gastrointestinal effects and headaches were reported in < 2% of patients in the controlled clinical trials.[1] A surveillance study observed 72 side effects in 1.3% of 3664 patients with mild CHF; 26 of these appeared to be related to the use of the extract.[3] The most common side effects were stomach upset, palpitations, headache, and dizziness. A mild but significant lowering of blood pressure and heart rate also has been observed in some trials[18,20]; this may have been an appropriate response to therapy in heart failure patients with initial hypertension and tachycardia.[1]

Interactions: Hawthorn extract may potentiate the action of digoxin, but the effect has not been well characterized. This combination was employed to decrease a dosage of cardiac glycosides.[3] Close monitoring is warranted if used concurrently with digoxin, other inotropes, and antiarrhythmic drugs.

Cautions: Hawthorn has mixed effects on platelet aggregation *in vitro*[17]; however, there are no reports of clinical hematologic effects, and none are expected *in vivo*. There are no data on safety during pregnancy or lactation.

Preparations & Doses: The two extracts most often employed in the European controlled clinical trials were WS 1442 (Crataegutt) and LI 132 (Faros). Crataegutt is a leaf and flower extract standardized to 18.75% OPCs. Faros is prepared from the leaves, flowers, and berry and is standardized to 2.2% flavonoids.[1-3] Only Crataegutt is marketed in the U.S., as HeartCare (Nature's Way).[2] Doses in the clinical trials ranged widely from 160 to 900 mg/day, usually in 2–3 divided doses. These daily doses represent about 4–30 mg of flavonoids and 30–160 mg of OPCs, respectively.[2]

––––––––––––– **Summary Evaluation** –––––––––––––

Objective improvements for patients with mild CHF have been consistently reported in many short-term controlled trials, implying promising effects for this herb. However, methodologic quality cannot be assured because the majority of clinical trials are not available in English. Moreover, unlike standard pharmaceutical treatments for CHF that have been well documented to reduce morbidity and mortality when used chronically, hawthorn has not been studied beyond 2 months of use, and results of one study demonstrated hawthorn to be equivalent to a very low dose of an ACE inhibitor. Thus, patients should be discouraged from using hawthorn alone, even for the treatment of mild CHF. In addition, heart failure should be managed by experienced clinicians, and poorly supervised use of hawthorn may expose the patient to unneeded risks.

---

references

1. Schulz V, Hänsel R, Tyler VE: Rational Phytotherapy: A Physicians' Guide to Herbal Medicine, 4th ed. New York, Springer, 2001.
2. Blumenthal M, Goldberg A, Brinckmann J (eds): Herbal Medicine: Expanded Commission E Monographs. Newton, MA, Integrative Medicine Communications, 2000.
3. Upton R (ed): Hawthorn leaf with flower. American Herbal Pharmacopoeia and Therapeutic Compendium. Santa Cruz, CA, American Herbal Pharmacopoeia, 1999.
4. Schüssler M, Hölzl J, Rump AFE, Fricke U: Functional and anti-ischemic effects of monoacetyl-vitexinrhamnoside in different *in vitro* models. Gen Pharmacol 26:1565–1570, 1995.
5. Chen ZY, Zhang ZS, Kwan KY, et al: Endothelium-dependent relaxation by hawthorn extract in rat mesenteric artery. Life Sci 63:1983–1991, 1998.
6. Schwinger RHG, Pietsch M, Frank K, Brixius K: Crataegus special extract WS 1442 increases force of contraction in human myocardium cAMP independently. J Cardiovasc Pharmacol 35:700–707, 2000.
7. Müller A, Linke W, Klaus W: Crataegus extract blocks potassium currents in guinea pig ventricular cardiac myocytes. Planta Med 65:335–339, 1999.
8. Pöpping S, Rose I, Ionescu Y, et al: Effect of a hawthorn extract on contraction and energy turnover of isolated rat cardiomyocytes. Arzneim-Forsch/Drug Res 45:1157–1161, 1995.
9. Joseph G, Zhao Y, Klaus W: Pharmakologisches wirkprofil von Crataegus extrakt im vergleich zu epinephrin, amrinon, milrinon, digoxin am isolierten perfundierten meerschweinchenherzen [Pharmacologic profile of Crataegus extract compared to epinephrine, amrinone, milrinone, and digoxin in isolated guinea pig hearts]. Arzneim-Forsch/Drug Res 45:1261–1265, 1995.
10. Müller A, Linke W, Zhao Y, Klaus W: Crataegus extract prolongs action potential duration in guinea-pig papillary muscle. Phytomed 3:257–261, 1996.
11. Al Makdessi S, Sweidan H, Dietz K, Jacob R: Protective effect of *Crataegus oxyacantha* against reperfusion arrhythmias after global no-flow ischemia in the rat heart. Basic Cardiol Res 94:71–77, 1999.
12. Krzeminski T, Chatterjee SS: Ischemia and early reperfusion arrhythmias: Beneficial effects of an extract of *Crataegus oxyacantha* L. Pharm Pharmacol Lett 3:45–48, 1993.
13. Al Makdessi S, Sweidan H, Müllner S, Jacob R. Myocardial protection by pretreatment with *Crataegus oxyacantha*. Arzneim-Forsch/Drug Res 46:25–27, 1996.

14. Rothfuss MA, Pascht U, Kissling G: Effect of long-term application of *Crataegus oxyacantha* on ischemia and reperfusion induced arrhythmias in rats. Arzneim-Forsch/Drug Res 51:24–28, 2001.

15. Shanthi R, Parasakthy K, Deepalakshmi PD, Niranjali DS: Protective effect of tincture of Crataegus on oxidative stress in experimental atherosclerosis in rats. J Clin Biochem 20:211–223, 1996.

16. Chatterjee SS, Koch E, Jaggy H, Krzeminski T: In-vitro und in-vivo untersuchungen zur kardioprotektiven wirkung von oligomeren procyanidinen in einem Crataegus-extrakt aus blattern mit bluten. [In vitro and in vivo investigations on the cardioprotective effects of oligomeric procyanidins in a Crataegus extract from leaves with flowers.] Arzneim-Forsch/Drug Res 47:821–825, 1997.

17. Vibes J, Lasserre J, Gleye J: Effects of a methanolic extract from *Crataegus oxyacantha* blossoms on TXA2 and PGI2 synthesizing activities of cardiac tissue. Med Sci Res 21:435–436, 1993.

18. Schmidt U, Kuhn U, Ploch M, Hübner WD. Efficacy of hawthorn (Crataegus) preparation LI132 in 78 patients with chronic congestive heart failure defined as NYHA functional class II. Phytomed 1:17–24, 1994.

19. Mills S, Bone K: Principles and Practice of Phytotherapy: Modern Herbal Medicine. Edinburgh, UK, Churchill Livingstone, 2000.

20. Von Eiff M, Brunner H, Haegeli A et al: Hawthorn/passion flower extract and improvement in physical exercise capacity of patients with dyspnea class II of the NYHA functional classification. Acta Therapeutica 20:47–63, 1994.

Horehound (*Marrubium vulgare*)

rating: 🐾

> - Used for many indications, primarily for cough suppression and expectoration
> - Has not been subjected to clinical evaluation

Marrubium vulgare—white horehound or horehound—is a member of the mint family. This wild herb is indigenous to Europe and Morocco. The woolly, hairy (hoary) leaves and white flowers have been used in herbal medicines.

Uses: Horehound is used mainly as an expectorant and antitussive[1]; it has been employed as therapy for coughs, bronchitis, respiratory infections, and sore throats, and used as a tonic.[2–4] It has also been taken for cardiac arrhythmias and diabetes; as a bowel and uterine stimulant; for loss of appetite and flatulence; and externally for sores and wounds.[5,6] Horehound is alleged to have antioxidant, anti-inflammatory, vasodilator, and diuretic properties.[1]

Horehound may have been used as a bitter confection or food since ancient times. It was chosen as one of the bitter herbs (maror) of the Jewish Passover feast[2,3] and is still used in confectionary, teas, ales, and other items as a bitter flavor.

Pharmacology: White horehound contains flavonoids (such as quercetin) and diterpenes, including the lactone premarrubiin which is a precursor of the bitter marrubiin. It also contains alcohols (e.g., marrubenol, marrubiol), mucilage, saponins, and the alkaloids betonicine and stachydine; a number of less important chemicals have also been identified.[1,4] It is claimed that marrubinic acid works as an appetite stimulant and as a choleretic.[5] Horehound, like other bitter substances, may function as a nonspecific expectorant by stimulating the gastro-pulmonary mucokinetic reflex.[7,8] It has demonstrated hypoglycemic effects in rabbits; this may support its use as an antidiabetic medicine in Mexico.[9]

Clinical Trials: There are no clinical trials that demonstrate the various alleged medical uses of horehound or its main constituent, marrubiin.[10]

Adverse Effects: The herb appears well tolerated in usual doses. However, some individuals may experience difficulty with its bitter quality. Large doses cause nausea and vomiting, and have a laxative effect.[7]

Interactions: No drug interactions are recognized.

Cautions: It has not been proved to be safe in pregnancy, but no restrictions are known during lactation.[5]

Preparations & Doses: Horehound can be prepared in liquid extracts and teas, and is commonly found in tablet form, such as medicinal candies or throat pastilles. The usual therapeutic dose is 4.5 g/day of the herb, or 30–100 ml of the juice; dosing is recommended three times a day.[5] The taste may need to be disguised to make it palatable.

Summary Evaluation

Horehound may have minor expectorant properties since, in common with all bitter agents, it may stimulate the gastropulmonary expectorant reflex. However, it has not been evaluated clinically, and it cannot be recommended for serious or persistent respiratory disorders. Other alleged health benefits lack evidence. Nevertheless, this ancient herb remains popular for sore throats and other minor conditions.

---

references

1. Horehound. The Review of National Products. St. Louis, MO, Facts and Comparisons, September 1996.
2. Grieve M: A Modern Herbal. Harmondsworth, England, Penguin Handbooks, 1984.
3. Wren RC: Potter's New Cyclopaedia of Medicinal Herbs and Preparations. New York, Harper & Row, 1972.
4. Newall CA, Anderson LA, Phillipson JD: Herbal Medicines: A Guide for Health-Care Professionals. London, The Pharmaceutical Press, 1996.
5. Blumenthal M, Goldberg A, Brinckmann J: Herbal Medicine: Expanded Commission E Monographs. Newton, MA, Integrative Medicine Communications, 2000.
6. Foster S, Tyler VE: Tyler's Honest Herbal, 4th ed. New York, The Haworth Press, 1999.
7. Ziment I: Respiratory Pharmacology and Therapeutics. Philadelphia, WB Saunders Company, 1978.
8. Ziment I: What to expect from expectorants. JAMA 236:193–194, 1976.
9. Roman RR, Alarcon-Aguilar F, Lara-Lemus A, Flores-Saenz JL: Hypoglycemic effect of plants used in Mexico as antidiabetics. Arch Med Res 23:59–64, 1992.
10. Leung AY, Foster S: Encyclopedia of Common Natural Ingredients used in Foods, Drugs and Cosmetics, 2nd ed. New York, John Wiley, 1996.

Horse Chestnut Seed*
(*Aesculus hippocastanum*)
rating: 🐾🐾🐾 +

> - Used for the treatment of chronic venous insufficiency
> - Clinical evidence in favor of beneficial effects
> - Processed seed extract well tolerated, with minimal to no side effects

The fruit of the horse chestnut tree contains large seeds with a shiny, brown coat. The unprocessed seeds are toxic when ingested, and are not to be confused with the edible fruit of the sweet chestnut, *Castanea sativa*.

Uses: The processed seeds are employed in a standardized horse chestnut seed extract (HCSE), which is a popular oral therapy in European countries for chronic venous insufficiency and localized edema.[1,2] Aescin, the active constituent of HCSE, is a registered drug in Germany and other European countries and is used topically and intravenously.[3] Topical HCSE and aescin preparations are alleged to decrease symptoms of varicose veins, superficial thrombophlebitis, lymphatic edema, hemorrhoids, hematomas, and a variety of sports injuries and other traumas.[2–4]

Traditionally, horse chestnut seeds have been used for arthritis and rheumatic conditions, neuralgia, rectal complaints, and other related disorders of inflammatory congestion and engorgement .[2] The bark and leaves of the plant have also been used medicinally.

Pharmacology: The primary active constituent of horse chestnut seeds is aescin (also spelled escin), which is a complex mixture of over 30 triterpene saponin glycosides.[4,5] Other constituents include flavonoids, condensed tannins, sterols, and fatty acids. Saponin glycosides are poorly absorbed; aescin's oral bioavailability is less than 1% of its intravenous dose.[6] In a number of animal and human pharmacologic studies, aescin and HCSE have been demonstrated to decrease capillary permeability and

---

* The standardized extract product is rated.

increase venous tone and flow.[2–4,7,8] They reduce lysosymal enzyme activity, which may reduce capillary protein leakage by inhibiting proteogylcan degradation of capillary walls.[9] Animal studies have also demonstrated that aescin has anti-inflammatory properties, reduces cerebral edema, inhibits experimental gastric ulcer formation, and may enhance ACTH and cortisol secretion.[3,4]

Clinical Trials: A systematic review of the literature uncovered 13 randomized controlled trials (RCTs) of HCSE for chronic venous insufficiency. All were double-blinded and fulfilled a majority of standard inclusion criteria to reduce bias.[10] None of these trials, however, were completely flawless.

Eight studies were placebo-controlled, and three were controlled against other European phytotherapy agents (rutosides or oxerutins). In the eight trials, an oral HCSE significantly (P values all < 0.05) decreased venous insufficiency–related symptoms (leg pain, pruritus, and leg fatigue or tenseness) or objective criteria for lower extremity edema (leg volume, circumference at ankle, and capillary filtration rate), compared to placebo.[10] Studies lasted 2–8 weeks, and mainly included patients with mild to moderate chronic venous insufficiency.

Similar benefits were found in RCTs of pregnant women with lower extremity edema[11] and in healthy subjects on a long-distance plane flight.[12] Although not adequately blinded, an RCT of 240 patients with chronic venous insufficiency found HCSE and compression stockings to have equivalent activity in decreasing leg volume measured by plethysmography (−43.8 ml and −46.7 ml, respectively, compared to +9.8 ml with placebo) after 12 weeks of therapy.[13]

In a well-designed U.S. double-blind RCT of 70 healthy volunteers, a 2% aescin topical gel significantly reduced tenderness of experimentally induced hematomas compared to placebo (P < 0.001).[14]

Adverse Effects: The side effects of oral HCSE are mild and infrequent. Incidence of mild gastrointestinal symptoms, headache, dizziness, and allergic reactions ranged from 0.9% to 3% in the controlled clinical trials, and the frequency was not significantly different from that of placebo in three trials.[10] Products that are not controlled-release or enteric coated may produce more gastrointestinal upset.[6]

Interactions: There are no recognized drug interactions with HCSE.

Cautions: Parenteral administration of aescin or horse chestnut products on rare occasions has been associated with severe renal, hepatic, and anaphylactic reactions.[15] Unprocessed horse chestnut seeds are poisonous and can cause severe gastrointestinal and neurotoxic reactions.[16] There are no embryotoxic or teratogenic effects of aescin in animal models[3]; however, safety of HCSE has not been established in pregnant or breast feeding women.

Preparations & Doses: Oral HCSE products based on German standards contain 16–20% triterpene glycosides, calculated as aescin. The usual recommended daily dose, and the most common dose used in the clinical trials, is 50 mg b.i.d. of aescin; this is equivalent to 600 mg/day of the standardized HCSE.[10] The standardized commercial preparation employed in most of the European controlled trials (Venostasin) is marketed in the U.S. as Venostat (Pharmaton/Boehringer Ingelheim).[1]

Summary Evaluation

Standardized HCSE is a well-tolerated herbal medicine that appears to be useful for the treatment of chronic venous insufficiency based on a number of controlled clinical trials. Benefits have not been adequately compared to standard therapies such as compression stockings and/or diuretics, but oral HCSE could be tried as an adjunctive or alternative therapy. Topical aescin or HCSE may be useful for localized areas of inflammation or edema, but controlled clinical studies are lacking.

---

references

1. Blumenthal M, Goldberg A, Brinckmann J: Herbal Medicine: Expanded Commission E Monographs. Newton, MA, Integrative Medicine Communications, 2000.
2. Mills S, Bone K: Principles and Practice of Phytotherapy: Modern Herbal Medicine. Edinburgh, Churchill Livingstone, 2000.
3. McLellan MC: Horse Chestnut (*Aesculus hippocastanum*), revised June 15, 2000. The Longwood Herbal Task Force. Accessed February 4, 2001 at www.mcp.edu/herbal/
4. Bombardelli E, Morazzoni P, Griffini A: *Aesculus hippocastanum* L. Fitoterapia 67:483–511, 1996.
5. Yoshikawa M, Murakami T, Matsuda H, et al: Bioactive saponins and glycosides. III. Horse chestnut. (1) The structures, inhibitory effects of ethanol absorption, and hypoglycemic activity of escins Ia, Ib, IIa, and IIIa from the seeds of *Aesculus hippocastanum* L. Chem Pharmaceut Bull 44:1454–1465, 1996.

6. Schulz V, Hänsel R, Tyler VE: Rational Phytotherapy: A Physicians' Guide to Herbal Medicine, 4th ed. NewYork, Springer, 2001.

7. Matsuda H, Li Y, Murakami T, et al: Effects of escins Ia, Ib, IIa, IIb from the horse chestnut, the seeds of *Aesculus hippocastanum* L., on acute inflammation in animals. Biol Pharmaceut Bull 20:1092–1095, 1997.

8. Guillaume M, Padioleau F: Veinotonic effect, vascular protection, anti-inflammatory and free radical scavenging properties of horse chestnut extract. Arzneim-Forsch 44:25–35, 1994.

9. Kreysel HW, Nissen HP, Enghofer E: A possible role of lysosomal enzymes in the pathogenesis of varicosis and the reduction in their serum activity by Venostasin. VASA 12:377–382, 1983.

10. Pittler MH, Ernst E: Horse-chestnut seed extract for chronic venous insufficiency: A criteria-based systematic review. Arch Dermatol 134:1356–1360, 1998.

11. Steiner M, Hillemanns HG: Venostasin retard in the management of venous problems during pregnancy. Phlebology 5:41–44, 1990.

12. Marshall M, Dormandy JA: Oedema of long distance flights. Phlebology 2:123–124, 1987.

13. Diehm C, Trampisch HJ, Lange S, Schmidt C: Comparison of leg compression stocking and oral horse-chestnut seed extract therapy in patients with chronic venous insufficiency. Lancet 347:292–294, 1996.

14. Calabrese C, Preston P: Report of the results of a double-blind, randomized, single-dose trial of a topical 2% escin gel versus placebo in the acute treatment of experimentally-induced hematoma in volunteers. Planta Med 59:394–397, 1993.

15. Newall CA, Anderson LA, Phillipson JD: Herbal Medicines—A Guide for Health-Care Professionals. London, Pharmaceutical Press, 1996.

16. Chestnut. The Lawrence Review of Natural Products, St. Louis, MO, Facts and Comparisons, February 1995.

Ivy (*Hedera helix*)
rating: 🐾 🐾

> - Used primarily for coughs; rheumatic disorders and skin diseases
> - Limited evidence for effectiveness

Common or English ivy is an evergreen climbing vine; it differs from ground ivy (*Glechoma hederacea*) and from American ivy (*Parthenocissus quinquefolia*) and the related Virginian creeper. Ivy is grown widely, but the commercial product is obtained mainly from Eastern Europe. The leaf is the part that is applied medicinally.

Uses: The European indications that are currently in favor are primarily for the respiratory tract.[1,2] In Germany, ivy is recommended for its expectorant effect in dry cough, common cold, and chronic respiratory tract disorders.[3,4] Extracts have been used as antispasmodics and as topical treatments of dermal infections and itching, as well as for weight loss. Common ivy also has been traditionally used for arthritis, scrofula, fevers, skin parasites, burns, and infections.[1,2]

Pharmacology: The main components of interest are saponins (3–6% content, including hederin and hederacosides), flavonol glycosides (including rutin and kaempferol), sterols (including stigmasterol and sitosterol), sesquiterpenes, and polyalkanes (including falcarinol).[2–4] The constituents in ivy are considered to have a mucokinetic effect, and they are reported to help loosen abnormal mucus in the respiratory tree.[3] There is some evidence from animal experiments that ivy' s saponins can increase respiratory tract secretions and can prevent acetylcholine-induced bronchospasm in guinea pigs.[4,5] A product containing its chief constituent, hederasaponin C (hederacoside C), has been shown to have antifungal properties and to be toxic to some parasites and bacteria.[6,7]

Clinical Trials: Several controlled clinical trials have been carried out in Germany with Prospan, an ivy extract product.[3] In one double-blind, randomized, placebo-controlled trial of short duration in 24 children with asthma, findings suggested a bronchospasmolytic effect as shown by statistically significant and clinically relevant improvement in airway resistance and intrathoracic gas volume.[3] A few other double-blind controlled studies on patients with chronic obstructive pulmonary disease suggest that ivy has clinical and physiologic value. The largest of these involved 99 patients given ivy extract or an established mucus-loosening drug, ambroxol; the benefits after 4 weeks of therapy were similar.[3] Unfortunately, the study lacked a placebo control, and since it is difficult to demonstrate the value of any mucokinetic agent, the clinical effectiveness of ivy remains uncertain.

Adverse Effects: There are no known side effects of common ivy products.

Interactions: No drug interactions are recognized.

Cautions: There are no data on ivy leaf in pregnant or breast-feeding women. Falcarinol, which is found mainly in the leaves, can cause contact dermatitis.[3,4] Oral ingestion of the bitter ivy berries can be toxic.[6]

Preparations & Doses: In Europe, preparations are available as teas, skin products, cosmetics, shampoos, anticellulite creams, and in proprietary mixtures such as those used for bronchitis. The typical daily dose is 0.3 g of crude herb or equivalent extract for bronchitis.[5,7]

Summary Evaluation

Products containing ivy leaf are among the many herbal remedies that may appeal to patients with coughs, sinus problems and bronchitis. Several controlled clinical trials in Germany showed possible benefits, but the value of these or any mucus-loosening agents are difficult to prove.

---

references

1. English Ivy. Accessed April 14, 2001 at http://www.webmd.com
2. Bisset NG, Wichtl M (eds): Herbal Drugs and Phytopharmaceuticals. Boca Raton, CRC Press, 1994.
3. Schulz V, Hänsel R, Tyler VE: Rational Phytotherapy. A Physicians' Guide to Herbal Medicine, 4th ed. Berlin, Springer, 2001.
4. März RW: Evaluation of a Phytomedicine. Clinical, Pharmacologic, and Toxicological Data of Sinupret. Dissertation, University of Utrecht, 1998.
5. Huntley A, Ernst E: Herbal medicines for asthma: A systematic review. Thorax 55:925–929, 2000.
6. Bruneton J: Pharmacognosy, Phytochemistry, Medicinal Plants. Secaucus, NY, Lavoisier Publishing Inc, 1995.
7. Blumenthal M, Goldberg A, Brinckmann J (eds): Herbal Medicine. Expanded Commission E Monographs. Newton, MA, Integrative Medicine Communications, 2000.

Kava (*Piper methysticum*)

rating: 🐾 🐾 🐾 –

- Has mild psychoactive and antianxiety properties
- Low toxicity with therapeutic doses
- Potential for drug and disease interactions, and CNS side effects may occur at higher doses

---

The kava plant (*Piper methysticum*) is a member of the pepper family, and is widely cultivated throughout the Pacific Islands.

Uses: As an herbal product in North America (and as a phytomedicine in Europe), kava extracts are commonly used for anxiety, stress, tension, and insomnia. A mildly psychoactive beverage made from the rhizome of the kava plant has been used for centuries by South Pacific Islanders, both ceremonially and socially, reportedly with relaxing or calming properties.[1]

Pharmacology: A lipid-soluble extract from the plant rhizome contains the main active constituents, called kava pyrones (or kava lactones). The primary kava pyrones include kawain, dihydrokawain, methysticum, and dihydromethysticum, which have been extensively studied *in vitro* and in *in vivo* animal models.[1–4] These substances appear to have local anesthetic properties by blocking voltage-dependent sodium channels, which explains why chewing the kava root causes numbness and tingling of the tongue and mucosa. The kava pyrones also have sedative, muscle relaxant, and anticonvulsant properties in animals.[1–4]

Clinical Trials: Six randomized, double-blind, placebo-controlled trials of standardized European kava extract products used for anxiety have been published in Germany.[5] In general, the methodologic quality of these German trials was good, but the sample sizes were small in most studies. Double-blinding and randomization procedures were described in most, but not all, studies.[5]

Four of these trials were chronic, lasting 1–6 months, and included 40–101 patients each.[5–8] Two studies included patients with a variety of anxiety disorders, while the other two evaluated women with primarily perimenopausal anxiety complaints.

In the two acute trials, 59 patients were given 2 preoperative doses prior to surgery in one study; in the other, 20 women were treated for 1 week while waiting for a tissue sample diagnosis.[5]

The kava extract products statistically reduced anxiety symptoms relative to placebo in all six studies. In the chronic trials, effects were usually observed within 1 week (the first measurement point in the studies), but the longest trial found effects to be statistically significant only after 2 months.[8]

Kava was also compared with relatively low doses of benzodiazepines in a randomized, double-blind, European trial of 172 moderately anxious patients over 6 weeks.[9] Kava's anxiolytic effects were similar to that of oxazepam 5 mg t.i.d. and bromazepam 3 mg t.i.d. (there was no placebo control). A number of controlled clinical trials of the isolated kava pyrone compound dl-kawain in Germany reportedly demonstrated similar therapeutic results to kava extracts.[2]

One randomized, double-blind trial (published in abstract form only) used a U.S. kava supplement, given to 60 patients for 1 month.[10] Kava's effect on mild day-to-day stress was reportedly better than that of placebo.

Adverse Effects: Side effects of the standardized preparations were infrequent and mild in the controlled trials. There were isolated reports of stomach complaints, restlessness, drowsiness, tremor, and headache.[5] Gastrointestinal discomfort, headache, dizziness, and allergic skin reactions have been reported in < 2.3% of patients in open trials.[2] Several studies suggest that therapeutic doses of European kava preparations do not affect intellectual and motor function[2,4,11,12] (kava is commonly believed to act like alcohol). After one 6-month clinical trial, withdrawal effects were reportedly not observed when therapy was discontinued.[8] A kava dermopathy characterized by yellowing of the skin and a scaly dermatitis is common in chronic heavy kava drinkers in the South Pacific; the effects are reversible after discontinuation of the herb.[13]

Kava may have dopamine antagonist properties. Three patients allegedly developed extrapyramidal-like dystonic reactions, and one developed worsening of Parkinson's disease when using European kava preparations.[14] Severe choreoathetosis developed in an Aboriginal Australian man in association with excessive kava beverage bingeing.[15] Excessive amounts of traditionally prepared beverages also may produce CNS depressant or intoxicating effects.[16,17] There are two reports of U.S. motorists found weaving between lanes who were arrested for "driving under the influence" after drinking 8–16 cups of a kava beverage.[18,19] Lastly, several patients with acute necrotizing hepatitis who were using kava products have been reported; one patient required a liver transplant.[20,21] The relationship of acute necrotizing hepatitis to kava use is unclear, but the disorder may represent a rare, idiosyncratic adverse reaction.

Interactions: There is limited data on drug interactions with kava. Severe disorientation has been reported in a patient using a U.S. kava product in conjunction with alprazolam, cimetidine, and terazosin; whether his symptoms were actually due to a drug-herb interaction is unclear.[22] Therapeutic doses of a European kava preparation reportedly did not affect safety-related performance when administered with alcohol,[23] but a liquid kava preparation did potentiate the CNS-depressant properties of alcohol in a separate study.[24]

Cautions: The German Commission E recommends that duration of administration not exceed 3 months without medical advice, presumably due to concerns of dependence and/or dermopathy. Patients should be warned that kava may adversely affect driving and/or operating heavy machinery.[25] Concomitant use with alcohol or other CNS depressants may have potentiating effects, especially if either is used in high doses. It is not clear if usual therapeutic doses of kava actually warrant these warnings, but caution seems prudent, especially for kava beverage products, which are more likely to be ingested in excess. Kava is not recommended for pregnant or nursing women due to lack of data.

Preparations & Doses: The usual recommended dose of kava is 140–250 mg/day of the kava pyrone constituents, in 2–3 divided doses. In European studies, the most common dose was 70 mg t.i.d. (210 mg/day), but ranged from 60–210 mg/day.[5] In the U.S. clinical trial, 120 mg kava pyrones (Kavatrol, by Natrol) was given b.i.d.[10] One major European formulation (WS 1490, also called Laitan) is standardized to 70% kava pyrones (100-mg tablet of kava = 70 mg kava pyrones). In contrast, kava pyrone content of U.S. brands usually varies between 30% and 55%. Kava extracts are commonly available in capsules, tablets, and liquid forms.

--------- **Summary Evaluation** ---------

Based on several European randomized controlled trials, kava appears to be beneficial for mild anxiety or stress. The relative efficacy of kava compared to usual doses of pharmaceutical anxiolytic drugs is unknown. Kava appears to be well tolerated at recommended therapeutic doses, but there is potential for adverse effects with higher than recommended doses and for drug interactions. Rare, serious reactions such as hepatitis may occur, and the herb should not be used in patients with liver disease. It would be prudent for patients susceptible to extrapyramidal side effects, such as those with Parkinson's disease or those taking drugs such as antipsychotics or metoclopramide, to avoid kava until interactions have been more clearly defined. Likewise, kava should not be mixed with CNS depressants such as benzodiazepines or alcohol.

references

1. Singh YN, Blumenthal M: Kava: An overview. HerbalGram 39:34–56, 1997.
2. Schulz V, Hänsel R, Tyler VE: Rational Phytotherapy: A Physicians' Guide to Herbal Medicine, 4th ed. New York, Springer, 2001.
3. Hänsel R: Kava-kava (*Piper methysticum* G. Forster) in contemporary medical research: Portrait of a medicinal plant. Eur J Herbal Med 3(3):17–23, 1997–1998.
4. Mills S, Bone K: Principles and Practice of Phytotherapy: Modern Herbal Medicine. Edinburgh, Churchill Livingstone, 2000.
5. Pittler MH, Ernst E: Efficacy of kava extract for treating anxiety: Systematic review and meta-analysis. J Clin Psychopharmacol 20:84–89, 2000.
6. Lehmann E, Kinzler E, Friedemann J: Efficacy of a special kava extract (*Piper methysticum*) in patients with states of anxiety, tension, and excitedness of non-mental origin: A double-blind placebo-controlled study of 4-week treatment. Phytomed 3:113–119, 1996.
7. Warnecke V: Psychosomatische dysfunktionen im weiblichen klimakterium [Neurovegative dysdonia in the female climacteric]. Fortschr Med 109: 119–122 (65–70) [English translation], 1991.
8. Volz HP, Kieser M: Kava-kava extract WS 1490 versus placebo in anxiety disorders: A randomized placebo-controlled 25-week outpatient trial. Pharmacopsychiat 30:1–5, 1997.
9. Woelk H, Kapoula O, Lehrl S, et al: A comparison of Kava special extract WS 1490 and benzodiazepines in patients with anxiety. Z Allg Med 69:271–277, 1993. [German; translated into English and published in Healthnotes Rev Complem Integr Med 6:265–270, 1999.]
10. Singh NN, Ellis CR, Singh YN: A double-blind, placebo controlled study of the effects of kava (Kavatrol) on daily stress and anxiety in adults. (Symposium abstracts) Alternat Therap 4:97–98, 1998.

11. Münte TF, Heinze HJ, Matzke M, Steitz J: Effects of oxazepam and an extract of kava roots (*Piper methysticum*) on event-related potentials in a word recognition task. Neuropsychobiol 27:46–53, 1993.

12. Gessner B, Cnota P, Steinbach TS: The effects of kava-kava extract on mental alertness in comparison with diazepam and placebo. Eur J Herbal Med 3(3):24–28, 1997–1998.

13. Norton SA, Ruze P: Kava dermopathy. J Am Acad Dermatol 31:89–97, 1994.

14. Schelosky L, Raffauf C, Jendroska K, Poewe W: Kava and dopamine antagonism (correspondence). J Neurol Neurosurg Psych 58:639–640, 1995.

15. Spillane PK, Fisher DA, Currie BJ: Neurological manifestations of kava intoxication. Med J Australia 167:172–173, 1997.

16. Prescott J, Jamieson D, Emdur N, Duffield P: Acute effects of kava on measures of cognitive performance, physiological function, and mood. Drug Alcohol Rev 12:49–58, 1993.

17. Norton SA: Herbal medicines in Hawaii: From tradition to convention. Hawaii Med J 57:382–385, 1998.

18. Swensen J: Man convicted of driving under influence of kava. Desert News, Salt Lake City, UT, August 5, 1996.

19. de Turenne V: Kava tea DUI case puts spotlight on community steeped in tradition. Los Angeles Times, May 7, 2000, p A28.

20. Escher M, Desmeules J: Hepatitis associated with kava, an herbal remedy for anxiety. BMJ 322:139, 2001.

21. Strahl S, Ehret V, Dahm HH, Maier KP: Nekrotisierende hepatitis nach einnahme pflanzlicher heilmittel. [Necrotizing hepatitis after taking herbal medication.] Dtsch Med Wschr 123:1410–1414, 1998. [German; English abstract]

22. Almeida JC, Grimsley EW: Coma from the health food store: Interaction between kava and alprazolam. Ann Intern Med 125:940–941, 1996.

23. Herberg KW: [Effect of kava-special extract WS 1490 combined with ethyl alcohol on safey-relevant performance parameters.] Blutalkohol 30:96–105, 1993. [German; English abstract from PUBMED]

24. Foo H, Lemon J: Acute effects of kava, alone or in combination with alcohol, on subjective measures of impairment and intoxication and on cognitive performance. Drug Alcohol Rev 16:147–155, 1997.

25. Blumenthal M, Goldberg A, Brinckmann J (eds): Herbal Medicine: Expanded Commission E Monographs. Newton, MA, Integrative Medicine Communications, 2000.

Lemon Balm (*Melissa officinalis*)

rating: 🐾🐾

- Traditionally used as a sedative and for dyspepsia; value is unproven
- Mild beneficial effects for herpes simplex infections demonstrated with topical use
- Safe and well tolerated in usual doses

Melissa officinalis, commonly known as lemon balm or melissa, is a member of the mint family. The leaves, which emit a fragrant lemony odor when bruised, are used medicinally.

Uses: Lemon balm has traditionally been employed as a mild anxiolytic, sedative, or hypnotic herb, and is commonly taken in combination with other herbs. It is also used for mild gastrointestinal dyspepsia or spasms, especially associated with anxiety, and is considered a carminative (helps expel gas from the stomach). Topically, it is promoted for herpes simplex infections and cold sores. Historically, lemon balm steeped in wine was used for wound dressings, to treat venomous bites and stings, and for other topical uses.[1,2]

Pharmacology: Important constituents include an essential oil (containing citronellal and other compounds), rosmarinic acid, flavonoids, polyphenols, and tannins.[1,2] The essential oil extract has spasmolytic or relaxant activity on isolated smooth muscles in animal models.[2] Limited studies of hydroalcoholic extracts given intraperitoneally or orally to mice have shown sedative-hypnotic effects.[2–4] *In vitro*, the essential oil has antimicrobial activity against various bacteria, fungi, and yeasts,[5] while the aqueous extracts have antiviral activity against herpes simplex virus, HIV, influenza virus, and others.[2,6,7] The rosmarinic acid constituent inhibits complement-dependent inflammatory reactions *in vitro* and in animal models.[2,3,8]

Extracts of *M. officinalis* have been demonstrated to bind *in vitro* to thyroid-stimulating hormone (TSH) and Grave's thyroid-stimulating immunoglobulin, thus blocking TSH-receptor activation.[3,9]

Clinical Trials: Oral preparations of lemon balm, alone, have not been studied in human clinical trials for any indication. Several controlled studies of lemon balm combined with other herbs (such as valerian) have suggested mild anxiolytic or hypnotic properties, but the specific role of lemon balm is not known.[10–12]

Based on *in vitro* antiviral activity, a 1% topical cream (Lomaherpan) was evaluated in two randomized, double-blind, placebo-controlled European trials for cutaneous herpes simplex infections.[13,14] Both trials demonstrated statistically significant improvements, but the clinical benefits were minimal. For example, one study (n = 66) found mean symptom scores were slightly decreased in the treatment group on day 2 (P = 0.42), but no difference was found in the total scores over 5 days of use, and global physician assessments were not statistically significant.[13] In the other study (n = 116), a statistical improvement on day 2 was demonstrated for swelling and redness, but not for other symptoms such as pain, erosion, scabbing, or vesication. However, the active treatment was favored in global assessment ratings by both patients and physicians.[14]

Although herbalists have suggested that lemon balm may be beneficial for hyperthyroidism, there is no published clinical experience.

Adverse effects: There are no known or reported side effects.[1,2]

Interactions: There are no recognized drug interactions, although caution is advisable if used in combination with other sedative-hypnotic agents.

Cautions: There is no data in pregnant or breast-feeding women. Although antithyroid effects have only been established *in vitro*, patients with thyroid disorders should probably have more frequent laboratory monitoring after initiating or discontinuing the herb.

Preparations & Doses: About 1.5–4.5 g of crude herb or liquid extract is generally administered 2–3 times daily as needed.[1,2] Solid extracts are usually administered in doses of 300–900 mg. A topical cream containing a 1% lyophilized aqueous 70:1 extract (Lomaherpan) was administered 2–4 times daily in the European clinical trials, starting early in an acute herpes outbreak.[13,14] This cream is available in the U.S. as Herpalieve (by PhytoPharmica) and Herpilyn (Enzymatic Therapy, Inc.).[15]

───────────── **Summary Evaluation** ─────────────

Lemon balm has a long history of use as a mild anxiolytic and sedative, and for relief of dyspepsia, but clinical studies have not been done to verify these properties. The herb may have some mild benefits as a topical agent for symptoms of herpes simplex infections. Lemon balm appears well tolerated, with no reported adverse effects.

references

1. Blumenthal M, Goldberg A, Brinckmann J (eds): Herbal Medicine: Expanded Commission E Monographs. Newton, MA, Integrative Medicine Communications, 2000.
2. *Melissae folium:* Melissa leaf. European Scientific Cooperative on Phytotherapy (ESCOP). Monographs on the medicinal uses of plant drugs. Exeter, UK, ESCOP, 1996.
3. Lemon balm. The Review of Natural Products. St. Louis, MO, Facts and Comparisons, February 1999.
4. Soulimani R, Fleurentin J, Mortier F, et al: Neurotropic action of the hydroalcoholic extract of *Melissa officinalis* in the mouse. Planta Med 57:105–109, 1991.
5. Larrondo JV, Agut M, Calvo-Torras MA: Antimicrobial activity of essences from labiates. Microbios 82:171–172, 1995.
6. Dimitrova Z, Dimov B, Manolova N, et al: Antiherpes effect of *Melissa officinalis* L. extracts. Acta Microbiol Bulg 29:65–72, 1993.
7. Yamasaki K, Nakano M, Kawahata T, et al: Anti-HIV-1 activity of herbs in Labiatae. Biol Pharm Bull 21:829–833, 1998.
8. Peake PW, Pussell BA, Martyn P, et al: The inhibitory effect of rosmarinic acid on complement involves the C5 convertase. Int J Immunopharm 13:853–857, 1991.
9. Auf'mkolk M, Ingbar JC, Kubota K, et al: Extracts and auto-oxidized constituents of certain plants inhibit the receptor-binding and the biological activity of Graves' immunoglobulins. Endocrinol 116:1687–1693, 1985.
10. Cerny A, Schmid K: Tolerability and efficacy of valerian/lemon balm in healthy volunteers (a double-blind, placebo-controlled, multicentre study). Fitoterapia 70:221–228, 1999.
11. Bourin M, Bougerol T, Guitton B, Broutin E: A combination of plant extracts in the treatment of outpatients with adjustment disorder with anxious mood: Controlled study versus placebo. Fundam Clin Pharmacol 11:127–132, 1997.
12. Dressing H, Riemann D, Low H, et al: Insomnia: Are valerian/balm combinations of equal value to benzodiazepine? Therapiewoche 42:726–736, 1992.
13. Koytchev R, Alken RG, Dundarov S: Balm mint extract (Lo-701) for topical treatment of recurring Herpes labialis. Phytomed 6:225–230, 1999.
14. Wöbling RH, Leonhardt K: Local therapy of herpes simplex with dried extract from *Melissa officinalis.* Phytomed 1:25–31, 1994.
15. Tyler VE: A guide to clinically tested herbal products in the U.S. Market. Healthnotes Rev Complem Integ Med 7:279–287, 2000.

Licorice (*Glycyrrhiza glabra*)

rating: 🐾 🐾 –

- An ancient, flavorful herb used for respiratory disorders, hepatitis, inflammatory diseases, and infections
- No evidence in support of the pure herb as a beneficial clinical agent
- Deglycyrrhizinated licorice (DGL) used for peptic disorders; is regarded as an allopathic drug outside the U.S.
- Risk of pseudo-hyperaldosteronism from large doses of licorice

---

There are several flowering plants whose roots provide the well-known product known as licorice or liquorice. *Glycyrrhiza* means sweet root, a tribute to the plant's intense sweetness. The best and sweetest product comes from warmer countries in Europe, such as Italy and Spain. The main commercial plant is *Glycyrrhiza glabra* (also called *Liquiritiae officinalis* or *L. radix*). Less sweet products come from *G. uralensis* (Chinese licorice),[1,2] which grows in Asia and Turkey, and *G. glandulifera*, the source of Russian licorice.[3,4]

Uses: Licorice has been in use for thousands of years in major medical systems as a confection and flavoring, as well as an herbal medicine.[5] In traditional Chinese formulations, licorice (*gan cao* or *kan tsiao*) is a frequent component; it is used as a "harmonizer" to integrate and reduce toxicity of the other herbs in prescribed mixtures. It has been used in both Chinese and Western medicine for respiratory problems, including allergies, colds, coughs, sore throat, bronchitis, asthma, and tuberculosis. It has also been a popular agent for treating stomach and bowel disorders, including dyspepsia, bowel spasm, and constipation. Licorice and derivatives, such as carbenoxalone, have been used for many years in Europe and Japan as allopathic drugs for treating peptic ulcer disease. Although use has declined because of the superiority of pharmaceutical drugs, many herbalists still favor licorice products.

Other indications include infectious diseases, aphthous ulcers, rheumatic disorders, and skin diseases.[1,4,5] Licorice has been employed by many herbalists for inflammatory disorders. In several countries, but particularly Japan, it has a reputation of being able to prevent the adverse effects of hepatotoxic agents; it has been used for treating various forms of poisoning and in the management of viral hepatitis. It is also regarded as an antioxidant and adaptogen, and numerous other uses have been described.

Pharmacology: The terpenoids of licorice are thought to contribute to many of its healing properties. The main constituent, glycyrrhizin, is a very sweet, saponin-like triterpene glycoside that is present in a concentration of at least 4%. Glycyrrhizin (also known as glycyrrhizic acid or glycyrrhizinic acid)[2] can be hydrolyzed in the bowel to yield the more active aglycone, glycyrrhetic acid (also known as glycyrrhetinic acid or enoxolone).[5] Enoxolone is the source of a synthetic succinate derivative, carbenoxolone, which has been used in Europe and Japan to treat gastric ulcers; it has less side-effects than other licorice constituents. Glycyrrhizin can be removed during the pharmaceutical preparation of licorice, and the resulting deglycyrrhizinated licorice (DGL) has been used to treat peptic ulcers. It is not entirely free of the side effects of pure licorice, since DGL may contain some glycyrrhizin.[5]

The effects of licorice and its derivatives on the stomach and duodenum are complex. The derivatives may inhibit 15-hydroxy-prostaglandin dehydrogenase and delta-13-prostaglandin reductase, thus increasing the concentration of prostaglandins in the stomach lining.[5,6] This may result in increased mucus production and cell proliferation, thereby favoring the healing of gastric ulcers. However, other actions have been invoked, including a decrease of acid production, protection against the damage caused by anti-inflammatory agents such as aspirin and ibuprofen, and an increase in plasma secretin release.[5]

The other major active constituents of licorice root are various flavonoids, including flavanones (e.g., liquiritin, liquiritigenin), isoflavones (e.g., formononetin), and chalcones (e.g., isoliquiritin). The leaves of the plant contain kaempferol and quercetin.[1,2,5] Volatile oils obtained from licorice plants include anethole, eugenol, and fenchone. Other chemicals in licorice are coumarins, sterols, amino acids, and sugars. The flavonoids are thought to provide antioxidant properties and may contribute to the alleged antispasmodic effects of licorice.[2]

Some licorice components, such as beta-glycyrrhetinic acid, act on the liver to increase glucuronidation of toxic metabolites. This compound can also induce cytochrome P-450-dependent enzyme activities in animal models.[5] Glycyrrhizin, when given intravenously to laboratory animals, can modify the expression of hepatitis B virus–related antigens on the hepatocytes and suppress sialylation of HbsAg.[7]

One of the most important pharmacologic effects found for licorice is that glycyrrhizin and glycyrrhetic acid (GA) inhibit 11β–hydroxysteroid dehydrogenase (11βOHSD), which serves to convert active cortisol to inactive forms.[5] The inhibition of 11βOHSD leads to an increase in cortisol, while other licorice derivatives act directly on mineralocorticoid receptors; as a result, there is an increased mineralocorticoid effect.[1,5] Glycyrrhetic acid can also inhibit the metabolism of prednisolone,[8] and both GA and glycyrrhizin bind to glucocorticoid and mineralocorticoid receptors. Licorice may thereby potentiate the activity of administered corticosteroids.

Clinical Trials:

• Liver Disease—Licorice products have been used in China and Japan for more than 25 years to treat chronic hepatitis.[7,9] An open Japanese study[9] evaluated a popular product, Stronger Neo-Minophagen, which has been used for many years to treat hepatitis C. It consists of 0.2% glycyrrhizin, 0.1% cysteine, and 2% glycine. Eighty-four patients were treated with 100 mg/day given intravenously for 8 weeks, followed by 2–7 times a week infusion for 2 to 16 (median 10) years. A comparable group of 109 patients was given a nonactive infusion. After 15 years, the incidence of cirrhosis was reported as 21% in the treated group, and 37% in the control group (p = 0.07). The Japanese investigators claimed that the glycyrrhizin helped prevent cirrhosis and hepatocellular carcinoma; its effectiveness was shown by a significant reduction in liver enzymes as well as cirrhosis incidence.

In a study in Europe, glycyrrhizin in doses of 80,160, or 240 mg was given intravenously three times a week for 4 weeks to patients with hepatitis C.[10] Fifty seven patients completed this double-blind, randomized, placebo-controlled study. The authors found significant improvement in liver function compared to placebo, as measured by serum alanine transaminase (ALT), but no reduction in viral load.

Since the findings of the very demanding Japanese studies are not likely to be subjected to evaluation by other investigators, the value of extremely long-term administration of intravenous licorice and its derivatives in hepatitis will probably remain unconfirmed.

• Peptic Ulcer Disease—Many controlled trials over the years have supported the clinical value of licorice derivatives in the treatment of gastric ulcers. A typical report from England of one such product, Caved-S (containing glycyrrhizin), involved 100 patients with gastric ulcer treated for 8 weeks in a double-blind, endoscopically monitored study comparing the licorice derivative with ranitidine. The two drugs were found to be of equal benefit.[11] A similar 8-week double-blind study was reported on 29 patients with esophagitis treated with carbenoxolone in a preparation containing an antacid and an alginate (Pyrogastrone) vs. a similar formulation lacking carbenoxolone. The active agent resulted in 82% improvement in symptoms versus 63%, with better healing revealed by endoscopy ($p < 0.05$).[12] Although the value of carbenoxolone is less certain for duodenal ulcer, a healing-rate comparable to that resulting from cimetidine has been shown in other studies.[13] There is, however, an unresolved dispute in the literature as to the value and side effects of carbenoxolone and other licorice products.[14]

• Other Indications—There is a lack of consistent findings to substantiate scattered reports on the value of licorice or its derivatives in other diseases, such as apthous ulcers, herpes, and AIDS.[1,5] Thus, although a preliminary report suggested that HIV replication was temporarily inhibited by intravenous glycyrrhizin in hemophiliacs,[15] this publication was not followed by further information on these patients, and the benefit of licorice in AIDS has not been substantiated during the past 10 years. Formerly, it was believed that licorice could be useful in Addison's disease, but its electrolyte-maintaining properties have not proved adequate, and there is no evidence that it was ever used as a successful treatment for hypoadrenal states.[16] In general, reports are of limited value, and they are contradictory as to licorice's value in hypoadrenalism. Anti-asthmatic, anti-inflammatory, antitumorogenic, and other purported effects have not been adequately evaluated in the clinical setting.[17]

Adverse Effects: The most important concern about licorice, and particularly glycyrrhizin, is that susceptible people can develop pseudo-hyperaldosteronism with chronic intake of large amounts (e.g., more than about 20 g/day). This can result from using herbal licorice; excessive dosing with flavored medicines; or over-indulgence in confectionary, chewing gum, or tobacco containing real licorice as a flavor.[5,18] The mineralocorticoid-potentiating properties of the herb can result in serious adverse effects such as hypernatremia, hypertension, peripheral edema, pulmonary edema, or other evidence of cardiac failure.[5,18]

Some patients are susceptible to developing hypokalemia, and this can result in profound muscle weakness or paralysis, which may be accompanied by rhabdomyolysis and myoglobinuria.[5,18] Hypokalemic alkalosis can occur, and sometimes arrhythmias may be precipitated.

Licorice and even safer derivatives, such as carbenoxolone, have lost favor in medical practice because of these serious side effects.

Interactions: Licorice derivatives, in large amounts, could adversely interact with drugs affecting electrolyte balance (such as diuretics and corticosteroids), and with antihypertension, antiarrhythmic, and cardiac failure medications. One of the constituents of licorice (isoliquiritigenin) has been reported to have antiplatelet activities,[5] but no significant clinical interactions affecting clotting have been recognized.

Cautions: Licorice is contraindicated in patients with hypertension, heart failure, renal insufficiency, and disorders of potassium regulation. Despite claims that it can cause hypoglycemia, there is no evidence in humans to support this contention. Excessive intake should be avoided in pregnancy and lactation since it may have effects on estrogenic and progestin balance,[19] and its safety in pregnancy has not been established. One study suggested that licorice in a dose of 7 g/day (0.5 g glycyrrhizin) could inhibit the enzymatic conversion of 17-hydroxy-progesterone to androstenedione, and could thus, in theory, impair gonadal function.[20]

Licorice products should not be taken in excessive dosages, and a course of treatment of no more than 20 g/day should probably be limited to 4–6 weeks. Low dosages of the herb and the use of licorice in cosmetic creams or gels are unlikely to cause harm and may be taken indefinitely. DGL is less likely to be harmful, even with chronic intake.

Preparations & Doses: Licorice is used in candies and chewing gum, and in many other products including tobaccos. However, so-called licorice confection in the U.S. usually contains very little real licorice; most of these products are based on molasses and corn oil, with anise flavoring and coloration added.

Licorice is marketed as the raw root and it is made available in many healthcare products.

The raw root is made available as chewing sticks; cut or powdered root is more uniform, with 5 g containing about 200 mg glycyrrhizin. Products are marketed in liquid or solid forms. The typical doses are 0.5–4 ml of a 1:1 liquid extract, or more commonly as 2–4 g t.i.d. of a solid dosage form, although up to 15 g/day can be used.[1] DGL is available in tablets of 350 mg, and 2–4 tablets can be taken before each meal. Carbenoxolone (sold by Sanofi Winthrop under the name Biogastrone) is used in a dosage of 50-100 mg t.i.d. It is not marketed in the U.S.

Summary Evaluation

Licorice is an ancient drug that is particularly popular in traditional Chinese medical practice. It has been used in many cultures as an expectorant and antitussive, although these properties have not been proved. Glycyrrhizin can increase cortisol effects and thus may have anti-inflammatory properties, but this has not been well studied clinically. Overuse of licorice products can, however, cause pseudo-hyperaldosteronism. Licorice and derivatives have been approved in some countries for use as a treatment of peptic ulcer disease, but they are less acceptable as orthodox remedies currently. Many additional uses have been described, but the claimed benefits are of dubious clinical relevance; claims of value in serious diseases such as viral hepatitis, AIDS, and cancer have not been adequately established. Overall, in spite of its popularity, it appears that licorice has very little benefit to offer as a medication. Nevertheless, reported studies showing benefit in hepatitis suggest that further clinical investigations would be justified.

references

1. Blumenthal M, Goldberg A, Brinckmann J (eds). Herbal Medicine. Expanded Commision E Monographs. Newton, MA, Integrative Medicine Communications, 2000.
2. Bisset NG, Wicht M (eds). Herbal Drugs and Phytopharmaceuticals, 2nd ed. Boca Raton, CRC Press, 1994.
3. Bruneton J. Pharmacognosy, Phytochemistry, Medicinal Plants. Secaucus, NY, Lavoisier Publishing, Inc., 1995.
4. Leung AY, Foster S. Encyclopedia of Common Natural Ingredients Used in Food, Drugs and Cosmetics, 2nd ed. New York, John Wiley & Sons, Inc., 1996.

5. Mills S, Bone K. Principles and Practice of Phytotherapy. Modern Herbal Medicine. Edinburgh, Churchill Livingstone, 2000.

6. Baker ME, Fanestil DD. Liquorice as a regulator of steroid and prostaglandin metabolism. Lancet 1991;337:428–429.

7. Sato H, Goti W, Yamamura J, et al. Therapeutic basis of glycyrrhizin on chronic hepatitis B. Antiviral Res 1996;30:171–177.

8. Chen M-F, Schimada F, Kato H, et al. Effect of oral administration of glycyrrhizin on the pharmacokinetics of prednisolone. Endocrinol Japon 1991;38:167–174.

9. Arase Y, Ideda K, Murashima N, et al. The long-term efficacy of glycyrrhizin in chronic hepatitis C patients. Cancer 1997;79:1494–1500.

10. van Rossum TG, Vulto AG, Hop WC, et al. Intravenous glycyrrhizin for the treatment of chronic hepatitis C: A double-blind, randomized, placebo-controlled phase I/II trial. J Gastroenterol Hepatol 1999;14:1093–1099.

11. Morgan AG, Pacsoo C, McAdam WAF. Comparison between ranitidine and ranitidine plus Caved-S in the treatment of gastric ulceration. Gut 1985;26:1377–1379.

12. Young GP, Nagy GS, Myren J, et al. Treatment of reflux esophagitis with a carbenoxolone/antacid/alginate preparation. A double-blind controlled trial. Scand J Gastroenterol 1986;21:1098–1104.

13. Schenk J, Schmack B, Rosch W, Domschke W. Controlled trial of carbenoxolone sodium vs. cimetidine in duodenal ulcer. Scand J Gastroenterol Suppl 1980;65:103–107.

14. DerMarderosian A (ed). The Review of Natural Products. St. Louis, MO, Facts and Comparisons, 2001, pp 369–370.

15. Hattori T, Ikematsu S, Koito A, et al. Preliminary evidence for inhibitory effect of glycyrrhizin on HIV replication in patients with AIDS. Antiviral Res 1989;11:255–261.

16. WHO Monographs on Selected Medicinal Plants. Vol. 1. Geneva, World Health Organization, 1999.

17. Shibata S. A drug over the millennia: Pharmacognosy, chemistry and pharmacology of licorice. Yakugaku Zasshi 2000;120:849–862.

18. Shepherd S. Plant poisoning, herbs. Licorice. http://www.emedicine.com/emerg/topic 450.htm

19. Zava DT, Dollbaum CM, Blen M. Estrogen and progestin bioactivity of foods, herbs and spices. Proc Soc Exp Biol Med 1998;217:369–378.

20. Armanini D, Bonanni G, Palermo M. Reduction of serum testosterone in men by licorice. N Engl J Med 1999;341:1158.

Lobelia (*Lobelia inflata*)

rating: 🐾 –

- Used in respiratory conditions and as an emetic
- Contains a nicotine-like alkaloid, which can be toxic in even moderate doses

---

This North American plant is known as Indian tobacco because of its taste and suitability for smoke inhalation via burning in pipes or cigarettes. It is also known as puke weed, as it can induce vomiting. Both the herb and seeds are used as medicines.

Uses: *Lobelia inflata* gained an inflated reputation as a respiratory drug, and when commonly used to treat asthma it was known as asthma weed. Its relaxing properties were praised by 19th century herbalists, who employed it for bowel disorders and diseases such as epilepsy and angina.[1,2] Lobelia is still recommended by some herbalists for treating asthma and bronchitis, and to induce vomiting.[3] A major use of lobeline (an alkaloid from the plant that has nicotine-like effects) was as a nicotine substitute in preparations to break the smoking habit (e.g., Nikoban); however, since such products are ineffective,[4] the FDA proscribed the use of lobeline and similar anti-smoking, over-the-counter cigarette substitutes.

Pharmacology: Lobelia is the source of piperidine alkaloids, including lobeline, lobelanine, and lobelanidine. It also provides a pungent volatile oil, resins, lipids, and gum.[5,6] The alkaloids, particularly lobeline, account for its pharmacologic effect on the nicotine receptors in the nervous system; initial stimulation is followed by depression.[2,8] Lobeline can stimulate the vomiting and respiratory centers, and it may act as a weak bronchodilator.[7] It also may act as a nonspecific expectorant, with a subemetic dose inducing a gastro-pulmonary secretory response. Although no modern clinical studies have demonstrated this effect, former experience suggests that this response does occur.[2] Lobelia is alleged to have a euphoriant effect, but its use for this purpose should be discouraged since its actions are irregular and too toxic to be condoned.[7]

Clinical Trials: Although lobeline has been used in asthma therapy, there are no good studies to support claims that it acts as a bronchodilator. Similarly, its value as an aid to smoking cessation has never been proved.[4]

Adverse effects: Lobelia is a potentially toxic herb. Although it can be safely used in subclinical amounts, even small doses can cause dry mouth, nausea, diarrhea, and dizziness.[2,7] In large systemic doses, lobelia extracts have a nicotinic effect, which can make patients feel very ill with sweating, vomiting, coughing, tremors, tachycardia, hypothermia, paresis, convulsions, and coma, leading to death.[7]

Interactions: Lobeline may potentiate the adverse effects of nicotine-containing products.

Cautions: Dosages that can induce vomiting run the risk of causing severe toxic responses. Patients with gastrointestinal or cardiovascular disease, especially if severe or unstable, should avoid this herb.

Preparations & Doses: The herb is still available in various preparations, but the formerly popular salts of lobeline are no longer manufactured. Tablets, lozenges, infusions, tinctures, tobaccos, and liniments have been used. A typical oral dose of lobelia is 0.5–8 mg; a total of 20 mg/day should not be exceeded.[5,8] Doses in excess of 500 mg are very toxic, and could be fatal.

Summary Evaluation

Lobelia should be considered of doubtful value and certain toxicity. Nevertheless, it is still marketed in combination products to treat asthma. The use of lobelia can no longer be condoned, since safer and more effective agents are readily available.

---

references

1. Kloss J: Back to Eden: The Classic Guide to Herbal Medicine, Natural Foods, and Home Remedies. Santa Barbara, CA, Woodbridge Press, 1975.
2. Felter HW, Lloyd JU: King's American Dispensatory, 18th ed., 1898. Accessed March 5, 2001 on Henriette's Herbal Homepage, http://www.ibiblio.org/ herbmed
3. Ziment I: Respiratory Pharmacology and Therapeutics. Philadelphia, W.B. Saunders Company, 1978.
4. Stead LF, Hughes JR: Lobeline for smoking cessation (Cochrane Review). In The Cochrane Library, Volume 2. Oxford, Update Software, 2001.
5. Bruneton J: Pharmacognosy, Phytochemistry, Medicinal Plants. Secaucus, NY, Lavoisier Publishing Inc, 1995.

6. Newall CA, Anderson LA, Phillipson JD: Herbal Medicines: A Guide for Health-Care Professionals. London, The Pharmaceutical Press, 1996.
7. Foster S, Tyler VE: Tyler's Honest Herbal, 4th ed. New York, The Haworth Press, 1999.
8. Parfitt K (ed): Martindale. The Extra Pharmacopoeia, 32nd ed. London, The Pharmaceutical Press, 1999.

Melatonin*

rating: 🐾🐾

> - Effective for short-term use in sleep-onset insomnia; unknown effectiveness for sleep-maintenance insomnia
> - Unclear if melatonin is effective in improving symptoms of jet lag
> - Mild adverse effects; short acting and unlikely to cause morning sedation

Melatonin, N-acetyl-5-methoxytryptamine, is an endogenous indolamine hormone that is released by the pineal gland in significant quantities in a circadian pattern.

Uses: Melatonin is most often used for insomnia and jet lag. It is also used by night-shift workers and for blind entrainment (to regulate sleep patterns in those who are blind). It has been researched as an oral contraceptive, antioxidant, and anticancer agent.

Pharmacology: Regulation of melatonin secretion corresponds to the habitual sleep-wake hours in humans. Thus, melatonin secretion increases during nightfall, 9 PM–4 AM, and levels gradually decline until daylight.[1] Exogenous melatonin has been used to supplement endogenous melatonin production for a number of indications.

Clinical Trials:

- Insomnia—Several randomized, double-blind clinical trials have been conducted evaluating the role of oral melatonin in patients with insomnia.[2-6] These studies all suggest melatonin improves the quality of sleep, sleep onset, and sleep duration. These trials were small (usually involving 6–20 patients) and used subjective assessments of sleep. Dosing, patient age, timing of drug administration, method of randomization, study duration, and type of monitoring varied greatly. More recently, a randomized, double-blind, placebo-controlled clinical trial, using objective

---

* *Editor's Note:* Although not an herb, melatonin is a dietary supplement that is included here because of its current popularity.

sleep measurements, assessed the effects of immediate- and sustained-release melatonin in 14 patients with sleep-onset and sleep-maintenance insomnia.[7] According to polysomnography readings, 0.5 mg immediate-release melatonin improved sleep onset significantly. Neither the 0.5 mg sustained-release melatonin nor the immediate-release melatonin was effective in those patients suffering from sleep-maintenance insomnia. Since the elderly tend to suffer from sleep-maintenance insomnia, such as early-morning awakenings and decreased total sleep time, these findings suggest that melatonin is not likely to be effective in older adults.

• Jet Lag—Jet lag occurs when the environmental time changes before the internal circadian rhythms can compensate. The results of the initial placebo-controlled, double-blind clinical trials of melatonin were all favorable, showing improvements in symptoms of daytime fatigue, mood, and recovery time (restoring normal sleep patterns, energy, and alertness).[8–11] In these trials, however, dosing, duration of therapy, and time of drug administration were not consistent, and only subjective reports of symptoms were evaluated. The largest (n = 257) and most recent clinical trial found no improvement with melatonin given in variable doses (0.5 and 5 mg) and at varying times, and used an objective rating scale to assess jet lag symptoms.[12] Thus, the role of melatonin for jet lag is still in question.

Adverse Effects: Melatonin is well tolerated, and its use can avoid the daytime somnolence commonly experienced with over-the-counter hypnotics. In clinical trials, melatonin has been associated with daytime drowsiness, tachycardia, dysthymia, and headache—but rarely.[8–12] Reversible cases of acute psychosis, acute amnesia, and erythematous plaques have been reported.[13–15]

Interactions: No drug interactions have been reported with melatonin. Many drugs, however, have been shown to increase and decrease endogenous melatonin levels[16–18]; the clinical significance of this effect is unknown.

Cautions: Patients with mania or bipolar disease may be at risk since melatonin may worsen mania.[13,19] High-dose melatonin (up to 300 mg) has suppressed luteinizing hormone (LH) surge and partially inhibited ovulation when combined with a progestin.[20] Therefore, melatonin should be avoided in women who are attempting to conceive. Long-term use of melatonin is not recommended due to a lack of data. A negative feedback effect on endogenous melatonin has *not* been observed in clinical trials of *short* duration.[21] However, chronic melatonin administration may decrease prolactin levels, and use should be discouraged while nursing.[22] Due to a lack of safety data, melatonin should be avoided during pregnancy.

Preparations & Doses: Dosing for melatonin varied widely in clinical studies, and products are available in a wide range of doses. Sustained-release products have not shown a significant benefit and generally cost more than immediate-release melatonin.

For insomnia, the lowest effective dose in clinical trials was 0.3 mg. If a low dose is ineffective, additional dosing up to a maximum of 10–20 mg may be required. Melatonin should be taken 30 minutes prior to the desired sleep time and lights should be turned off.

For jet lag, doses between 0.5 and 8 mg of the immediate-release formulation taken on the evening of departure have been used in the clinical trials. The most effective dose, timing of administration, and duration of use have not been determined. Typical jet lag symptoms usually resolve within 6 days after destination arrival.

To prevent potential viral transmission and contamination, products derived from animal pineal glands should be avoided; products that use a synthetic form of melatonin are preferable.

--- **Summary Evaluation** ---

Melatonin appears to be of value in alleviating sleep-onset insomnia. Currently, the literature does not support its use in sleep-maintenance insomnia. Melatonin may help reduce jet lag by facilitating sleep at the desired time upon arrival; however, study results are conflicting. Melatonin is well tolerated and is associated with less daytime drowsiness than other over-the-counter hypnotics. Thus, it is an acceptable alternative for sleep induction and for managing similar sleep disturbances.

references

1. Brzezinski A, Lynch HJ, Seibel MM, et al: The circadian rhythm of plasma melatonin during the normal menstrual cycle and in amenorrheic women. J Clin Endocrinol Metab 66:891–895, 1988.
2. Wurtman RJ, Zhdanova I: Improvement of sleep quality by melatonin. Lancet 346:1491, 1995.
3. Garfinkel D, Laudon M, Nof D, et al: Improvement of sleep quality in elderly people by controlled-release melatonin. Lancet 346:541–544, 1995.

4. Dahlitz M, Alvarez B, Vignau J, et al: Delayed sleep phase syndrome response to melatonin. Lancet 337:1121–1124, 1991.

5. Haimov I, Lavie P, Laudon M, et al: Melatonin replacement therapy of elderly insomniacs. Sleep 18:598–603, 1995.

6. James SP, Sack DA, Rosenthal NE, et al. Melatonin administration in insomnia. Neuropsychopharmacol 3:19–23, 1990.

7. Hughes RJ, Sack RL, Lewy AJ, et al: The role of melatonin and circadian phase in age-related sleep-maintenance insomnia: Assessment in a clinical trial of melatonin replacement. Sleep 21:52–68, 1998.

8. Petrie K, Dawson AG, Thompson L, et al: A double-blind trial of melatonin as a treatment for jet lag in international cabin crew. Biol Psychiatry 33:526–530, 1993.

9. Petrie K, Conaglen JV, Thompson L, et al: Effect of melatonin on jet lag after long haul flights. BMJ 298:705–707, 1989.

10. Claustrat B, Brun J, David M, et al: Melatonin and jet lag: Confirmatory result using a simplified protocol. Biol Psychiatry 32:705–711, 1992.

11. Arendt J, Aldous M, Marks V, et al. Alleviation of jet lag by melatonin: Preliminary results of a controlled double blind study. BMJ 292:1170, 1986.

12. Spitzer RL, Terman M, Williams JB, et al: Jet lag: Clinical features, validation of a new syndrome specific scale, and lack of response to melatonin in a randomized, double-blind trial. Amer J Psychiatr 156:1392–1396, 1999.

13. Force RW, Hansen L, Bedell M, et al: Psychotic episode after melatonin. Ann Pharmacother 31:1408, 1997.

14. Bardazzi F, Placucci F, Neri I, et al: Fixed drug eruption due to melatonin. Acta Derm Venereol 78:69–70, 1997.

15. Badia P, Hughes RJ, Wright KP, et al: Effects of exogenous melatonin on memory, sleepiness and performance after a 4-hour nap. J Sleep Res 5:11, 1996.

16. Murphy PJ, Myers BL, Badia P, et al: Nonsteroidal anti-inflammatory drugs alter body temperature and suppress melatonin in humans. Physiol Behav 59:133–139, 1996.

17. Monteleone P, Tortorella A, Borriello R, et al: Suppression of nocturnal plasma melatonin levels by evening administration of sodium valproate in healthy humans. Biol Psychiatry 41:336–341, 1997.

18. Cowen PJ, Fraser S, Sammons R, et al: Atenolol reduces plasma melatonin concentration in man. Br J Clin Pharmacol 15:579–581, 1983.

19. Maurizi CP: A preliminary understanding of mania: Roles for melatonin, vasotocin and rapid-eye-movement sleep. Med Hypothes 54:26–29, 2000.

20. Voordouw BCG, Euser R, Verdonk RE, et al: Melatonin and melatonin-progestin combinations alter pituitary-ovarian function in women and can inhibit ovulation. J Clin Endocrinol Metab 74:108–117, 1992.

21. Sack RL, Lewy AJ, Blood ML, et al: Melatonin administration to blind people phase advances and entrainment. J Biol Rhythms 6:249–261, 1991.

22. Arendt J: Chronic, timed, low-dose melatonin treatment in man: Effects on sleep, fatigue, mood and hormone rhythms. EPSG Newsl Suppl 5:51, 1984.

Milk Thistle (*Silybum marianum*)

rating: 🐝 🐝 +

> - Used primarily for protection against, or treatment of, liver disease
> - Decreased serum transaminases in some trials, but clinical benefits not clearly established
> - Appears safe and well-tolerated

Milk thistle is a member of the *Asteraceae* or daisy family. Generally, it is the fruit or seed that is used medicinally.

Uses: Milk thistle is typically employed as a hepato-protectant or to treat established liver disease. This application is based on a long tradition of use for liver, spleen, and biliary disorders.[1,2] A standardized formulation has been studied by European researchers and promoted for prevention or treatment of all types of liver damage.

Pharmacology: Milk thistle seeds contain silymarin, a mixture of three primary flavonolignans: silybin (also known as silybinin or silibinin), silychristin, and silydianin.[1,2] Silybin is the most abundant. There are several potential mechanisms by which these compounds may protect the liver from hepatotoxins, or treat established liver disease.

In vitro, silybin is an antioxidant that reduces lipid peroxidation and scavenges radicals in human platelets, white blood cells, and endothelial cells.[3] These antioxidant properties limit depletion of important endogenous antioxidants such as glutathione and superoxide dismutase *in vitro* and *in vivo*.[4,5] This effect has been demonstrated to reduce oxidative damage to liver cells by a variety of different hepatotoxins (e.g., *Amanita phalloides* mushrooms, acetaminophen, carbon tetrachloride, and alcohol).[4]

Silybin also strongly inhibits the enzyme 5-lipoxygenase, and thus reduces the formation of inflammatory leukotrienes.[3] The high concentrations required to inhibit cyclo-oxygenase, however, are unlikely to be achieved in clinical practice.[3] Lastly, silybin limits the activity of Kupffer cells in vitro, which may help to slow the progression of chronic liver disease.[7]

Silymarin enhances transcription of liver proteins *in vitro*, by stimulating a DNA-dependent RNA-polymerase I.[6] This action may contribute to cellular regeneration in the liver. Silymarin also slows collagen accumulation in experimental models of biliary fibrosis,[8] a mechanism that also may alter the course of chronic liver disease.

Clinical Trials: A comprehensive and systematic review sponsored by the U.S. Agency for Healthcare Research and Quality[9] identified 14 randomized, controlled trials (RCTs) involving milk thistle for the treatment of various forms of liver disease.[10–24] All were prospective, blinded, European studies; eight are published in the English language. Milk thistle was evaluated in patients with chronic alcoholic liver disease in seven trials; liver disease of mixed etiology in three trials; viral hepatitis in three trials; and treatment of drug-induced liver disease in one trial. Two RCTs also evaluated the prevention of drug-induced liver disease.[25,26] Legalon, a European standardized extract of milk thistle, was used in a majority of the trials. The results of most of these studies are limited by poor study design and quality of reporting.[9]

In pure **alcoholic liver disease**, two trials included patients with cirrhosis,[10,12] while the other five trials included patients whose disease was either of mixed or unknown severity.[11,13–16] Legalon was used in all these trials; dosing ranged from 280 to 450 mg/day, and lasted from 1 month to 2 years. Three trials reported no significant improvements in transaminases, histology, or survival.[12–14] Four trials reported improvements in at least one transaminase enzyme or histology, but also did not find improvements in survival.[10,11,15,16] The two trials with the highest methodologic quality[12,14] were among those noting no significant improvements. Both of these trials had study durations of at least 90 days and included patients with cirrhosis and alcoholic liver disease of mixed severity.

Three trials evaluated the effects of milk thistle for patients with **liver disease of mixed etiology**, not specified solely from alcohol; most subjects had cirrhosis.[17–20] The trial with the highest methodologic quality had a sample size of about 170 patients, and patients received 420 mg/day of Legalon. Results were analyzed at 2 and again at 4 years.[17,18] After 4 years, a nonsignificant trend toward improved survival was reported. A re-analysis of the data published 9 years later noted that for patients who had the mildest disease, Child's Class A, the improvement was statistically significant at the 2-year mark.[17,18] No improvement was found in transaminases, or for survival in patients with Child's Class B or C. The two trials with lower methodologic quality did not use Legalon preparations, and had sample sizes that ranged from 65 to 177 patients and study durations that ranged from 40 to 90 days.[19,20] In both of these trials, at least one or both of the two forms of transaminase improved significantly compared to placebo.

Patients with **viral hepatitis** were evaluated in three trials. In one study, 59 patients with acute hepatitis A and B were given 420 mg of Legalon daily for 25 days. Both aspartate aminotransferase (AST) and bilirubin were significantly reduced at the study endpoint, while alanine aminotransferase (ALT) and alkaline phosphatase were not.[21] Two trials enrolled patients with chronic viral hepatitis; in one, patients had either hepatitis B and/or C, and in the other, the viral type was not stated.[22,23] Dosing ranged from 240 mg of Silipide for 7 days, to 420 mg of Legalon for 1 year. In the year-long trial there was a nonsignificant trend toward improved liver histology.[23] In the other trial, both AST and ALT were significantly reduced at 7 days, but alkaline phosphatase was not.[22]

In an RCT of **drug-induced hepatitis**, milk thistle was given to patients with liver disease caused by phenothiazines. A subset of patients also had serology-confirmed hepatitis B. At 90 days, there was no significant change in transaminase levels for patients receiving silymarin or placebo, with or without continuation of psychotropic medication.[24] Two RCTs evaluated the use of milk thistle for prophylaxis of drug-induced liver disease. One 8-week, unblinded trial in 172 patients found that significantly fewer patients had elevations of transaminases when a silymarin/*Fumaria officinalis* herbal combination was administered with antituberculosis drugs, compared to antituberculosis drugs administered alone.[25] In contrast, a 12-week, double-blinded trial in 222 patients observed no significant differences in transaminases when silymarin was given in combination with tacrine, compared to tacrine alone.[26]

Case series of intravenous silybin used for Amanita mushroom poisoning have been published in Europe.[27] Typically, the silybin was given in daily doses of 20–50 mg/kg, depending on the disease severity, and in combination with other treatments used at the time such as gastric lavage and penicillin. In general, when silybin was administered within 48 hours of the ingestion and the disease severity was mild to moderate, a benign clinical course was reported. When silybin was administered to patients with severe disease, a decline in mortality was also observed when compared to historical controls. However, prospective controlled trials for this use have not been published.

Adverse Effects: No major side effects have been reported for patients using milk thistle.[9] Loose stools and other mild gastrointestinal effects occur rarely.[1,2]

Interactions: There are no reported drug interactions with milk thistle.[1,2] Silybin does not interact with most hepatic cytochrome P450 (CYP) enzyme systems, but inhibition of CYP3A4 (as well as UGT1A6/9 and possibly CYP2C9) enzymes has been demonstrated in several *in vitro* studies.[28–30] Caution is thus warranted in using the herb in combination with other drugs metabolized in the liver.

Cautions: People with allergies to plants of the Asteraceae family (e.g., daisy, sunflower, chrysanthemum, ragweed) may be allergic to milk thistle as well. Milk thistle's safety in pregnant and breast-feeding women has not been established.

Preparations & Doses: A daily dose of 200–400 mg of silymarin in 2–3 divided doses is usually recommended; this range of dosage was employed in the clinical trials.[1,2] Milk thistle products are usually standardized to contain no less than 70–80% silymarin. The product used in most of the European trials, Legalon, is marketed in the U.S. as Thisylin (Nature's Way).[2] Silipide, or IdB 1016, a silymarin-phosphatidylcholine complex that has enhanced bioavailability,[22] is not marketed in the U.S.

Summary Evaluation

The efficacy of milk thistle in alleviating symptoms of viral and alcohol-related liver disease is not established. Improved liver transaminases and improved survival in mild alcoholic liver disease have been demonstrated in limited studies, but are not consistently found among the many clinical trials. It is doubtful that milk thistle is beneficial in severe liver disease such as cirrhosis. Prophylactic use of milk thistle to protect the liver against hepatotoxins (e.g., alcohol) is based primarily on laboratory and animal data, with inadequate clinical evidence. Milk thistle has not been compared with interferon or other pharmaceutical options for viral hepatitis, nor has an effect on viral loads been evaluated. Although clinically relevant benefits are not clearly established, because milk thistle has no major side effects and there is a lack of well-tolerated orthodox drugs, it is tempting for patients to try milk thistle for preventing or treating established liver disease. If used, efficacy can be monitored with appropriate laboratory testing.

references

1. Schulz V, Hänsel R, Tyler VE: Rational Phytotherapy: A Physicians' Guide to Herbal Medicine, 4th ed. New York, Springer, 2001.

2. Blumenthal M, Goldberg A, Brinckmann J (eds): Herbal Medicine: Expanded Commission E Monographs. Newton, MA, Integrative Medicine Communications, 2000.

3. Dehmlow C, Murawski N, deGroot H: Scavenging of reactive oxygen species and inhibition of arachidonic acid metabolism by silybinin in human cells. Life Sci 58:1591–1600, 1996.

4. Shear NH, Malkiewicz IM, Klein D, et al: Acetaminophen-induced toxicity to human epidermoid cell line A431 and hepatoblastoma cell line Hep G2, in vitro, is diminished by silymarin. Skin Pharmacol 8:279–291, 1995.

5. Feher J, Lang I, Nekam K, et al: In vivo effect of free radical scavenger hepatoprotective agents on superoxide dismutase (SOD) activity in patients. Tokai J Exp Clin Med 15:129–134, 1990.

6. Sonnenbichler J, Goldberg M, Hane L, et al: Stimulatory effect of silybinin on the DNA synthesis in partially hepatectomized rat livers: Non-response in hepatoma and other malignant cell lines. Biochem Pharmacol 35:538–541, 1986.

7. Dehmlow C, Erhard J, deGroot H: Inhibition of Kupffer cell functions as an explanation for the hepatoprotective properties of silibinin. Hepatology 23:749–754, 1996.

8. Boigk G, Stroedter L, Herbst H, et al: Silymarin retards collagen accumulation in early and advanced biliary fibrosis secondary to complete bile duct obliteration in rats. Hepatology 26:643–649, 1997.

9. Mulrow C, Lawrence V, Jacobs B, et al: Milk thistle: Effects on liver disease and cirrhosis and clinical adverse effects. Evidence Report/Technology Assessment No. 21. AHRQ Publication No. 01-E025. Rockville, MD, Agency for Healthcare Research and Quality, October 2000.

10. Lang I, Nekam K, Deak G, et al: Immunomodulatory and hepatoprotective effects of in vivo treatment with free radical scavengers. Ital J Gastroenterol 22:283–287, 1990.

11. Salmi HA, Sarna S: Effect of silymarin on chemical, functional and morphological alterations of the liver. A double-blind controlled study. Scand J Gastroenterol 17:517–521, 1982.

12. Pares A, Planas R, Torres M, et al: Effect of silymarin in alcoholic patients with cirrhosis of the liver: Results of a controlled, double-blind, randomized and multicenter trial. J Hepatol 28:615–621, 1998

13. Bunout D, Hirsch S, Petermann M, et al: Estudio controlado sobre el efecto de la silimarina en la enfermedad hepatica alcoholica [Controlled study of the effect of silymarin on alcoholic liver disease]. Rev Med Chil 120:1370–1375, 1992.

14. Trinchet JC, Coste T, Levy VG, et al: Traitement de l'hepatite alcoolique par la silymarine. Une etude comparative en double insu chez 116 malades [Treatment of alcoholic hepatitis with silymarin. A double-blind comparative study in 116 patients]. Gastroenterol Clin Biol 13:120–124, 1989.

15. Feher JDG, Muzes G, Lang I, et al: Silymarin kezeles majvedo hatasa idult alkoholos majbetegsegben [Hepatoprotective activity of silymarin (Legalon) therapy in patients with chronic alcoholic liver disease]. Orv Hetil 130:2723–2727, 1989.

16. Fintelmann V, Albert A: Nachweis der therapeutischen wirksamkeit von legalon bei toxischen lebererkrankungen im doppelblindversuch [Double-blind trial of silymarin sodium in toxic liver damage]. Therapiewoche 30:5589–5594, 1980.

17. Benda L, Dittrich H, Ferenchi P, et al: Zur wirksamkeit von silymarin auf die uberlebensrate von patienten mit leberzirrhose [The influence of therapy with silymarin on the survival rate of patients with liver cirrhosis]. Wien Klin Wochenschr 92:678–683, 1980.

18. Ferenchi P, Dragosics B, Dittrich H, et al: Randomized controlled trial of silymarin treatment in patients with cirrhosis of the liver. J Hepatol 9:105–113, 1989.

19. Tanasescu C, Petrea S, Baldescu R, et al. Use of the Romanian product Silimarina in the treatment of chronic liver disease. Rev Roum Med 26:311–322, 1988.

20. Marcelli R, Bizzoni P, Conte D, et al: Randomized controlled study of the efficacy and tolerability of a short course of IdB 1016 in the treatment of chronic persistent hepatitis. Eur Bull Drug Res 1:131–135, 1992.

21. Magliulo E, Gagliardi B, Fiori GP: Zur wirkung von silymarin bei der behandlung der akuten virushepatitis [Results of a double-blind study on the effect of silymarin in the treatment of acute viral hepatitis, carried out at two medical centers]. Med Klin 73:1060–1065, 1978.

22. Buzzelli G, Moscarella S, Giusti A, et al: A pilot study on the liver protective effect of silybin-phosphatidylcholine complex (IdB 1016) in chronic active hepatitis. Int J Clin Pharmacol Ther Toxicol 31:456–460, 1993.

23. Kiesewetter E, Leodolter I, Thaler H: Ergebnisse zweier doppelblindstudien zur wirksamkeit von silymarin bei chronischer hepatits [Results of two double-blind studies on the effect of silymarin in chronic hepatitis]. Leber Magen Darm 7:318–323, 1977.

24. Palasciano G, Portincasa P, Palmieri V, et al: The effect of silymarin on plasma levels of malon-dialdehyde in patients receiving long-term treatment with psychotropic drugs. Curr Ther Res Clin Exp 55:537–545, 1994.

25. Magula D, Galisova Z, Iliev N, et al: [Effect of silymarine and Fumaria alkaloids in the prophylaxis of drug-induced liver injury during antituberculotic treatment]. Stud Pneumol Phtiseol 56:206–209, 1996.

26. Allain H, Shuck S, Lebreton S, et al: Aminotransferase levels and silymarin in de novo tacrine-treated patients with Alzheimer's disease. Dement Geriatr Cogn Disord 10:181–185, 1999.

27. Hruby K, Csomos G, Fuhrmann M, Thaler H: Chemotherapy of Amanita phalloides poisoning with intravenous silibinin. Human Toxicol 2:183–195, 1983.

28. Budzinski JW, Foster BC, Vandenhoek S, Arnason JT: An in vitro evaluation of human cytochrome P450 3A4 inhibition by selected commercial herbal extracts and tinctures. Phytomed 7:273–282, 2000.

29. Beckmann-Knopp S, Rietbrock S, Weyhenmeyer R, et al: Inhibitory effects of silibinin on cytochrome P-450 enzymes in human liver microsomes. Pharmacol Toxicol 86:250–256, 2000.

30. Venkataramanan R, Ramachandran V, Komoroski BJ, et al: Milk thistle, an herbal supplement, decreases the activity of CYP3A4 and uridine diphospho-glucuronosyl trasferase in human hepatocyte cultures. Drug Metab Dispos 28:1270–1273, 2000.

Mints (*Mentha* species)

rating: 🐾🐾🐾 −

> - Minor calcium channel antagonists
> - Used for upper respiratory problems, irritable bowel syndrome, dyspepsia, and colonic spasm, and as a topical counterirritant
> - Supportive clinical evidence

Spearmint (*Mentha spicata*) and the related horsemint were well known in the Graeco-Roman era, and mint was used in biblical times. Peppermint (*M. piperita*) appeared in the 18th century in England as a hybrid between spearmint and watermint. It is less flavorful than spearmint, while Japanese mint or cornmint (*M. arvensis*) is more flavorful.

Uses: Over the ages, spearmint, peppermint, and other mints have been used as flavors, aromas, and medications.[1,2] They have been taken mainly for digestive symptoms such as dyspepsia and irritable bowel, and for respiratory and dermatologic conditions. In general, all of the common mints have similar effects and are best known because of the popularity of their characteristic taste in candies, foods, and medications and for the refreshing effect they give to skin and mouth preparations. *M. pulegium*, pennyroyal, is a dangerous member of the mint family, and its oil should not be used in herbal therapeutics.

Pharmacology: The most important of the over 80 compounds in mints is the essential oil menthol,[3] also known as peppermint camphor. The l-isomer of menthol is found mainly in Japanese mint, constituting 70–95% of the essential oil; in peppermint, it may constitute 29–48%.[2] Menthol, which can be synthesized from thymol, is a terpenoid alcohol; menthone, another major constituent, is a terpenoid ketone.[4] Spearmint contains less menthol than peppermint, and its oil is used mainly as a flavoring agent. The related pennyroyal oil contains the characteristic toxic compound pulegone; this constitutes 90–95% of the content of the oil. Pulegone can be synthetically hydrogenated to l-menthone, which can then be reduced to give l-menthol.

Some of the effects of mints may be due to tannins or other components. Other volatile oils and chemicals that are extracted from mints include cineole, limonene, and flavonoids.[2-4]

Peppermint oil acts on the smooth muscle of the bowel.[5] It relaxes the gastroesophageal sphincter, and thus serves as a carminative, facilitating eructation.[6] It can relax hypermotile or spasmodic intestinal muscle, and its flavonoids may have a cholagogic effect and stimulate bile secretion.[5] Laboratory studies show that peppermint oil and menthol inhibit depolarization-induced calcium uptake into nerves. They relax the smooth muscles by acting as calcium channel antagonists.[3,5,7] The effect of mint oil on the skin is tingly, refreshing and antipruritic; the oil is a mild anesthetic or counterirritant.[8]

The pharmacologic actions of peppermint are attributed mainly to menthol, but several other constituents may cause these effects.[6] *In vitro* studies suggest that mint oils may have minor antiviral and antibacterial properties[6]; cytotoxic and anti-inflammatory effects have also been reported.[2]

Although menthol vapor subjectively appears to open congested nasal passages, studies have shown that this is not a physical effect.[5] Indeed, concentrated menthol can increase congestion and impair ciliary motion.[3] Menthol has, however, shown benefits in the treatment of experimentally-induced cough. In one careful study, 20 healthy volunteers were challenged with inhaled citric acid; a preparation of menthol in eucalyptus oil was found to significantly reduce the induced cough ($p < 0.0005$).[9]

Clinical Trials:

• Gastrointestinal Uses—Most studies have been carried out in Germany. The European commercial products Colpermin and Pepogest, which are enteric-coated, delayed-release, pH-sensitive capsules containing 0.2 ml peppermint oil, have been evaluated. They release the herbal chemical in the colon to treat spasm.[10] Eight randomized, controlled studies involving a total of 265 patients were critically reviewed in a meta-analysis to determine the outcome of treatment for gastric distress, flatulence, hyperactive intestines, and other symptoms that constitute irritable bowel syndrome (IBS).[3,5] Only five placebo-controlled, double blind trials were satisfactory for analysis, and overall there was a positive effect ($p < 0.001$). However, the criteria for diagnosing IBS in the eight trials were not judged to be satisfactory in 91.5% of the patients,[5] although all had symptoms suggestive of colonic spasm.

In a subsequent randomized, double-blind, placebo-controlled trial, 101 patients were treated 3 to 4 times a day for one month with Colpermin or placebo.[11] A significant symptomatic response to peppermint oil was reported, with 79% effectiveness for pain relief and reduced lower bowel symptoms compared to 43% for placebo (p < 0.05). A similar randomized, double-blind, 2-week study of 42 children who met criteria for IBS suggested peppermint was more effective than placebo, with 76% improving vs. 19% respectively (p < 0.001).[12]

A double-blind, randomized study on 141 patients undergoing barium enema examination showed that the addition of peppermint oil to the barium suspension reduced colonic muscle spasm (no spasm in 60% vs. 35% in the placebo group).[13] In another study, 405 patients were given intracolonic peppermint oil during colonoscopy, resulting in a spasmolytic effect in 88.5%; a group of 36 treated with placebos had a 33.3% response.[14]

A randomized, double-blind trial of 213 patients with dypepsia combined with IBS evaluated two different formulations of an enteric-coated, peppermint oil/carraway oil mixture given 3 times a day.[15] One product (Enteroplant) contained 90 mg peppermint oil with 50 mg carraway oil; the reference product contained 36 mg and 20 mg, respectively. Equivalent benefits were obtained with each preparation in reducing pain intensity, but the frequency of pain was significantly less (p = 0.04) for the test preparation compared to the lower-dose reference preparation. The same investigators subsequently studied 96 outpatients with functional dyspepsia in a randomized, double-blind evaluation using the same 90mg/50mg combination test formulation compared with a placebo.[16] Dosing was given only twice a day for 4 weeks. Statistically significant and clinically relevant improvements in symptoms were found in the test group (40% vs. 22%).

A similar study on 118 patients compared the same test formulation of Enteroplant with cisapride for functional dyspepsia.[17] Similar reductions in pain over the course of 4 weeks were found with both agents compared to baseline. One problem with these studies is that they did not evaluate peppermint alone.

• Headaches—Topical peppermint oil has also been evaluated for the treatment of headaches. In three randomized, double-blind, placebo-controlled trials in a total of 190 patients with tension headaches, there was a significant benefit of a 10% ethanol solution of peppermint oil applied to the forehead and temples, with 65% improving versus 25% on placebo.[3] All the headache studies were performed by the same group of investigators, and the findings have not been corroborated. In contrast, topical peppermint oil was not effective for migraine.[3]

Adverse Effects: Most clinical studies found peppermint oil products to be well tolerated, with only minor adverse effects. Side effects included heartburn, nausea, vomiting, and perianal burning.[5]

Interactions: There are no recognized drug interactions. Since menthol acts as a calcium-channel blocker, it theoretically should be used cautiously in patients who are receiving one of these drugs or are intolerant of the class. However, its wide use, without reported problems, suggests it has considerable safety and probably lacks significant interactions.

Cautions: Menthol ingested in amounts of 2 g has been fatal in some cases.[18] Large doses of peppermint oil can cause CNS stimulation; a dose of about 1 g/kg can be fatal.[6,19] Pennyroyal oil, which contains pulegone, was formerly taken to induce menstruation; it could also induce abortions, with concomitant severe liver toxicity and fatalities.[2,20] Pennyroyal oil can cause multiple organ failure in infants.[21] Menthol cannot be metabolized by neonates with G6PD deficiency and it may cause jaundice; neonates and other susceptible subjects should only use mints and their oils with extreme caution.[2]

Inhalation of menthol or its instillation into the nose can cause irritation and even nasal obstruction. Reflex gagging, apnea, and collapse can occur in infants, and cardiac arrhythmia in susceptible adults.[18,19] Allergy to mint oils results in rashes, headaches, flushing, and asthma.[18] Occasionally, asthma can be induced by minimal doses of menthol, such as occur in toothpaste.[22]

Some physicians advise that peppermint should be avoided in patients with esophagitis, hiatal hernia, or gastroesophageal reflux disease, since it can relax the gastroesophageal sphincter.[3] To prevent this problem, enteric-coated capsules are used for treating lower bowel disorders; they release the oil in the distal bowel where it has a local effect.[18] The safety of peppermint products during pregnancy and nursing has not been established for therapeutic ranges of dosing.

Preparations & Doses: Mint extracts, menthol, and related chemicals are found in numerous types of health products, varying from foods and cigarettes to creams and cough preparations.

Menthol can be given orally to adults in a dosage of 30–120 mg,[6] and is used in topical formulations in 1–10% concentrations. The typical oral dose of peppermint oil is 0.2–1.2 ml/day, usually given in 2–3 divided doses. One enteric-coated product evaluated in the European clinical trials, Pepogest, is marketed in the U.S. by BioTherapies and Nature's Way. It contains 0.2 ml of peppermint oil/capsule, and recommended dosing is 1–2 capsules t.i.d. between meals. Mint leaf products, which can be brewed in teas, are given in 1.5–6 g dosages.[6] The brewed product contains very low concentrations of menthol and menthone.[18]

Summary Evaluation

Peppermint and other mints and their natural and synthetic compounds, of which menthol is the most important, are frequently used in everyday life. Their main value is as flavorful aromatic products, and it is commonly accepted that they soothe skin, throat, respiratory, and bowel conditions. One major therapeutic indication for menthol and mint products is IBS; benefits have been found in several controlled clinical trials. These products may also relieve colonic spasm when introduced locally during endoscopy or enemas. There is evidence that topical use may relieve tension headaches. Preparations made from the herb have low toxicity for most people. However, small amounts of the essential oils from Mentha species can be harmful when given to neonates and infants.

references

1. Rosengarten F. The Book of Spices. New York, Pyramid Books, 1973.
2. Leung AY, Foster S. Encyclopedia of Common Natural Ingredients Used in Food, Drugs and Cosmetics, 2nd ed. New York, John Wiley & Sons, Inc, 1996.
3. Schulz V, Hänsel R, Tyler VE. Rational Phytotherapy: A Physicians' Guide to Herbal Medicine, 4th ed. Berlin, Springer, 2000.
4. Bruneton J. Pharmacognosy, Phytochemistry, Medicinal Plants. Secaucus, New York, Lavoisier Publishing, Inc, 1995.
5. Pittler MH, Ernst E. Peppermint for irritable bowel syndrome: A critical review and meta-analysis. Am J Gastroenterol 1998; 93:1131–1135.
6. Olsol A, Pratt R, Gennaro AR (eds). The United States Dispensatory, 27th ed. Philadelphia, JB Lippincott Company, 1973.
7. Koch TR. Peppermint oil and irritable bowel syndrome. Am J Gastroenterol 1998;93:2304–2305.
8. Göbel H, Schmidt G, Dworshak M, et al. Essential plant oils and headache mechanisms. Phytomed 1995;2:93–102.

9. Morice AH, Marshall AE, Higgins KS, Grattan TJ. Effect of inhaled menthol on citric acid induced cough in normal subjects. Thorax 1994;49:1024–1026.

10. Holt S. New formulations of dietary supplements can deliver new benefits. Altern Complement Therap 2000;6:15–19.

11. Liu J-H, Chen G-H, Yeh H-Z, et al. Enteric coated peppermint oil capsules in the treatment of irritable bowel syndrome: A prospective randomized trial. J Gastroenterol 1997;32:765–768.

12. Kline RM, Kline JJ, DiPalma J, Barbero GJ. Enteric-coated, pH-dependent peppermint oil capsules for the treatment of irritable bowel syndrome in children. J Pediatr 2001;138:125–128.

13. Sparks MJ, O'Sullivan P, Herrington AA, Morcos SK. Does peppermint oil relieve spasm during barium enema? Br J Radiol 1995;812:841–843.

14. Asao T, Mochiki E, Suzuki H, et al. An easy method for the intraluminal administration of peppermint oil before colonoscopy and its effectiveness in reducing colonic spasm. Gastrointest Endosc 2001;53:172–177.

15. Freise J, Kohler S. Peppermint oil-carraway oil fixed combination in non-ulcer dyspepsia: Comparison of the effects of enteric preparations. [German; Medline Abstract] Pharmazie 1999;54:210–215.

16. May B, Kohler S, Schneider B. Efficacy and tolerability of a fixed combination of peppermint oil and carraway oil in patients suffering from functional dyspepsia. Aliment Pharmacol Ther 2000;14:1671–1677.

17. Madisch A, Heydenreich CJ, Wieland V, et al. Treatment of functional dyspepsia with a fixed peppermint oil and carraway oil combination preparation as compared to cisapride. A multicenter, reference-controlled, double-blind equivalence trial. Arzneimittelforschung 1999;49:425–432.

18. Bowen IH, Cubbin IJ. *Mentha piperita* and *Mentha spicata*. In DeSmet PAGM, Keller K, Hänsel R, Chandler RF (eds): Adverse Effects of Herbal Drugs. Vol. 1, Berlin, Springer-Verlag, 1992, pp 171–178.

19. Tisserand R, Balacs T. Essential Oil Safety. A Guide for Health Care Professionals. Edinburgh, Churchill Livingstone, 1995.

20. Boyd EL. *Hedesma pulegioides* and *Mentha pulegium*. In DeSmet PAGM, Keller K, Hänsel R, Chandler RF (eds): Adverse Effects of Herbal Drugs. Vol. 1, Berlin, Springer-Verlag, 1992, pp 151–156.

21. Bakerink JA, Gospe SM, Dimand RJ, Eldridge MW. Multiple organ failure after ingestion of pennyroyal oil from herbal tea in two infants. Pediatrics 1996;98:944–947.

22. Kawane H. Menthol and aspirin-induced asthma. Respir Med 1996;90:247.

MSM*

rating: 🐝

> - Used for arthritis and other inflammatory
>   disorders
> - Little clinical research documenting effectiveness
> - Adverse effects not adequately defined

MSM, or methylsulfonylmethane, is the oxidation product of DMSO (dimethylsulfoxide). It is known by a variety of other names, including crystalline dimethylsulfoxide, $DMSO_2$, and dimethyl sulfone. MSM is naturally found in fruits, vegetables, grains, and a variety of green plants. It is also found in mammals and has been identified in human milk and urine.

Use: MSM has been employed as a food supplement in animals, and is now commonly advocated in humans for a number of indications, most notably rheumatoid arthritis and osteoarthritis.[1] Proponents also claim MSM can improve the symptoms of a wide variety of diseases including: non-migraine headache, tendinitis, carpal tunnel syndrome, fibromyalgia, asthma, sinusitis, pollen allergies, lupus erythematosus, interstitial cystitis, and scleroderma.[1]

Pharmacology: MSM can act as a sulfur donor in amino acid metabolism.[2] Sulfur is necessary in the formation of connective tissues,[1] and proponents of MSM claim that its sulfur-donating activity could be beneficial in arthritis and other connective tissue diseases. DMSO, initially used as an industrial solvent in paint thinners and antifreeze, was also advocated for a variety of inflammatory disorders in the 1970s and 1980s, although clinical trial results have been inconsistent.[3,4] DMSO is FDA-approved for interstitial cystitis.

The majority of the evidence for MSM comes from animal and *in vitro* studies, which suggests that MSM can reduce synovial proliferation and may have free radical scavenger properties.[1,5] While early animal studies did not support any anti-inflammatory effects,[6,7] one study in mice reported a decrease in inflammatory antibody titers.[5]

Editor's Note: Although not an herb, MSM is a dietary supplement that is included because of its current popularity.

Clinical Trials: Clinical research documenting the effectiveness of MSM in humans is lacking. Only one small, randomized, double-blind clinical trial has been conducted in patients with radiographic evidence of osteoarthritis.[8] MSM was compared to placebo for 4 months; improvements in pain were measured at 4 and 6 weeks. Initially, eight patients received MSM and four received placebo; the authors included additional patients 2 months later. A total of 10 patients received MSM and six placebo. An improvement in pain was reported in 60% of patients who received MSM compared to 20% of those receiving placebo at week 4. While this study is promising, its value is limited by the very small sample size, short monitoring period, and questionable methods of patient enrollment.

Adverse Effects: Anecdotal information suggests that MSM is associated with gastrointestinal upset, diarrhea, and abdominal cramping.[1] MSM does not share the adverse effects of DMSO, such as skin irritation, distinctive odor, ocular toxicity, and peripheral neuropathy,[9–11] but the side effects of MSM have not been adequately studied.

Interactions: There are no known drug interactions, but data is limited.

Cautions: Commercially available MSM is synthesized from DMSO. Since industrial-grade DMSO is often used in preparing MSM, the potential for impurity-induced toxicities exists.[1] Pharmaceutical-grade DMSO should be used (although it may not be) in preparing MSM for human consumption. There are no data with respect to pregnancy and lactation.

Preparations & Doses: Various MSM formulations are available, including tablets (e.g., 500 mg, 750 mg and 1000 mg), powder formulations, eyedrops, eardrops, and topical preparations. In the one available clinical trial, the daily oral dose of MSM was 2250 mg given in divided doses.[8] Two 750-mg capsules were given in the morning on an empty stomach and one 750-mg capsule before lunch. Often MSM is found in combination with other dietary supplements such as glucosamine sulfate and chondroitin sulfate; the value and safety of these combinations have not been studied.

Summary Evaluation

There is not enough evidence to support the use of MSM in patients with rheumatoid arthritis and osteoarthritis, or for any other indication. Adequate clinical assessment of safety and effectiveness has not been published. MSM is favored over DMSO because it is considered less toxic; however, DMSO, after considerable popularity 20 years ago, has failed to establish itself as a useful agent for similar indications.

---

references

1. Kolasinski SL. Dimethylsulfoxide (DMSO) and methylsulfonylmethane (MSM) and for the treatment of arthritis. Altern Med Alert 3:115–119, 2000.
2. Richmond VL. Incorporation of methylsulfonyl-methane sulfur into guinea pig serum proteins. Life Sci 39:263–268, 1986.
3. Cronin JR. Methylsulfonylmethane: Nutraceutical of the next century. Alt Complement Ther 12:386–389, 1999.
4. Bennett RM, Kappes J, Kessler S, et al. Dimethyl sulfoxide does not suppress an experimental model of arthritis in rabbits. J Rheumatol 10:533–538, 1983.
5. Trentham DE, Rowland D. Dimethyl sulfoxide does not suppress the clinical manifestations of collagen arthritis. J Rheumatol 10:114–116, 1983.
6. Freeman GR. DMSO in otology. Laryngoscope 86:921–929, 1976.
7. Percy EC, Carson JD. The use of DMSO in tennis elbow and rotator cuff tendinitis: A double-blind study. Med Sci Sports Exerc 13:215–219, 1981.
8. Lawrence RM. Methylsulfonylmethane: A double-blind study of its use in degenerative arthritis. Int J Anti Aging Med 1:50, 1998.
9. Reinstein L, Mahon R Jr, Russo GL. Peripheral neuropathy after concomitant dimethyl sulfoxide use and sulindac therapy. Arch Phys Med Rehabil 63:581–584, 1982.
10. Swanson BN, Ferguson RK, Raskin NH, Wolf BA. Peripheral neuropathy after concomitant administration of dimethyl sulfoxide and sulindac. Arthritis Rheum 26:791–793, 1983.
11. Noel PRB, Barnett KC, Davies RE, et al. The toxicity of dimethyl sulphoxide (DMSO) for the dog, pig, rat and rabbit. Toxicology 3:143–169, 1975.

Mullein (*Verbascum densiflorum*)

rating: 🐾

> - Used mainly for coughs and sore throats, and as an expectorant
> - Clinical value not established

Common mullein, *Verbascum densiflorum* or *V. thapsus*, is known by many names, such as flannel flower and lungwort. The herb is indigenous to Europe and North Africa, but is also found in Asia and America, where the spiked, flowering heads are visible at roadsides. The yellow flowers are popular in herbal preparations, but the flannel-like leaves and the roots are also employed.

Uses: Mullein has traditionally been used especially to treat coughs and to aid expectoration; these applications are similar to those for the better-known coltsfoot. Mullein also has been given for multiple other indications,[1] but currently it is of minor importance. It remains popular in some countries, including Mexico, as a soothing, demulcent treatment for asthma, bronchitis, throat irritation, and cough. It was formerly recommended for rheumatic disorders and wound therapy, and as a diuretic.[1] Other traditional uses include skin infections and inflammation, bruises, burns, gout, ear infections, and hemorrhoids.[2] It is allowed as a flavoring in alcoholic beverages in the United States.[3]

Pharmacology: The main constituent, a polysaccharide mucilage, may account for 2–3% of the herbal product. It is said to be soothing to the respiratory mucosa.[4] It may soothe the oropharyngeal receptors that mediate coughs in upper respiratory infections, but there is no evidence that tracheobronchial tree receptors are similarly affected. Other compounds include flavonoids, glycosides, tannins, and iridoids.[1] Verbascoside is a unique iridoid glycoside that can inhibit aldose reductase and 5-lipoxygenase; as a consequence, it may have anti-inflammatory and antioxidant properties.[5]

Other relevant components are various saponins (such as songarosaponins) and bitter amorphous substances.[2] These agents may cause reflex expectoration through gastric stimulation.[6]

In vitro studies suggest that mullein may have antiviral effects,[2,7] and it may potentiate the anti-influenza virus action of amantadine in tissue culture.[7]

Clinical Trials: No controlled clinical studies have been carried out on mullein or its individual constituents.

Adverse Effects: Adverse reactions have not been reported, and are unlikely to result when conventional doses are used.

Interactions: No drug interactions are recognized.[8]

Cautions: A mullein herbal preparation from the flowers, called gordolobo yerba in Mexico, was reported to have been contaminated with *Senecio longilobus*, which contains hepatotoxic pyrrolizidine alkaloids.[9]

Preparations & Doses: Infusions can be made from mullein, and a total dose of 3–4 g/day of the dried flowers or leaves has been recommended.[1] Similar or smaller amounts of mullein are recommended for herbal teas; fluid extracts and tinctures are also available.[8]

––––––––––––––– **Summary Evaluation** –––––––––––––––

Mullein is a harmless herb that is mainly used as a throat lozenge and mild cough suppressant, and for its possible expectorant effect. It has not been clinically studied, and it is unlikely to be of significant value.

references

1. Bisset NG, Wichtl M (eds): Herbal Drugs and Phytopharmaceuticals, 2nd ed. Boca Raton, CRC Press, 1994.
2. Mullein. The Review of Natural Products. St. Louis, MO, Facts and Comparisons, April 1998.
3. McGuffin M, Hobbs C, Upton R, Goldberg A (eds): Botanical Safety Handbook. Boca Raton, CRC Press, 1997.
4. Peirce A: The American Pharmaceutical Association Practical Guide to Natural Medicines. New York, William Morrow and Company, 1999.
5. Bruneton J: Pharmacognosy, Phytochemistry, Medicinal Plants. Secaucus, NY, Lavoisier Publishing Inc, 1995.
6. Ziment I (ed): Practical Pulmonary Disease. New York, John Wiley and Sons, 1983.
7. Serredjieva S: Combined anti-influenza virus activity of flos verbasci infusion and amantadine derivatives. Phytother Res 14:571–574, 2000.
8. Blumenthal M, Goldberg A, Brinckmann J (eds): Herbal Medicine. Expanded Commission E Monographs. Newton, MA, Integrative Medicine Communications, 2000.
9. De Smet PAGM: Toxicological outlook on the quality assurance of herbal remedies. In De Smet PAGM, Keller K, Hänsel R, Chandler RF (eds): Adverse Effects of Herbal Drugs. Vol. 1. Berlin, Springer Verlag 1992, pp 1–72.

Nettle (*Urtica dioica*)

rating: 🐿️🐿️ +

- Commonly used for arthritis pains, allergies, BPH, or as a diuretic
- Results of clinical trials promising, but benefits unproven
- Appears to be safe and well tolerated

Urtica dioica, commonly called nettle, nettles, or stinging nettle, is often regarded as a noxious weed. *Urtica* comes from the latin *urere*, meaning "to burn," and is the source of the medical term urticaria. Direct contact with the mature plant can break off tiny trichomes or hairs on the leaves and stems, injecting chemicals into the skin that cause long-lasting irritation and stinging. The flowering plant and its roots are used medicinally, and the toxic trichomes are destroyed in processing.

Uses: Nettle is predominately employed in Western cultures for the treatment of arthritis pain, allergies, and benign prostatic hypertrophy (BPH). In European herbal traditions, it is also considered to have diuretic properties. Historical and folk uses of nettle include treatment for diarrhea, constipation, asthma, pleurisy, and eczema; it has also been used as an astringent or hemostatic for nose bleeds, uterine hemorrhage, and the like.[1-4] The leaves are used for their analgesic, anti-inflammatory, and diuretic properties, while the root is used for its antiproliferative effect on prostatic cells.

Pharmacology: The major constituents of the leaves include organic acids (e.g., carbonic, formic, citric), amines, and flavonoid compounds.[2] The stinging source of nettle is in the leaf and stem glandular hairs, which contain acetylcholine, serotonin, formic acid, and histamine.[5] The roots contain β-sitosterol and other sterols, lectins, polysaccharides, hydroxycoumarins and lignans.[1–2] In addition, the plant is rich in amino acids, vitamins, and other nutrients.[6]

Nettle extracts can partially inhibit prostaglandin and leukotriene synthesis *in vitro*,[2,3] and have been found to inhibit specific inflammatory mediators such as IL-2, IFN-gamma, and NF-kappaB.[7,8]

A decreased release of lipopolysaccharide-stimulated TNF-alpha and IL-1 was demonstrated in blood from human volunteers taking a nettle leaf extract, but other *in vitro* effects were not validated.[4]

Hormonally responsive prostate tissue is altered in subjects using nettle root extracts, and this has been attributed to several compounds present in the root.[2,3] A steroidal-like hydrophobic compound inhibits Na^+/K^+-ATPase, which can suppress prostatic cell growth.[9] Lignans inhibit the binding of sex hormone–binding globulin (SHBG) to androgens,[10,11] and nettle decreases SHBG serum levels in controlled studies.[2] Specific compounds may also inhibit 5-alpha-reductase or aromatase activity in the prostate, blocking the formation of dihydrotestosterone or estradiol, respectively.[2,3] Further, polysaccharide fractions of methanolic extracts have anti-proliferative effects on prostate epithelia.[12,13]

A diuretic effect was observed in rats after intravenous or intraperitoneal injections of a nettle extract,[14,15] but no effect was observed after oral administration.[15] Parenteral administration of nettle extracts can also cause depression of the central nervous system (CNS), hypotension, and bradycardia in animals.[1,14,15]

Clinical Trials: Many of these studies have been performed in Germany.

• Arthritis—The anti-inflammatory/analgesic property of nettle leaf has been used for arthritis symptoms.[16] Topical application appeared to be beneficial in a randomized controlled trial (RCT) for base-of-thumb osteoarthritis; however, the double-blinding (which is difficult to provide for a stinging preparation) was incomplete.[17] Oral preparations were reported to be beneficial in four German studies, primarily in terms of NSAID dose reduction. However, the quality of these studies is questionable because only two were controlled, one randomized, and none blinded.[4,18]

• Allergies—For the treatment of allergic rhinitis, a double-blind RCT in the U.S. evaluated the effect of an orally administered freeze-dried preparation for 1 week.[19] Global assessments of subjective effectiveness were favorable after therapy was completed, but personal diary data revealed only a slightly better outcome than placebo. The large drop-out rate (mainly in the nettle group), unclear dosing, and lack of statistical analysis weaken the results of this study.

• Benign Prostatic Hypertrophy—For the treatment of BPH symptoms, root extracts have been reported to be beneficial in at least 8 uncontrolled studies, lasting from 3 weeks to 20 months.[4,6]

Five double-blind placebo-controlled trials published in German have been summarized by others.[2,4,20] The first study, published in 1982, found that objective improvements from nettle were no better than placebo. However, four subsequent studies found nettle products to be more effective than placebo in increasing urine flow, decreasing residual urine volume, and decreasing urinary frequency. Beneficial effects were usually observed in a few weeks to months, but methodologic strengths or weaknesses of these studies have not been evaluated. Two long-term European double-blind RCTs of products combined with saw palmetto also found beneficial effects for BPH.[21,22] In contrast, a recent U.S. double-blind RCT of a combination saw palmetto-nettle root extract (80 mg) taken t.i.d. for 6 months found no symptomatic benefits in men with BPH compared to placebo.[23] The dose of nettle root extract was significantly less than in the positive studies.

• Diuresis—Although nettle has been widely considered to have diuretic properties, only one German study has evaluated this effect clinically. In an uncontrolled trial of 32 patients with heart failure or venous insufficiency, the oral use of nettle's fresh sap or juice over a 14 day-period was reported to significantly increase urine output.[24] The details and methods of this study are not available in English.

Adverse Effects: Nettle is well tolerated; side effects are generally similar to placebo in the controlled studies. Mild gastrointestinal irritation has been reported, but is uncommon.[1,2,4]

Interactions: Because nettle extract has CNS-depressant effects in rodent toxicity studies, some authorities warn against concomitant use with CNS depressants. However, it is doubtful that these results apply to humans; there are no reported adverse CNS effects or drug interactions with nettle in the herbal or medical literature.

Cautions: Uteroactivity has been reported in pregnant and non-pregnant mice,[1] so caution is warranted in pregnant and breast-feeding women. Herbalists have generally found no adverse effects in these populations, however.[3]

Preparations & Doses: Multiple preparations and formulations of nettle are available, and controlled studies have examined different oral dosing regimens. For the anti-inflammatory effect in acute arthritis, 1340 mg/day of a powdered extract or 50 g/day of stewed nettle leaf was used.[4] For allergic rhinitis, two 300-mg capsules of freeze-dried stinging nettle were dosed 1–7 times per day (mean t.i.d.).[19] For BPH, typical doses are 300–600 mg b.i.d. of a methanol extract of the root.[4] In the herbalist literature, 2–5 g t.i.d. of dried herb is usually taken as an infusion or extract.[1,24] Topical application of the fresh leaf can be an effective analgesic, as long as the nettle produces a stinging sensation with wheals (it may act as a simple counterirritant), and treatment is repeated daily for several days.[16]

Summary Evaluation

Several clinical trials have found nettle to be beneficial for arthritis pain and BPH symptoms, but poorly designed or unknown study methodology limits the potential benefits reported in these investigations. Minimal clinical evidence is available for the use of nettle in allergic rhinitis and as a diuretic. As the use of nettle appears to be safe and well tolerated, it is acceptable for patients to try this herb for mild arthritic, allergic, or BPH symptoms. However, the efficacy for any indication remains unproven.

references

1. Newall CA, Anderson LA, Phillipson JD: Herbal Medicines: A Guide for Health-Care Professionals. London, The Pharmaceutical Press, 1996.
2. European Scientific Cooperative on Phytotherapy: *Urticae radix:* Nettle Exeter, UK, ESCOP, March 1996.
3. Yarnell E: Stinging nettle: A modern view of an ancient healing plant. Altern Complem Ther (June):180–186, 1998.
4. Mills S, Bone K: Principles and Practice of Phytotherapy: Modern Herbal Medicine. Edinburgh, UK, Churchill Livingstone, 2000.
5. McGovern TW, Barkley TM: Botanical briefs: Stinging nettle–*Urtica dioica* L. Cutis 62:63–64, 1998.
6. Bombardelli E, Morazzoni P: *Urtica dioica* L. Fitoterapia 68:387–401, 1997.
7. Klingelhoefer S, Obertreis B, Quast S, Behnke B: Antirheumatic effect of IDS 23, a stinging nettle leaf extract, on *in vitro* expression of T helper cytokines. J Rheumatol 26:2517–2522, 1999.
8. Riehemann K, Behnke B, Schulze-Osthoff K: Plant extracts from stinging nettle (*Urtica dioica*), an antirheumatic remedy, inhibit the proinflammatory transcription factor NF-kappaB. FEBS Lett 442:89–94, 1999.
9. Hirano T, Homma M, Oka K: Effects of stinging nettle root extracts and their steroidal components on the Na^+/K^+-ATPase of the benign prostatic hyperplasia. Planta Med 60:30-33, 1994.
10. Hryb DJ, Khan MS, Romas NA, Rosner W: The effect of extracts of the roots of the stinging nettle (*Urtica dioica*) on the interaction of SHBG with its receptor on human prostatic membranes. Planta Med 61:31–32, 1995.
11. Gansser D, Spiteller G: Plant constituents interfering with human sex hormone-binding globulin. Z Naturforsch 50:98-104, 1995.

12. Konrad L, Müller H-H, Lenz C, et al: Antiproliferative effect on human prostate cancer cells by a stinging nettle root (*Urtica dioica*) extract. Planta Med 66:44–47, 2000.

13. Lichius JJ, Lenz C, Lindemann P, et al. Antiproliferative effect of a polysaccharide fraction of a 20% methanolic extract of stinging nettle roots upon epithelial cells of the human prostate (LNCaP). Pharmazie 54:768–771, 1999.

14. Tahri A, Yamani S, Legssyer A, et al: Acute diuretic, natriuretic, and hypotensive effects of a continuous perfusion of aqueous extract of *Urtica dioica* in the rat. J Ethnopharmacol 73:95–100, 2000.

15. Tita B, Faccendini P, Bello U, et al: *Urtica dioica* L.: Pharmacological effect of ethanol extract. Pharmacol Res 27:21–22, 1993.

16. Randall C, Meethan K, Randall H, Dobbs F: Nettle sting of *Urtica dioica* for joint pain-An exploratory study of this complementary therapy. Complem Therap Med 7:126–131, 1999.

17. Randall C, Randall H, Dobbs F, et al: Randomized controlled trial of nettle sting for treatment of base-of-thumb pain. J Roy Soc Med 93:305–309, 2000.

18. Chrubasik S, Enderlein W, Bauer R, Grabner W: Evidence for antirheumatic effectiveness of herba *Urticae dioicae* in acute arthritis: A pilot study. Phytomed 4:105–108, 1997.

19. Mittman P: Randomized, double-blind study of freeze-dried *Urtica dioica* in the treatment of allergic rhinitis. Planta Med 56(10):44–47, 1990.

20. Schulz V, Hänsel R, Tyler VE: Rational Phytotherapy: A Physician's Guide to Herbal Medicine, 4th ed, New York, Springer, 2001.

21. Metzker H, Kieser M, Hölscher U. Efficacy of a combined Sabal-Urtica preparation in the treatment of benign prostatic hyperplasia. Urologe[B] 36:292–300, 1996. [English translation]

22. Sökeland J, Albrecht J: A combination of Sabal and Urtica extracts vs. finasteride in BPH (Stage I to II acc. to Alken): A comparison of therapeutic efficacy in a 1-year double-blind study. Urologe[A] 36:327–333, 1997.

23. Marks LS, Partin AW, Epstein JI, et al: Effects of a saw palmetto herbal blend in men with symptomatic benign prostatic hyperplasia. J Urol 163:1451–1456, 2000.

24. Blumenthal M, Goldberg A, Brinckmann J (eds): Herbal Medicine: Expanded Commission E Monographs. Newton, MA, Integrative Medicine Communications, 2000.

Papaya (*Carica papaya*)

rating: 🐾 🐾

- Used orally as a digestive aid, for dyspepsia, and for inflammation; topically applied to wounds
- Older clinical trials suggest benefits in post-traumatic inflammation and pain; studies require verification
- Relatively safe and well tolerated in usual doses

Found in tropical countries, the papaya tree is also known as the pawpaw or melon tree. The seeds, leaves, and fruit have all been used in folk medicine. The sap or latex, a milky fluid collected from the mature unripe fruit, is known as crude papain when dried.

Uses: Commercially available papain, a mixture of proteolytic enzymes, is the active ingredient in meat tenderizers; it softens the meat by partially digesting the proteins. Contained in contact lens cleansers, dentifrices, and cosmetics, the enzyme is also used to clarify beer.[1] Papain is available in FDA-approved topical preparations as an enzymatic debridement for necrotic tissue in burns, ulcers, and other wounds. A specific purified fraction, chymopapain, is approved for chemonucleosis (the treatment of herniated intervertebral discs by injection), which has largely fallen out of favor due to allergic and other adverse reactions.[2]

As an herbal dietary supplement, oral papain is most often recommended as a digestive aid (especially with protein-rich meals) and for dyspepsia.[1] Papaya preparations have also been used traditionally for inflammatory disorders, hemorrhoids, intestinal worms, diarrhea, tumors, and respiratory infections.[1,3,4] It is used in some cultures to induce abortion and labor, and is employed topically for psoriasis, ringworm, wounds, ulcers, and infections.[5]

Pharmacology: Crude papain, also called "vegetable pepsin," is an enzyme mixture from the dried latex of the fruit, and is also found in the leaves and trunk.[1] It is composed of related proteolytic enzymes: papain, chymopapain A and B, and papaya peptidase.[1,3] The purified papain enzyme is a thiol protease, obtaining enzymatic activity from the sulfhydryl group of the cysteine residue.[1] It is poorly active in extreme acidic or basic media, can be digested by pepsin, and is poorly absorbed when ingested orally[3,4]; thus, it may have unpredictable activity when exposed to gastric contents. Papain hydrolyzes proteins, small peptidases, amides, and some esters.[1]

Papaya latex has fungicidal activity: isolated enzymes with fungicidal properties include alpha-D-mannosidase and N-acetyl-ß -D-glucosaminidase.[6,7] The latex has been studied in combination with fluconazole, demonstrating a synergistic effect *in vitro* against *Candida albicans*.[8] Antihelminthic properties have been demonstrated for both the seeds and latex *in vitro*[9,10] and in animal models.[11,12] The chief antihelminthic constituent in the seeds appears to be benzyl isothiocyanate.[13] Variable antibacterial activity *in vitro* has also been found in the leaves, seeds, and fruit.[14,15]

In animal models, diuretic and hypotensive activity has been reported for the root and unripened fruit extracts, respectively.[16,17] Papain preparations protect against experimental ulcers.[18] Seed extracts affect sperm viability and have antifertility properties in various male animal models; extracts are being evaluated for their potential as a male contraceptive.[19,20]

Clinical Trials: The use of oral papain tablets has been evaluated in several older, controlled clinical trials for post-traumatic inflammation. In double-blind trials of patients undergoing oral or head and neck surgeries,[21–25] abdominal surgeries,[26] and episiotomies,[27] papaya proteolytic enzyme tablets appeared to reduce postoperative edema, inflammation, or pain when compared to placebo. In a randomized, single-blind study in 129 patients undergoing oral surgery, papaya enzyme tablets were more effective than placebo, but less effective than prednisolone 20 mg/day for postsurgical pain and trismus.[28] In a randomized, double-blind trial of 125 college athletes with contusions or related injuries, papaya enzyme tablets produced a better therapeutic response and less disability than placebo tablets.[29] The results of several of these studies are questionable, however, because the criteria for the inflammatory signs or pain were subjective, and the study methodologies or results were not well described. In addition, there have been no confirmatory studies in several decades.

In a recent trial from India, patients undergoing radiation therapy for head and neck cancer were given an oral proprietary product (Wobe-Mugos; 3 tablets t.i.d. for 7 weeks), which contained 60 mg of papain along with other enzymes such as bromelain, trypsin, chymotrypsin, and pancreatin.[30] Compared to a control group who received no supplements, significantly less mucositis and dysphagia from radiation therapy was reported in the treatment group. In German controlled clinical trials, enzyme mixtures containing papain given as throat lozenges were reported to be beneficial for pharyngitis, and one study demonstrated benefits of a papain mixture for herpes zoster infection.[31] Oral papain enzymes, most commonly administered as a dilute solution of Adolph's meat tenderizer, have been used with some success in the medical treatment of gastric bezoars,[32,33] but have not been evaluated in controlled trials.

Papaya extracts administered topically or by injection have been evaluated in limited clinical trials. In a study from Gambia, a crude topical papaya paste (mashed pulp of the papaya fruit) was applied to the dressings of 32 children with full-thickness or infected burns once or twice daily.[34] In this uncontrolled study, the papaya paste was reported to effectively debride the wounds, obviating the need for surgical debridement prior to surgery. In another uncontrolled study, 10 patients received intralesional injections of papaya latex into their keloid scars every 21 days; a marked regression of up to 90% in keloid size was reported.[35]

Adverse Effects: There are no significant side effects reported from the clinical studies using oral papaya enzyme tablets. Griping and "intestinal inflammation" from ingestion of the fresh latex has been reported in older accounts.[4]

Interactions: A papaya extract used as a slimming aid was reported to possibly enhance the effect of warfarin.[36] The patient was admitted for cardiac surgery and found to have an INR of 7.4, which declined after withdrawal of both warfarin and the extract. Further details of the case are unknown.

Cautions: Allergic reactions, including angioedema and anaphylaxis, have been reported with a variety of papain products.[4,37] Positive skin tests and allergic reactions to papain can be demonstrated in 1% of individuals with allergies to other substances.[38] Solutions of meat tenderizer used for gastric bezoars, which may not have been sufficiently dilute, have been reported to cause gastric ulcer, esophageal perforation, and hypernatremia.[32,39] Crude papain orally administered to rats has been reported to be embryotoxic and teratogenic,[40] while no detrimental effects were observed with a purified papain enzyme.[41] Use during pregnancy and lactation is not recommended due to the limited data.

Preparations & Doses: A typical dose of 1–2 papaya/papain enzyme tablets administered q.i.d. for about 3–7 days was used in the clinical studies to reduce inflammation. Several of these older studies used Papase, a product formerly manufactured by Warner-Chilcott Laboratories, which contained 5 mg or 10,000 Warner-Chilcott units (of milk-clotting activity) per tablet. Activity of papain is expressed in many ways, depending on the supplier.[1,2] Doses of commercial papain products, often recommended as a digestive aid, vary widely between 10 and 1000 mg per day, usually given as 1–4 pills with or after meals. The fresh fruit juice or leaf infusions are also advocated.

Summary Evaluation

Papaya enzymes can hydrolyze protein and are commonly employed as meat tenderizers and wound cleansers. As a dietary supplement, papaya enzymes are used as a digestive aid or to treat dyspepsia, but there are no clinical trials to substantiate these effects. There is *in vitro* and animal data to support some of papaya's traditional indications, such as for helminthic and fungal infections; these potential properties have also not been evaluated in clinical studies. A number of controlled clinical trials suggest that orally administered papaya enzymes can help to reduce post-traumatic pain and inflammation; however, these older studies (as well as other reported uses) require validation. Papain is poorly active in the gastric contents and may not be appreciably absorbed.

references

1. Leung AY, Foster S. Encyclopedia of Common Natural Ingredients used in Food, Drugs, and Cosmetics, 2nd ed. New York, John Wiley & Sons, Inc, 1996.
2. Parfitt K (ed). Martindale: The Complete Drug Reference. London, Pharmaceutical Press, 1999.
3. Blumenthal M (ed). The Complete German Commission E Monographs: Therapeutic Guide to Herbal Medicines. Boston, Integrative Medicine Communications, 1998.
4. Hwang K, Ivy AC. A review of the literature on the potential therapeutic significance of papain. Ann NY Acad Sci 1951;54:161–207.
5. Hewitt H, Whittle S, Lopez S, et al. Topical use of papaya in chronic skin ulcer therapy in Jamaica. West Indian Med J 2000;49:32–33.

6. Giordani R, Siepaio M, Moulin-Traffort J, Régli P. Antifungal action of *Carica papaya* latex: Isolation of fungal cell wall hydrolysing enzymes. Mycoses 1991;34:469–477.

7. Giordani R, Cardenas ML, Moulin-Traffort J, Régli P . Fungicidal activity of latex sap from *Carica papaya* and antifungal effect of D(+)-glucosamine on *Candida albicans* growth. Mycoses 1996;39:103–110.

8. Giordani R, Gachon C, Moulin-Traffort J, Régli P. A synergistic effect of *Carica papaya* latex sap and fluconazole on *Candida albicans* growth. Mycoses 1997;40:429–437.

9. Lal J, Chandra S, Raviprakash V, Sabir M. *In vitro* anthelmintic action of some indigenous medicinal plants on *Ascaridia galli* worms. Ind J Physiol Pharmac 1976;20(2):64–68.

10. Tona L, Kambu K, Ngimbi N, et al. Antiamoebic and phytochemical screening of some Congolese medicinal plants. J Ethnopharmacol 1998;61:57-65.

11. Satrija F, Nansen P, Bjørn H, et al. Effect of papaya latex against *Ascaris suum* in naturally infected pigs. J Helminthol 1994;68:343-346.

12. Satrija F, Nansen P, Murtini S, He S. Anthelminthic activity of papaya latex against patent *Heligmosomoides polygyrus* infections in mice. J Ethnopharmacol 1995;48:161–164.

13. Kermanshai R, McCarry BE, Rosenfeld J, et al. Benzyl isothiocyanate is the chief or sole anthelmintic in papaya seed extracts. Phytochem 2001;57:427–435.

14. Osato JA, Santiago LA, Remo GM, et al. Antimicrobial and antioxidant activities of unripe papaya. Life Sci 1993;53:1383–1389.

15. Thomas OO. Re-examination of the antimicrobial activities of *Xylopia aethiopica*, *Carica papaya*, *Ocimum gratissimum* and *Jatropha curcas*. Fitoterapia 1989;60:147–155.

16. Sripanidkulchai B, Wongpanich V, Laupattarakasem P, et al. Diuretic effects of selected Thai indigenous medicinal plants in rats. J Ethnopharmacol 2001;75:185–190.

17. Eno AE, Owo OI, Itam EH, Konya RS. Blood pressure depression by the fruit juice of *Carica papaya* (L.) in renal and DOCA-induced hypertension in the rat. Phytother Res 2000;14:235–239.

18. Chen C-F, Chen S-M, Chow S-Y, Han PW. Protective effects of *Carica papaya* Linn. on the exogenous gastric ulcer in rats. Am J Chin Med 1981;9:205–212.

19. Lohiya NK, Pathak N, Mishra PK, Manivannan B. Reversible contraception with chloroform extract of *Carica papaya* Linn. seeds in male rabbits. Reprod Toxicol 1999;13:59–66.

20. Pathak N, Mishra PK, Manivannan B, Lohiya NK. Sterility due to inhibition of sperm motility by oral administration of benzene chromatographic fraction of the chloroform extract of the seeds of *Carica papaya* in rats. Phytomed 2000;7:325–333.

21. Vallis CP, Lund MH. Effect of treatment with *Carica papaya* on resolution of edema and ecchymosis following rhinoplasty. Curr Therap Res 1969;11:356–359.

22. Lund MH, Royer RR. *Carica papaya* in head and neck surrgery. Arch Surg 1969;98:180–182.

23. Magnes GD. Proteolytic enzymes in oral surgery. J Am Dental Assoc 1966;72:1420–1425.

24. Metro PS, Horton RB. Plant enzymes in oral surgery. Oral Surg Oral Med Oral Path 1965;19:309–316.

25. Yarrington CT, Bestler JM. A double-blind evaluation of enzyme preparation in postoperative patients. Clin Med 1964;71:710–712.

26. Thorek P, Pandit JK. Proteolytic enzymes in wound repair: Immediate postoperative effects. Applied Therapeut 1964;6:323–325.

27. Boutselis JG, Sollars RJ. The effect of proteolytic enzymes on episiotomy pain and swelling. Ohio State Med J 1964;60:551–553.

28. Caci F, Gluck GM. Double-blind study of prednisolone and papase as inhibitors of complications after oral surgery. J Am Dental Assoc 1976;93: 325–327.

29. Holt HT. *Carica papaya* as ancillary therapy for athletic injuries. Curr Therap Res 1969;11:621–624.

30. Kaul R, Mishra BK, Sutradar P, et al. The role of Wobe-Mugos in reducing acute sequele of radiation in head and neck cancers: A clinical phase III randomized trial. Ind J Cancer 1999;36:141–148.

31. Papain. Natural Medicines Comprehensive Database. Accessed July 8, 2001 at www.naturaldatabase.com/monograph

32. Zarling EJ, Moeller DD. Bezoar therapy: Complication using Adolph's meat tenderizer and alternatives from literature review. Arch Intern Med 1981; 141:1669–1670.

33. Dwivedi AJ, Chahin F, Agrawal S, et al. Gastric phytobezoar treatment using meat tenderizer. Dig Dis Sci 2001;46:1013–1015.

34. Starley IF, Mohammed P, Schneider G, Bickler SW. The treatment of paediatric burns using topical papaya. Burns 1999;25:636–639.

35. Ahmad K. Regression in keloid scar by intralesional injection of papaya milk. Br J Plast Surg 1998;51:261.

36. Shaw D, Leon C, Kolev S, Murray V. Traditional remedies and food supplements: A 5-year toxicological study (1991–1995). Drug Safety 1997;17: 342–356.

37. Bernstein DI, Gallagher JS, Grad M, Bernstein IL. Local ocular anaphylaxis to papain enzyme contained in a contact lens cleansing solution. J Allergy Clin Immunol 1984;74:258–260.

38. Mansfield LE, Ting S, Haverly RW, Yoo TJ. The incidence and clinical implications of hypersensitivity to papain in an allergic population, confirmed by blinded oral challenge. Ann Allergy 1985;55:541–543.

39. Holsinger JW, Fuson RL, Sealy WC. Esophageal perforation following meat impaction and papain ingestion. JAMA 1968;204:188–189.

40. Singh S, Devi S. Teratogenic and embryotoxic effect of papain in rat. Indian J Med Res 1978;67:499–510.

41. Schmidt H. Effect of papain on different phases of prenatal ontogenesis in rats. Reprod Toxicol 1995;9:49–55.

Passion Flower (*Passiflora incarnata*)

rating: 🐌

> - Commonly used as a sedative-hypnotic or anxiolytic herb; clinical trials not performed
> - Considered mild and safe with usual doses, but isolated adverse reactions reported

There are over 400 species of passion flower (genus Passiflora), which are also known as maypop, apricot vine, or passion vine. The dried, leafy, aerial parts of the *P. incarnata* species have been most frequently used medicinally.

Uses: Passion flower is promoted as a mild herbal anxiolytic, sedative, and hypnotic. It is a popular ingredient in many European sedative-hypnotic herbal combination products (often with valerian, lemon balm, and other herbs).[1–4] Herbalists have also used passion flower for neuralgia, seizures, hysteria, and various physiologic disorders of presumed nervous origin—whenever a "calming" action is desired. Passion flower was included in over-the-counter (OTC) sedative and sleep aids in the United States until 1978, when the FDA banned it due to lack of proven effectiveness.

Pharmacology: *P. incarnata* contains flavonoids (e.g., vitexin and isovitexin), small amounts of indole or harmala alkaloids (harman and related compounds), and maltol, all of which have pharmacologic activity in animal models.[1,2,4] In most rodent studies, herbal extracts administered orally and by injection have sedative or hypnotic activity.[1,5] Harmala alkaloids have CNS activity (including psychedelic properties when given in large amounts); interact with a variety of neuroreceptor systems; and are inhibitors of the monoamine oxidase (MAO) enzyme.[6,7] Chrysin, thought to be a flavonoid component of a related Passiflora species (*P. coerulea*), binds to benzodiazepine receptors and has anxiolytic actions in mice[8–10]; however, chrysin may not be found in *P. incarnata*.[11]

Clinical Trials: Passion flower has only been studied in combination products with other potentially sedative-hypnotic herbs or drugs; thus, the efficacy of passion flower itself is unknown. Euphytose, a European product that combines *P. incarnata* with several other herbal sedatives (including valerian), was found to have statistically beneficial anxiolytic properties in a double-blind, placebo-controlled study.[12] In contrast, a European controlled study comparing a single oral dose of Valverde (*P. incarnata*, valerian, balm, and pestilence wort) with 3 mg of bromazepam found that both were no more effective than placebo.[13]

Compoz, formerly a popular U.S. OTC product that contained *P. incarnata* (as well as scopolamine and antihistamines), was found to have equivalent anxiolytic effects to placebo in one study; however, the amount of Passiflora in 3 tablets of Compoz was 22.5 mg, a daily dose that was probably negligible.[14] Compoz has been removed from the market.

Despite having CNS effects in rodents, an aqueous extract from a related Passiflora species, *P. edulis*, had no sedative-hypnotic effects in nine healthy volunteers.[15]

Adverse Effects: In general, passion flower is considered to be safe and nontoxic, and dependence and withdrawal have not been reported.[1–3] However, there are isolated case reports of adverse reactions. Five patients required hospitalization due to unresponsiveness or altered consciousness associated with overdoses (100–600 ml) of a *P. incarnata* product (Relaxir; usual dose 2 teaspoons) used in Norway.[16] One patient appeared to respond to flumazenil. In Australia, a 34-year-old female developed severe nausea, vomiting, drowsiness, prolonged QTc on EKG, and episodes of nonsustained ventricular tachycardia associated with initiation of a *P. incarnata* product (Sedacalm) at therapeutic doses.[17] Lastly, a patient with rheumatoid arthritis developed a cutaneous hypersensitivity reaction associated with the use of an oral extract.[18] Product adulteration or contamination may have been responsible for these disparate reactions.

Other species of Passiflora have been implicated in toxicities. An aqueous extract of *P. edulis* caused abnormal elevations of aspartate aminotransferase (AST) and amylase in several healthy volunteers.[15] Old reports that passion flower contains toxic cyanogenic glycosides are probably referring to the ornamental blue passion flower, *P. coerulea*, and not to *P. incarnata*.[19]

Interactions: Although pure harmala alkaloids have MAO inhibitor activity in animal experiments,[7] adverse reactions or interactions in humans using passion flower have not been reported. Newer studies have shown that only trace amounts of the alkaloids are contained in the herb (< 0.1 ppm),[20] and thus doses used clinically should not have MAO inhibitor activity.

Cautions: Safety in pregnant and breast-feeding women has not been evaluated.

Preparations & Doses: The usual recommended dose is about 500–2000 mg of dried herb, or 300–400 mg of commonly prepared extracts, 3–4 times daily, or as needed.[1–3]

--- **Summary Evaluation** ---

Passion flower is commonly used as a mild anxiolytic, sedative, and hypnotic herb, properties which have been demonstrated only with large doses in animal studies. Beneficial activity in humans has not been adequately evaluated at therapeutic doses, and evidence-based recommendations cannot be made. Available information suggests that effects are likely to be mild in usual doses, and can only be regarded as possibly beneficial for minor problems of anxiety or insomnia.

references

1. European Scientific Cooperative on Phytotherapy (ESCOP): Passiflorae herba: Passiflora. Monographs on the medicinal uses of plant drugs. Exeter, UK, ESCOP, July 1997.
2. Newall CA, Anderson LA, Phillipson JD: Herbal Medicines: A Guide for Health-Care Professionals. London, The Pharmaceutical Press, 1996.
3. Blumenthal M, Goldberg A, Brinckmann J (eds): Herbal Medicine: Expanded Commission E Monographs. Newton, MA, Integrative Medical Communications, 2000.
4. Passion Flower. The Review of Natural Products. St. Louis, MO, Facts and Comparisons, March 1999.
5. Speroni E, Billi R, Mercati V, et al: Sedative effects of crude extract of *Passiflora incarnata* after oral administration. Phytotherapy Res 10:S92–S94, 1996.
6. Ergene E, Schoener EP: Effects of harmane (1-methyl-beta-carboline) on neurons in the nucleus accumbens of the rat. Pharmacol Biochem Behav 44:951–957, 1993.
7. Rommelspacher H, May T, Salewski B: Harman (1-methyl-beta-carboline) is a natural inhibitor of monoamine oxidase type A in rats. Eur J Pharmacol 252:51–59, 1994.
8. Medina JH, Paladini AC, Wolfman C, et al: Chrysin (5,7-di-OH-flavone), a naturally occurring ligand for benzodiazepine receptors, with anticonvulsant properties. Biochem Pharmacol 40:2227–2231, 1990.
9. Wolfman C, Viola H, Paladini A, et al: Possible anxiolytic effects of chrysin, a central benzodiazepine receptor ligand isolated from *Passiflora coerulea*. Pharmacol Biochem Behav 47:1–4, 1994.
10. Zanoli P, Avallone R, Baraldi M: Behavioral characterisation of the flavonoids apigenin and chrysin. Fitoterapia 71:S117-S123, 2000.

11. Speroni E, Billi R, Perellino NC, Minghetti A: Role of chrysin in the sedative effects of *Passiflora incarnata* L. Phytotherapy Res 10:S98–S100, 1996.
12. Bourin M, Bougerol T, Guitton B, Broutin E: A combination of plant extracts in the treatment of outpatients with adjustment disorder with anxious mood: controlled study versus placebo. Fundam Clin Pharmacol 11:127–132, 1997.
13. Gerhard U, Hobi V, Kocher R, König C: Die sedative akutwirkung eines pflanzlichen entspannungsdragées im vergleich zu bromazepam. [The acute sedating effect of a herbal tranquilizer compared to that of bromazepam.] Schweiz Rundsch Med Prax 80:1481–1486, 1991 [English abstract].
14. Rickels K, Hesbacher PT: Over-the-counter daytime sedatives: a controlled study. JAMA 223:29–33, 1973.
15. Maluf E, Borros HMT, Frochtengarten ML, et al. Assessment of the hypnotic/sedative effects and toxicity of *Passiflora edulis* aqueous extract in rodents and humans. Phytotherapy Res 1991;5:262–266.
16. Solbakken AN, Rorbakken G, Gundersen T: Naturmedisin som rusmiddel. [An herbal product used for intoxication.] Tidsskr Nor Laegeforen 117:1140–1141, 1997 [English translation].
17. Fisher AA, Purcell P, Le Couteur DG: Toxicity of *Passiflora incarnata* L. Clin Toxicol 38:63–66, 2000.
18. Smith GW, Chalmers TM, Nuki G: Vasculitis associated with herbal preparation containing Passiflora extract. Br J Rheum 32:87–88, 1993.
19. Foster S, Tyler VE: Tyler's Honest Herbal, 4th ed. Binghamton, NY, Haworth Herbal Press, 1999.
20. Rehwald A, Sticher O, Meier B: Trace analysis of harman alkaloids in *Passiflora incarnata* by reversed-phase high performance liquid chromatography. Phytochem Analysis 6:96–100, 1995.

PC-SPES

rating: 🐾🐾 −

> - A mixture of eight Chinese herbs used for prostate cancer
> - Well documented PSA-lowering effects in clinical studies
> - Adverse effects similar to estrogen or androgen-ablation therapy; include infrequent thromboembolic events

PC-SPES (PC stands for prostate cancer; SPES is the Latin root for hope) is a mixture of concentrated extracts of eight primarily Chinese herbs: *Dendranthema morifolium* (chrysanthemum; ju hua), *Ganoderma lucidum* (reishi mushroom; ling zhi), *Glycyrrhiza glabra* (licorice; gan cao), *Isatis indigotica* (dyer's woad; da ging ye), *Panax pseudoginseng* (sanchi ginseng; san qi), *Rabdosia rubescens* (rabdosia; dong ling cao), *Scutellaria baicalensis* (baikal skullcap; huang qin), and *Serenoa repens* (saw palmetto).

Uses: In the early 1990s, Dr. Sophie Chen, a chemist, formulated PC-SPES with the help of Dr. Allan Wang and colleagues. The herbal remedy was reportedly derived from a recipe handed down by Wang's great-grandfather, a court physician to the emperor of China.[1,2] It was marketed commercially in the U.S. in 1996, and its popularity was initially prompted by anecdotes and testimonials from prostate cancer support groups and internet bulletin boards.[3,4] PC-SPES is specifically used to treat prostate cancer.

Pharmacology: PC-SPES contains many active plant chemicals, including flavonoids, alkaloids, terpenoids, and saponins. Each individual herb has specific anti-neoplastic, anti-inflammatory, or immunomodulatory properties reported in experimental *in vitro* studies. Anti-proliferative effects include inhibition of DNA polymerases, topoisomerases, and signal transduction pathways.[5,6]

Anti-tumor effects of whole PC-SPES extracts have been demonstrated *in vitro* and in animals. These effects include increased apoptotic rate of prostate cancer cells (reduction in cellular viability and growth rate) and suppressed proliferation of other human tumor cell lines; a reduction of prostate tumors in rodents has been found.[1,5,7–9] PC-SPES also has estrogenic activity *in vitro* and in animals[10]; in prostate cancer patients, the herbal mixture can reduce testosterone levels to anorchid levels.[11] Anti-neoplastic activity seems to be greatest in androgen-sensitive tumors, but PC-SPES is also active against some tumors that are refractory to hormones.[5–7] Thus, its estrogenic or hormonal effect may not be its sole mechanism of action. The combination of different herbs may have additive or synergistic anti-neoplastic or phytoestrogenic effects. It is currently unknown which of the eight constituents of PC-SPES are most important.

Clinical Trials: To date, PC-SPES has been evaluated in six relatively small (n = 8–70), uncontrolled, observational studies of prostate cancer patients with both hormone-sensitive and hormone-refractory tumors.[8–13] All trials found significant reductions in PSA serum levels compared to baseline, and most demonstrated treatment-related PSA declines of > 50%, which are known to be associated with improved survival in other studies of prostate cancer treatment.[14]

In hormone-sensitive prostate cancer, PC-SPES appears to be especially effective in reducing PSA levels.[9–11] PSA reductions of > 50% were observed in up to two-thirds of hormone-naive patients in one study using low-doses (3 capsules/day).[9] PSA reductions of > 80% were observed in all 32 patients in another study (to undetectable levels in 81%) using a high dose of 9 capsules/day.[11] No progression of cancer (i.e., new abnormality on bone scan or other evidence of tumor growth) was observed in either study at a median follow-up of 8.5 and 16 months, respectively. In the latter study, 31 of 32 patients also had declines of testosterone to the anorchid range, usually by 2 months.[11]

In hormone-refractory prostate cancer, which typically has a poor prognosis with few therapeutic options, outcomes are not as significant, but are positive for many patients.[9,11–13] In one retrospective study, PSA reductions of > 50% were observed in 12 of 23 patients, with a median duration of PSA response of 2.5 months, and median time to PSA progression of 6 months (time from treatment initiation to PSA increase of more than 50% above the nadir level).[13] In the trial with the longest observation period, PSA reductions of > 50% were observed in 19 of 35 patients with hormone refractory cancer.[11] Median time for the PSA to nadir was 2.5 months, and median time to PSA progression was 4 months; 86 % of patients had disease progression. In a 5-month study of 16 patients with hormone-refractory prostate cancer, PSA reductions of > 50% were observed in 13 patients.[12] Quality-of-life indicators also improved in this latter study, including declines in pain; however, this study was not controlled.

PC-SPES has not been compared to standard therapeutic regimens for prostate cancer. Nevertheless, the PSA reductions appear similar to those demonstrated with conventional chemotherapy for this disease.

Adverse Effects: Side effects are characterized as relatively mild and well tolerated relative to other cancer therapies, and are similar to standard oral estrogen treatment or androgen-ablation therapy.[1] Common adverse effects observed in the clinical trials, which appear to be dose-dependent, include gynecomastia or nipple tenderness (35–100%), decreased libido or erectile dysfunction (100% in two studies), and hot flashes (4–42%).[1,8–13] Mild gastrointestinal effects, leg cramps, and occasional allergic reactions also occur.

Less frequently, thromboembolic events such as superficial phlebitis, deep vein thrombosis (DVT), and pulmonary emboli have been observed (2–6% of patients in the larger studies).[1,8–13] The actual cause-and-effect relationship of this side effect is unknown, as patients with prostate cancer may be at increased baseline risk of hypercoagulable events.

Unlike conventional androgen deprivation therapy, PC-SPES was not associated with a reduction in bone mineral density in a small 1-year study of 15 patients.[15]

Interactions: Although there are no reported drug interactions with PC-SPES, interactions might be expected with other hormonal therapies. Certainly there is a greater potential for interactions compared to that of single herb products, because of the large number of herbs that constitute this preparation.

Cautions: PC-SPES is relatively contraindicated in patients with a history of thromboembolic or significant cardiovascular disease due to the risk of thromboembolic side effects. Some researchers or clinicians recommend aspirin or low-dose warfarin, especially in higher-risk patients, for prophylaxis of thromboembolic complications.[3,12,14] The effectiveness of this approach has not been clinically evaluated.

Preparations & Doses: PC-SPES is marketed (by BotanicLab) in 320-mg capsules containing a proprietary mixture of the eight herbal extracts. The dose administered in the clinical trials is 3–9 capsules/day, typically administered as 1–3 capsules t.i.d. on an empty stomach. Patients and clinicians typically adjust the dosage depending on the severity of the disease, the PSA response, and the side effects of the therapy. The cost of PC-SPES treatment is significant. A bottle of 60 capsules costs $108 when ordered from the manufacturer; at 6–9 capsules/day the monthly cost is $324–486.

———————————— **Summary Evaluation** ————————————

PC-SPES is an herbal mixture that can significantly reduce PSA serum levels and may reduce disease progression in patients with prostate cancer. At least part of its mechanism of action is due to estrogenic or androgen-antagonist activity, which also causes predictable side effects. Significant reductions in PSA are especially observed for patients with hormone-responsive prostate cancer, but the risk of thromboembolism, while small, poses a concern. The risks may be more acceptable for hormone-refractory prostate cancer, in which PC-SPES has less reliable effects on the PSA, but in which conventional options are limited.

However, trials to date have not been controlled, and efficacy compared to other chemotherapeutic regimens, including estrogenic agents, is unknown. Data on long-term survival outcomes and side effects, impact on quality of life, and optimum dosage is limited. This potent herbal therapy, which may offer significant benefits to selected patients with prostate cancer, should be used under the supervision of a qualified physician specialist.

references
1. Ades T, Gansler T, Miller M, Rosenthal DS. PC-SPES: Current evidence and remaining questions. CA Cancer J Clin 2001;51:199–204.
2. Anon. Chinese herbs: The formulation that means hope. PC-SPES for prostate cancer. Integrat Med Consult, Newton, MA, Integrative Medicine Communications, 1999;1(Aug 1):108.
3. Porterfield H. UsToo PC-SPES surveys: Review of studies and update of previous survey results. Molec Urol 2000;4:289-291. [Updated data at www.rootsandsprouts.com/ustoo_survey.htm]
4. PC-SPES Online Support Group. www.pcspes.com.
5. Darzynkiewicz Z, Traganos F, Wu JM, Chen S. Chinese herbal mixture PC SPES in treatment of prostate cancer (review). Intl J Oncology 2000;17:729–736.

6. Geliebter J, Mittelman A, Tiwari RK. PC-SPES and prostate cancer. J Nutr 2001;131:164S–166S.
7. Kubota T, Hisatake J, Hisatake Y, et al. PC-SPES: A unique inhibitor of proliferation of prostate cancer cells in vitro and in vivo. Prostate 2000;42:163–171.
8. de la Taille A, Hayek OR, Buttyan R, et al. Effects of a phytotherapeutic agent, PC-SPES, on prostate cancer: A preliminary investigation on human cell lines and patients. BJU Intl 1999;84:845–850.
9. de la Taille A, Buttyan R, Hayek O, et al. Herbal therapy PC-SPES: In vitro effects and evaluation of its efficacy in 69 patients with prostate cancer. J Urology 2000;164:1229–1234.
10. DiPaola RS, Zhang H, Lambert GH, et al. Clinical and biologic activity of an estrogenic herbal combination (PC-SPES) in prostate cancer. N Engl J Med 1998;339:785–791.
11. Small EJ, Frohlich MW, Bok R, et al. Prospective trial of the herbal supplement PC-SPES in patients with progressive prostate cancer. J Clin Oncol 2000;18:3595–3603.
12. Pfeifer BL, Pirani JF, Hamann SR, Klippel KF. PC-SPES, a dietary supplement for the treatment of hormone-refractory prostate cancer. BJU Intl 2000;85:481–485.
13. Oh WK, George DJ, Hackmann K, et al. Activity of the herbal combination, PC-SPES, in the treatment of patients with androgen-independent prostate cancer. Urology 2001;57:122–126.
14. Stein CA. Medical treatment of hormone refractory disease (In Advances in Prostate Cancer Therapy. Federal Forum). U.S. Med 2000(Suppl):36:8–13, 19–22.
15. Ross RW, Kussmaul S, Small EJ. The effect of the herbal supplement PC-SPES on bone mineral density in men with prostate cancer. Am Soc Clin Oncol, abstract no. 2355, accessed July 4, 2001 at www.asco.org/prof/me/html/01astracts/0020/2355.htm

Pokeroot (*Phytolacca americana*)

rating: 🦠 −

> - An American folk remedy for inflammatory conditions; also used as an emetic/cathartic
> - May cause severe gastrointestinal toxicity; should not be used

Pokeroot, *P. americana* or *P. decandra*, is also referred to as pokeweed, poke, pokeberry, inkberry, and American nightshade. This ubiquitous perennial shrub is found throughout the United States, often in roadside ditches and damp fields.

Uses: Pokeroot was once a popular folk remedy, used orally or topically for inflammatory and rheumatic conditions, itching, headache, lymphadenitis, edema, cancer, and infectious syndromes.[1–4] The dried root was listed in U.S. pharmacopoeias as an official emetic and purgative in the early part of the 20th century. Because this plant can cause severe gastrointestinal toxicity, however, its medicinal use has appropriately waned. Pokeroot accounts for a significant number of plant poisonings each year, and has been on the "top 20" list of the most frequently ingested plants reported to poison control centers.[5]

Pharmacology: Pokeroot contains triterpene saponins, tannins, resins, glycoproteins, and many other components.[1–3] An active glycoprotein lectin called pokeweed mitogen stimulates lymphocytes and can cause hemagglutination. Plasmacytosis, eosinophilia, and platelet phagocytosis can follow internal ingestion or cutaneous exposure through cuts or abrasions.[6–8] An isolated pokeweed antiviral protein has activity against a number of plant and mammalian viruses (including herpes simplex, influenza, and HIV-1) and is being studied in animal models for HIV disease.[9,10] This cytotoxin, covalently linked to specific antibodies to form an immunotoxin, is also being investigated against osteosarcomas and other malignancies.[11]

The saponin fractions have anti-inflammatory activity in animal models, which supports its traditional use for inflammatory conditions.[1,2] However, the saponin content (e.g., phytolaccine) also leads to the adverse gastrointestinal effects of pokeroot, such as vomiting, diarrhea, and abdominal cramping.[6,12] The root itself contains the most active and toxic components, but the leaves, berries, and other plant parts can be toxic as well.[4]

Clinical Trials: The potential medicinal uses of pokeroot as a traditional herbal remedy are historical and anecdotal. Pokeroot has never been studied in controlled clinical trials.

Adverse Effects: Pokeroot poisoning causing acute, self-limited gastroenteritis has been well documented.[6] Emesis and diarrhea have been reported after eating salad discovered to contain pokeroot leaves.[12,13] Pokeroot tea has caused nausea, vomiting, hematemesis, bloody diarrhea, hypotension, and syncope.[14,15] Chewing or ingesting the raw root can cause a similar presentation.[4,16] One patient who ingested raw leaves developed a second-degree heart block (Mobitz type 1), possibly caused by a vagal effect.[17] Rarely, deaths have occurred.[4]

Interactions: No drug interactions are recognized.

Cautions: Young, tender greens that have been parboiled (boiled twice and the water discarded) and mature berries are considered less toxic. However, even these precautions may not eliminate toxicity.[4,12]

Preparations & Doses: Doses of dried root preparations up to 0.2–1 g/day and dilute tinctures and teas have been used in the past.[1,2] A distinction between safe and toxic dosages is difficult, and oral use in general should be considered potentially toxic.

Summary Evaluation

As early as 1979, the Herb Trade Association recognized the toxicity of pokeroot, and recommended that it not be sold without appropriate warnings.[18] It is currently accepted that pokeroot *should not be sold or recommended for any indication*, since the potential for harm outweighs any likely benefit.

references

1. Mills S, Bone K: Principles and Practice of Phytotherapy: Modern Herbal Medicine. Edinburgh, Churchill Livingstone, 2000.
2. Newall CA, Anderson LA, Phillipson JD: Herbal Medicines: A Guide for Health-Care Professionals. London, The Pharmaceutical Press, 1996.
3. Pokeweed. The Lawrence Review of Natural Products. St. Louis, MO, Facts and Comparisons, April 1991.
4. Roberge R, Brader E, Martin ML, et al: The root of evil—pokeweed intoxication. Ann Emerg Med 15:470–473, 1986.

5. Litovitz TL, Holm KC, Bailey KM, Schmitz BF: 1991 annual report of the American Association of Poison Control Centers national data collection system. Am J Emerg Med 10:452–505, 1992.

6. Furbee B, Wermuth M: Life-threatening plant poisoning. Crit Care Clin 13:849–888, 1997.

7. Barker BE, Farnes P, LaMarche PH: Peripheral blood plasmacytosis following systemic exposure to *Phytolacca americana* (pokeweed). Pediatrics 38:490–493, 1966.

8. Barker BE, Farnes P, LaMarche PH: Haematological effects of pokeweed. Lancet 1:437, 1967.

9. Tumer NE, Hudak K, Di R, et al: Pokeweed antiviral protein and its applications. Curr Top Microbiol Immun 240:139–158, 1999.

10. Uckun FM, Chelstrom LM, Tuel-Ahlgren L, et al: TXU (anti-CD7)-pokeweed antiviral protein as a potent inhibitor of human immunodeficiency virus. Antimicrob Agents Chemother 42:382–388, 1998.

11. Anderson PM, Meyers DE, Hasz DE, et al: *In vitro* and *in vivo* cytotoxicity of an anti-osteosarcoma immunotoxin containing pokeweed antiviral protein. Cancer Res 55:1321–1327, 1995.

12. Centers for Disease Control: Plant poisonings—New Jersey. MMWR 30(6): 65–67, 1981.

13. Stein ZLG: Pokeweed-induced gastroenteritis. Am J Hosp Pharm 36: 1303, 1979.

14. Lewis WH, Smith PR: Poke root herbal tea poisoning. JAMA 242:2759–2760, 1979.

15. Jaeckle KA, Freemon FR: Pokeweed poisoning. South Med J 74:639–640, 1981.

16. Goldfrank L, Kirstein R: The feast. Hosp Physician 12(8):34–38, 1976.

17. Hamilton RJ, Shih RD, Hoffman RS: Mobitz type 1 heart block after pokeweed ingestion. Vet Human Toxicol 37:66–67, 1995.

18. Herb Trade Association Policy on the Sale of Poke Root, April 18, 1979.

Pygeum (*Pygeum africanum*)

rating: 🐾🐾 +

> - May be beneficial for treating mild symptoms of benign prostatic hyperplasia
> - Safe and well tolerated

The African plum, *Prunus africana* or *Pygeum africanum*, is an evergreen tree native to the highland forests of central and southern Africa. It is commonly referred to as pygeum.

Uses: A powdered bark extract of pygeum, especially popular in France and Italy since the late 1960s, is commonly used to relieve symptoms associated with benign prostatic hyperplasia (BPH).[1-3] The powdered bark was traditionally mixed into a milk suspension and drunk to to relieve urinary problems.[2] Pygeum has also been used historically to relieve fever, inflammation, gastrointestinal upset, and kidney disease.[2]

Pharmacology: The exact chemicals and their mechanism of action responsible for the observed *in vivo* effects of pygeum remain unknown. The bark contains pentacyclic terpenes, ferulic esters of long-chain fatty acids such as n-docosanol, and phytosterols such as β-sitosterol, β-sitosterene, and campesterol.[1] Pygeum extracts inhibit prostatic fibroblast growth and the effects of certain growth factors, including basic fibroblast growth factor, epidermal growth factor, and insulin growth factor.[4-6] Oral pygeum extracts have also demonstrated anti-inflammatory effects in animal and in *in vitro* studies.[3,7] At high doses, pygeum preparations have weak anti-estrogenic effects in animals.[8] Pygeum extracts preserve bladder contractility and elasticity in several studies of partial bladder outlet obstruction in a rabbit model.[9,10] This effect may be due to protection against cellular or neuronal membrane damage from hydrolytic enzymes and ischemia.[9-11] Whether these pharmacologic effects are clinically significant in humans is unknown.

Clinical Trials: Over 30 clinical trials have reported a variety of beneficial effects for BPH.[3,12] Many of these studies were uncontrolled or had other methodologic flaws, and only a few are available in English.[12] The largest, most rigorously designed study conducted to date was published in 1990.[13] This randomized, multinational, double-blind, and placebo-controlled study evaluated 50 mg of a standardized pygeum extract (Tadenan) given twice daily with meals for 60 days in 255 patients with BPH. The researchers reported that the pygeum extract significantly improved outcomes of maximum urine flow rate, residual urine volume, voided volume, nocturia, and daytime urinary frequency ($p < 0.025$). However, the researchers did not use a standardized symptom score index to measure subjective symptom improvement, and not all patient data was included in each analysis of individual outcomes. Similar criticisms apply to many other pygeum studies.

A high-quality meta-analysis of the worldwide literature reviewed the results of 18 studies that were randomized and placebo-controlled, and that enrolled a total of 1562 men.[12] All but one study were double-blinded, and 10 placebo-controlled studies employed a standardized *P. africanum* monopreparation (e.g., Tadenan). The dosage range was 75–200 mg daily. Differences in reporting methods between studies prohibited pooling of all outcome data for the four measures of pygeum effectiveness: overall symptoms, nocturia, peak urine flow, and residual volume. Nine of the ten placebo-controlled studies reported a beneficial effect of pygeum on at least one measure of effectiveness, but statistically significant improvements were inconsistently found for different outcomes. The authors concluded that the overall evidence suggests that pygeum modestly but significantly improves urologic symptoms and flow measures.

Nevertheless, the many deficiencies and methodologic variabilities of the individual studies limit the results. Only one of the 18 studies described their treatment allocation concealment method. Other limitations included small study size, relatively short duration for studies of BPH (none more than 4 months), and differences in outcome measurements. Most studies failed to report baseline patient demographics such as comorbid conditions and prostate size, and there was a lack of standardized urologic symptom score scales. None of the studies compared pygeum extracts to alpha-blockers or finasteride.

Adverse Effects: Pygeum is very well tolerated. Adverse effects are similar in frequency to placebo in the controlled studies. They include mild gastrointestinal upset, diarrhea, constipation, dizziness, and headache.[3,12,14]

Interactions: Pygeum has not been reported to interact with any other medication or supplement.

Cautions: Pygeum is rarely used in women; there are no data in pregnancy and lactation.

Preparations & Doses: Most of the clinical trials employed a European pygeum extract, Tadenan (currently unavailable in the U.S.), standardized to 14% triterpenes and 0.5% n-docosanol.[3] The usual oral dose was 50 mg taken twice daily. Another European product that has been clinically tested in a few trials, Pygenil, is available in the U.S. as Pygeum Extract (Solaray).[15] Most pygeum products available in the U.S. are combined with other herbs, such as saw palmetto, uva ursi, or pumpkin seed. The optimum dose, and dosing of other pygeum formulations and combination products, is unknown.

--------------------- Summary Evaluation ---------------------

Based on the beneficial results of clinical trials and its relative safety, pygeum may be a reasonable option for patients with mild BPH symptoms. However, due to deficiencies in the published literature, efficacy has not been proven beyond a reasonable doubt. There are no data on comparisons with other standard therapies for BPH.

references

1. Bombardelli E, Morazzoni P: *Prunus africana* (Hook. F.) Kalkm. Fitoterapia 68:205–218,1997.
2. Foster S, Tyler VE: The Honest Herbal, 4th ed. Binghamton, NY, Haworth Herbal Press, 1999.
3. Andro MC, Riffaud JP: *Pygeum africanum* extract for the treatment of patients with benign prostatic hyperplasia: A review of 25 years of published experience. Curr Ther Res 56:796–817, 1995.
4. Levin RM, Das AK: A scientific basis for the therapeutic effects of *Pygeum africanum* and *Serenoa repens*. Urol Res 28:201–209, 2000.
5. Yablonsky F, Nicolas V, Riffaud JP, Bellamy F: Antiproliferative effects of *Pygeum africanum* extract on rat prostatic fibroblasts. J Urol 157:2381–2387, 1997
6. Paubert-Braquet M, Monboisse JC, Servent-Saez N, et al: Inhibition of bFGF and EGF-induced proliferation of 3T3 fibroblasts by extract of *Pygeum africanum* (Tadenan). Biomed Pharmacother 48(Suppl1):43s–47s, 1994.
7. Paubert-Braquet M, Cave A, Hocquemiller R, et al: Effect of *Pygeum africanum* extract on A23187-stimulated production of lipoxygenase metabolites from human polymorphonuclear cells. J Lipid Mediators Cell Signal 9:285–290, 1994.

8. Mathe G, Orbach-Arbouys S, Bizi E, Court B: The so-called phyto-estrogenic action of *Pygeum africanum* extract. Biomed Pharmacother 49:339–340, 1995.

9. Levin RM, Das AK, Haugaard N, et al: Beneficial effects of Tadenan therapy after two weeks of partial obstruction in the rabbit. Neurourol Urodynam 16:583–599, 1997.

10. Levin RM, Levin SS, Zhao Y, Buttyan R: Cellular and molecular aspects of bladder hypertrophy. Eur Urol 32(Suppl1):15–21, 1997.

11. Chee MW, Levin RM, Buttyan R: Effect of Tadenan on the expression of HSP-68 following partial outlet obstruction (Abstract) J Urol 161(Suppl):229, 1999.

12. Ishani A, MacDonald R, Nelson D, et al: *Pygeum africanum* for the treatment of patients with benign prostatic hyperplasia: A systematic review and quantitative meta-analysis. Am J Med 109:654–664, 2000.

13. Barlet A, Albrecht J, Aubert A, et al: Wirksamkeit eines extraktes aus *Pygeum africanum* in der medikamentoesen therapie von miktionsstoerungen infolge einer benignen prostatahyperplasie. [Efficacy of a *Pygeum africanum* extract in the treatment of micturitional disorders due to benign prostatic hyperplasia.] Wien Klin Wochenschrift 102:667–673, 1990.

14. Chatelain C, Autet W, Brackman F: Comparison of once- and twice-daily dosage forms of *Pygeum africanum* extract in patients with benign prostatic hyperplasia: A randomized, double-blinded study, with long-term open label extension. Urol 54:473–478, 1999.

15. Tyler VE: A guide to clinically tested herbal products in the U.S. market. Healthnotes Rev Complem Integr Med 7:279–287, 2000.

Red Clover (*Trifolium pratense*)
rating: 🐾 🐾

> - Commonly used as a natural "estrogen-substitute" for women's health
> - Contains phytoestrogenic isoflavones similar to soy products
> - Beneficial claims not supported by results from placebo-controlled trials
> - Well tolerated without reported side effects

Red clover is a legume in the pea family often used for hay and as a nitrogen-fixing crop. This three-leaf clover is thought to be the model for the suit of clubs in playing cards, and perhaps for the Irish shamrock. The dried reddish flowers are used medicinally.

Uses: Red clover has gained widespread popularity as a phytoestrogen, along with other isoflavone-containing legumes such as soybeans. It is commonly used as a natural "estrogen-substitute" for menopausal symptoms and for the prevention of osteoporosis and cardiovascular disease in women.[1] It is also being marketed for benign prostatic hyperplasia (BPH) and prostate health in men. Traditionally, red clover has been used for dermatologic disorders such as eczema and psoriasis, for venereal disease, and as an expectorant, antispasmodic, and sedative.[2,3] Many supporters believe that red clover has anti-cancer properties, and this herb was included in the Hoxsey anti-cancer formula in the 1940s, which is still used in some alternative cancer clinics.[3]

Pharmacology: Red clover contains phytoestrogenic isoflavones (1.0–2.5%) such as genistein and daidzen, and especially their methylated precursers biochanin A and formononetin.[4,5] Other constituents include coumarins, saponins, and salicylic acid.[2] Whole red clover extracts increase uterine weight in rats and have significant estrogen-agonist and progesterone-antagonist activity *in vitro*.[4,6,7] This estrogenic activity is due to the isoflavonoid constituents, predominantly genistein.[7] These isoflavones also have anti-tumor properties in mice and inhibit human cancer cell lines *in vitro*.[8–11]

Clinical Trials: Red clover contains some of the same isoflavone phytoestrogens found in soy products (genistein and daidzen), but the potential health benefits of red clover extracts have not been demonstrated in high-quality, randomized, controlled trials (RCTs). The most heavily promoted product is Promensil, a standardized extract containing 40 mg of total isoflavones that has been evaluated in several studies (some are available only as unpublished abstracts from the manufacturer).

For menopausal symptoms, an uncontrolled trial initially reported significant reductions in hot flashes and night sweats in 23 postmenopausal women taking Promensil for 2–3 months.[12] However, two double-blind RCTs failed to validate these findings. Out of 51 peri- or post-menopausal women with at least three hot flashes per day, 43 completed a 30-week crossover study that compared 40 mg/day of Promensil with placebo.[13] No significant differences were found in symptoms. Similarly, in 37 postmenopausal women with at least three hot flashes per day, no statistically significant effects were observed with Promensil compared to placebo at daily doses of 40 mg and 160 mg over 12 weeks.[14] All three trials monitored for systemic estrogen activity and found no changes compared to baseline or placebo in estradiol, follicle stimulating hormone, or sex hormone–binding globulin concentrations in the blood, nor on endometrial thickness or vaginal maturation scores in the different studies.

For cardiovascular endpoints, one double-blind RCT indirectly studied the systemic arterial compliance (estimated by blood pressures and ultrasound measurements) in 26 postmenopausal women for 20 weeks. Daily doses of 40 and 80 mg of Promensil increased arterial compliance compared to baseline placebo run-in values in 14 patients who completed the study. Comparisons to a small placebo group (every fifth woman randomized) could not be done as only three patients completed the study in the placebo group. Plasma lipids were not significantly affected.[15] Two other RCTs of red clover isoflavone products also failed to find any effect on cholesterol levels; one trial of 40 mg/day in 93 postmenopausal women with moderately elevated cholesterol levels,[16] and another with 86 mg/day in 14 healthy pre-menopausal women.[17] Another RCT found that a 40-mg dose increased HDL cholesterol levels (by 18%) in a *post hoc* analysis; however, the 160-mg dose did not reach statistical significance, and total cholesterol levels were not measured.[14]

A few trials (available in abstract form) on bone density found promising but mixed results. Promensil at a dose of 40 mg/day was administered in a randomized, double-blind, placebo-controlled trial of 107 women. Reduced vertebral bone loss was observed in pre- and peri-menopausal subjects, but not in post-menopausal women at 1 year. Changes in hip bone loss were not observed in any subgroup.[18] Rimostil, a red clover isoflavone extract similar to Promensil, was administered at three different doses (28.5 mg, 57 mg, and 85.5 mg) to 50 post-menopausal women who were also taking 1200 mg/day of calcium. Significant increase in bone density was reported at the proximal (but not distal) radius and ulna at 6 months. For all three doses tested, statistical increases were seen in HDL cholesterol and decreases in apolipoprotein B concentrations at 6 months. This study, however, was not placebo-controlled.[19]

Adverse Effects: Adverse effects have not been reported with red clover extracts or supplements; no side effects have been reported in the controlled clinical trials.

Interactions: No drug interactions have been reported. Herbal medicine authorities often recommend that red clover should be avoided in patients at high risk of bleeding, such as those taking anticoagulants or soon to undergo surgery.[2] This recommendation is based on the natural coumarin constituents of red clover; these occur in many plants and are often confused with the drug Coumadin or warfarin. Although cattle can develop severe bleeding tendencies when grazing on moldy alfalfa hay (sweet clover), an anticoagulant compound is produced only when a mold converts a specific coumarin compound in alfalfa (4-hydroxycoumarin) to bishydroxycoumarin (dicoumarol).[20] The possibility of there being anticoagulant effects with red clover or any other coumarin-containing herb (there are over 1300 different natural coumarin compounds) is unlikely.

Cautions: Abundant feeding on red clover has caused infertility in animals, presumably due to the estrogenic isoflavones.[4,21] Although estrogenic effects have not been clearly demonstrated in controlled clinical trials, these effects may be dose-dependent, and excessive amounts should be avoided during pregnancy and lactation. The safety of red clover has not been established for patients with estrogen-dependent tumors such as breast cancer or for those on hormonal therapies. Usual recommended doses do not appear to have clinical estrogenic effects and are probably not contraindicated; however, the absolute risk of any dose is unknown, and therefore large amounts should be avoided.

Preparations & Doses: Products standardized to 40 mg total isoflavones are usually administered in 1–2 doses daily. The product tested in most of the clinical trials, Promensil (Novogen), contains 4 mg genistein, 3.5 mg daidzein, 24.5 mg biochanin A, and 8 mg formononetin. More traditional forms are less precisely administered as 4 g of dried flowertop, or by infusion, fluid extract, or tincture t.i.d.[1,2]

Summary Evaluation

Red clover contains isoflavone phytoestrogens, similar to soy products. The herb has estrogenic activity in animals and *in vitro*, but red clover products have not demonstrated systemic therapeutic estrogen effects in humans at usual doses. Claims that red clover isoflavones can benefit menopausal symptoms or cholesterol levels are not supported by evidence from placebo-controlled trials. Beneficial findings on bone density are promising, but require further study. Red clover is well tolerated, with no documented adverse effects.

references

1. McCaleb R, Leigh E, Morien K. The Encyclopedia of Popular Herbs. Roseville, CA, Prima Health, 2000.
2. Newall CA, Anderson LA, Phillipson JD. Herbal Medicines: A Guide for Health-Care Professionals. London, The Pharmaceutical Press, 1996.
3. Foster S, Tyler VE. Tyler's Honest Herbal, 4th ed. New York, Haworth Herbal Press, 1999.
4. Saloniemi H, Wähälä K, Nykänen-Kurki P, et al. Phytoestrogen content and estrogenic effect of legume fodder. Proc Soc Exp Biol Med 208:13–17, 1995.
5. Lundh T. Metabolism of estrogenic isoflavones in domestic animals. Proc Soc Exp Biol Med 208:33–39, 1995.
6. Zava DT, Dollbaum CM, Blen M. Estrogen and progestin bioactivity of foods, herbs, and spices. Proc Soc Exp Biol Med 217:369–378, 1998.
7. Liu J, Burdette JE, Xu H, et al. Evaluation of estrogenic activity of plant extracts for the potential treatment of menopausal symptoms. J Agric Food Chem 49:2472–2479, 2001.
8. Yanagihara K, Ito A, Toge T, Numoto M. Antiproliferative effects of isoflavones on human cancer cell lines established from the gastrointestinal tract. Cancer Res 53:5815–5821, 1993.
9. Cassady JM, Zennie TM, Chae Y-H, et al. Use of a mammalian cell culture benzo(a)pyrene metabolism assay for the detection of potential anticarcinogens from natural products: Inhibition of metabolism by biochanin A, an isoflavone from *Trifolium pratense* L. Cancer Res 48:6257–6261, 1988.

10. Peterson G, Barnes S. Genistein and biochanin A inhibit the growth of human prostate cancer cells but not epidermal growth factor receptor tyrosine autophosphorylation. Prostate 22:335–345, 1993.

11. Peterson G, Barnes S. Genistein inhibits both estrogen and growth factor-stimulated proliferation of human breast cancer cells. Cell Growth Differentiat 7:1345–1351, 1996.

12. Nachtigall LB, Fenichel R, La Grega L, et al. The effects of isoflavone derived from red clover on vasomotor symptoms, endometrial thickness, and reproductive hormone concentrations in menopausal women (Abstract). San Diego, 81st Annual Meeting of the Endocrine Society, June 12–15, 1999.

13. Baber RJ, Templeman C, Morton T, et al. Randomized placebo-controlled trial of an isoflavone supplement and menopausal symptoms in women. Climacteric 2:85–92, 1999.

14. Knight DC, Howes JB, Eden JA. The effect of Promensil, an isoflavone extract, on menopausal symptoms. Climacteric 2:79–284, 1999.

15. Nestel PJ, Pomeroy S, Kay S, et al. Isoflavones from red clover improve systemic arterial compliance but not plasma lipids in menopausal women. Clin Endocrinol Metab 84:895–898, 1999.

16. Howes JB, Sullivan D, Lai N, et al. The effects of dietary supplementation with isoflavones from red clover on the lipoprotein profiles of post-menopausal women with mild to moderate hypercholesterolaemia. Atherosclerosis 152:143–147, 2000.

17. Samman S, Wall PML, Chan GSM, et al. The effect of supplementation with isoflavones on plasma lipids and oxidisability of low density lipoprotein in pre-menopausal women. Atherosclerosis 147:277–283, 1999.

18. Atkinson C, Compston JE, Robins SP, Bingham SA. The effects of isoflavone phytoestrogens on bone; preliminary results from a large randomised controlled trial (Abstract 2359). Toronto, Canada, 82nd Annual Meeting of the Endocrine Society, June 21–24, 2000.

19. Baber R, Bligh PC, Fulcher G, et al. The effect of an isoflavone dietary supplement (Rimostil) on serum lipids, forearm bone density and endometrial thickness in post-menopausal women (Abstract). New York, 10th Annual Meeting of the North American Menopause Society, September 23–25, 1999.

20. DeSmet PAGM. Toxicological outlook on the quality assurance of herbal remedies. In: De Smet PAGM (ed): Adverse Effects of Herbal Drugs. Vol. 1. Berlin, Springer, 1992, pp 1–72.

St. John's Wort
(*Hypericum perforatum*)
rating: 🐿️🐿️🐿️ –

- Antidepressant effects are similar to those of pharmaceutical drugs for mild-moderate depression in short-term studies.
- Adverse effects are milder than with standard antidepressant drugs, but there are many important drug interactions.

The name, St. John's wort, is thought to refer to the blooming season of the flower around St. John's Day; another explanation is the reddish color produced when the buds and flowers are crushed, symbolizing the blood of St. John the Baptist. The flowering tops of St. John's wort are dried and used medicinally.

Uses: St. John's wort is widely promoted and used for the treatment of mild to moderate depression and dysthymia. Over several centuries, the traditional application has been relief of anxiety, melancholy, and other mood disorders. The plant also has been used as an antiviral and diuretic, and for diarrhea, dyspepsia, parasites, neuralgia, sciatica, and rheumatism.[1,2] An oily infusion is employed topically to treat wounds, burns, ulcers, and muscle pains.

Pharmacology: The primary constituents of St. John's wort include naphthodianthrones (e.g., hypericin, pseudohypericin), phloroglucinols (e.g., hyperforin), flavonoids (e.g., quercetin, hyperoside), proanthocyanidins (e.g. catechin), and essential oils.[3,4] Products have long been standardized to the plant's total hypericin content (made up of hypericin and pseudohypericin); however, recent pharmacologic and clinical studies have found that antidepressant activity is more closely correlated with hyperforin.[5,6] In animal models, St. John's wort affects behavior similarly to standard antidepressant drugs.[4] The biochemical mechanism of action also appears to be similar: hypericum extracts and hyperforin inhibit the synaptosomal reuptake of monoamines such as serotonin, norepinephrine, and dopamine with about equal affinity, which is unique among antidepressant agents.[4,6,7] In addition, the monoamine oxidase (MAO) enzyme is very weakly inhibited in animal and *in vitro* studies (doses needed are 100 times higher than for monoamine reuptake inhibition), and this action is not thought to be clinically significant.[4,6,7] Hypericin and pseudohypericin have *in vitro* and *in vivo* activity against certain bacteria and many enveloped viruses, including herpes viruses and retroviruses.[3,8]

Clinical Trials: In Europe, St. John's wort has been studied for the treatment of depression in approximately 35 randomized controlled trials (RCTs) since 1979. Linde et al published a 1996 systematic review and meta-analysis of 23 (updated in 1998 to include 27) RCTs for mild to moderate depression.[9,10] St. John's wort was found to be statistically superior to placebo, with response rates of 56% and 25%, respectively, and was as effective as low doses of tricyclic antidepressants (TCAs). Twenty four of the 27 studies were double-blinded. However, many of these studies can be criticized for small sample sizes, lack of intention-to-treat analyses, heterogeneity of diagnoses, short duration (mostly 4–6 weeks), smaller than expected placebo responses, and use of low doses of comparison medications (e.g., 75 mg/day of imipramine or maprotiline). There were no studies comparing St. John's wort to newer antidepressants such as the selective serotonin and norepinephrine reuptake inhibitors (SSRIs and SNRIs). Also, product type and doses (ranging from 350 to 1800 mg/day, mostly 500–900 mg/day) were not consistent across studies.

Similar but less convincing benefits were found in a separate meta-analysis that re-examined the published studies. With more stringent inclusion criteria, this review evaluated six RCTs. St. John's wort was 1.5 times more likely than placebo to improve depression, compared to about a 2.5-fold improvement reported by Linde et al.[11] A review of six similar RCTs published since the initial Linde meta-analyses found that four additional trials demonstrated benefits greater than placebo, but the evidence from the two trials showing similar benefits to TCAs were not as compelling.[12]

Several large, high-quality, double-blind RCTs have been published more recently that address some of the deficiencies of past studies regarding dosing and comparison drugs, although none were long term (all 6–8 weeks). In the first three-armed trial of St. John's wort, 1050 mg/day (350 mg t.i.d.) was found to be more effective than placebo and at least as effective as 100 mg/day of imipramine in 263 patients with moderate depression.[13] In 324 patients with mild-moderate depression, 500 mg/day (250 mg b.i.d.) was equivalent to a larger imipramine dose of 150 mg/day.[14] In a trial of 209 severely depressed patients, a large St. John's wort dose of 1800 mg/day (600 mg t.i.d.) was also found to have similar effects to imipramine 150 mg/day.[15] Lastly, three recent double-blind RCTs lasting 6–7 weeks have compared St. John's wort with SSRIs in patients with mild to moderate depression. Two studies of 149 elderly and 240 adult patients found different St. John's wort products (800 mg/day and 500 mg/day, respectively) to be equivalent to fluoxetine 20 mg daily.[16,17] A smaller trial of 30 patients also found equivalent benefits with St. John's wort 900 mg/day and sertraline 75 mg/day.[18]

In contrast, the first large, randomized, double-blind, and placebo-controlled trial conducted in the U.S. failed to demonstrate antidepressant effects in 200 patients with moderate depression using 900 mg/day (300 mg t.i.d., increased to q.i.d. if inadequate response at 4 weeks) of St. John's wort.[19] In the 8-week intention-to-treat analysis, a significant benefit was found compared to placebo only for the number reaching remission of illness, but the rates were very low (14.3% vs. 4.9%, respectively). The reason for the contrasting results of this well-designed trial is unknown, although this study did not enroll patients who had only mild depression.

Other claims for St. John's wort have not been validated in double-blind RCTs. Antiviral benefits have been reported in uncontrolled studies of HIV-infected patients using oral or intravenous hypericum extracts, presented at several AIDS conferences.[2,8] However, significant changes in antiviral endpoints were not demonstrated in a published, phase 1 clinical study using high doses of oral or IV hypericin, and dosing was limited in most patients due to significant phototoxic reactions.[8]

Adverse Effects: St. John's wort is generally well tolerated; occasional side effects include mild gastrointestinal symptoms, tiredness/sedation, dizziness/confusion, headache, dry mouth, and dermatitis.[20] In the controlled clinical trials, the frequency of side effects was about the same as placebo in placebo-controlled studies (4–12%), and was significantly less than standard antidepressant drugs.[9,10,12,17,20] Rarely, patients have developed a phototoxic dermatitis from oral or topical use due to the hypericins (which are photodynamic pigments); fair skinned individuals taking larger than usual doses are probably at higher risk.[20–22] A painful neuropathy after sun exposure (without dermatitis) occurred in one patient. It resolved several weeks after St. John's wort was withdrawn.[23] Like other antidepressants, St. John's wort appears to be able to induce mania or hypomania in susceptible individuals.[24–26]

Interactions: St. John's wort, like pharmaceutical antidepressants, can interact with a wide variety of drugs to affect their plasma concentrations and clinical effects. Reductions of indinavir, digoxin, and amitriptyline serum concentrations have been demonstrated in pharmacokinetic studies,[27–29] and clinical interactions have been reported with cyclosporin (> 35 patients, some of whom experienced transplant rejection), warfarin, theophylline, and oral contraceptives (breakthrough bleeding).[30–33] As with rifampin and barbiturates, St. John's wort appears to induce the 3A4 isozyme of the hepatic cytochrome P450 system (CYP3A4) to enhance drug metabolism. The actual mechanism is not conclusively elucidated, however, as studies have shown effects consistent with both induction and inhibition of this system,[34,35] and St. John's wort does not interact with all drugs that are metabolized by the CYP3A4 system (e.g., carbamazepine).[36] Induction of the intestinal P-glycoprotein drug transporter is also hypothesized to affect certain drugs.[28] Nevertheless, any drug metabolized by these mechanisms should be considered to potentially interact with St. John's wort. Patients combining St. John's wort with SSRI drugs may also be at risk of the serotonin-syndrome.[37,38]

Because of the *in vitro* evidence that St. John's wort weakly inhibits the MAO enzyme, there has been concern raised about the potential for clinical (*in vivo*) MAO inhibitor interactions. However, there is no documented evidence or clinical reports of interactions with tyramine-containing foods or other drugs. Based on current evidence, MAO inhibition appears quite unlikely at usual therapeutic doses.

Cautions: Transient hypotension with decreased responsiveness to vasopressors while undergoing general anesthesia was reported in a healthy young woman taking St. John's wort. The authors hypothesized that adrenergic desensitization could have occurred.[39] There are no data regarding the safety of St. John's wort during pregnancy. In a small study of 30 breast-feeding women using St. John's wort, there was no apparent affect on lactation. There was a statistically increased frequency of mild infant "side effects" in the St. John's wort group (5/30; one case of lethargy and two cases each of colic and drowsiness) versus the control groups (1/97; one case of colic). The clinical significance of these results is not clear.[40]

Preparations & Doses: Effective doses from clinical trials range from about 500 mg to 1800 mg daily. The usual oral dose of a standardized extract of St. John's wort is 900 mg/day in 2–3 divided doses. Most St. John's wort products used in the European clinical trials are standardized to 0.3% total hypericins, such that 900 mg/day of the extract is equivalent to 2.7 mg of hypericins and about 5 g of the dried herb.[1,2] The only clinically tested brand standardized to hypericin that is available on the U.S. market is Kira (Lichtwer Pharma). Other clinically tested products standardized to 2–6% hyperforin (now thought to be a more important constituent of the herb) are available in the U.S. as Movana (Pharmaton) and Perika (Nature's Way).[41]

-------------------- **Summary Evaluation** --------------------

In short-term studies, St. John's wort appears to have antidepressant properties similar to standard drugs used for mild to moderate depression, and with less adverse effects. St. John's wort also has many important drug interactions, which are of significant concern for many patients who use this herb. Concerns about its safety have resulted in a variety of prescribing restrictions in countries outside the U.S., and St. John's wort appears to be the first of the current herbs of mass popularity to have the potential to interact with numerous pharmaceutical drugs. *It is thus essential to monitor the potential effects of St. John's wort on any major drug that a patient is taking*, and to be able to counsel patients about both the advantages and disadvantages of using this herb.

references

1. Blumenthal M, Goldberg A, Brinckmann J (eds). Herbal Medicine: Expanded Commission E Monographs. Newton, MA, Integrative Medicine Communications, 2000.
2. Mills S, Bone K. Principles and Practice of Phytotherapy: Modern Herbal Medicine. Edinburgh, UK, Churchill Livingstone, 2000.
3. Upton R (ed). St. John's wort: *Hypericum perforatum*. American Herbal Pharmacopoeia and Therapeutic Compendium, July 1997.
4. Nathan PJ. The experimental and clinical pharmacology of St John's wort (*Hypericum perforatum* L.). Molec Psych 1999;4:333–338.
5. Laakmann G, Schüle C, Baghai T, Kieser M. St. John's wort in mild to moderate depression: The relevance of hyperforin for the clinical efficacy. Pharmacopsychiatry 1998;31(Suppl):54–59.

6. Chatterjee SS, Bhattacharya SD, Wonnemann M, et al. Hyperforin as a possible antidepressant component of hypericum extracts. Life Sciences 1998;63:499–510.

7. Müller WE, Rolli M, Schäfer C, Hafner U. Effects of hypericum extract (LI 160) in biochemical models of antidepressant activity. Pharmacopsychiatry 1997;30(Suppl):102–107.

8. Gulick RM, McAuliffe V, Holden-Wiltse J, et al. Phase I studies of hypericin, the active compound in St. John's wort, as an antiretroviral agent in HIV-infected adults: AIDS Clinical Trials Group Protocols 150 and 258. Ann Intern Med 1999;130:510–514.

9. Linde K, Ramirez G, Mulrow CD, et al. St. John's wort for depression—An overview and meta-analysis of randomized clinical trials. BMJ 1996;313: 253–258.

10. Linde K, Mulrow CD. St John's wort for depression (Cochrane Review). In The Cochrane Library, Issue 4. Oxford, Update Software, 2000.

11. Kim HL, Streltzer J, Goebert D. St. John's wort for depression: A meta-analysis of well-defined clinical trials. J Nerv Ment Dis 1999;187:532–539.

12. Stevinson C, Ernst E. Hypericum for depression: An update of the clinical evidence. Eur Neuropsychopharmacol 1999;9:501–505.

13. Philipp M, Kohnen R, Hiller K-O. Hypericum extract versus imipramine or placebo in patients with moderate depression: Randomised multicentre study of treatment for eight weeks. BMJ 1999;319:1534–1538.

14. Woelk H (for the Remotiv/Imipramine Study Group). Comparison of St John's wort and imipramine for treating depression: Randomised controlled trial. BMJ 2000;321:536–539.

15. Vorbach EU, Arnoldt KH, Hübner W-D. Efficacy and tolerability of St. John's wort extract LI 160 versus imipramine in patients with severe depressive episodes according to ICD-10. Pharmacopsychiatry 1997;30(Suppl):81–85.

16. Harrer G, Schmidt U, Kuhn U, Biller A. Comparison of equivalence between the St. John's wort extract LoHyp-57 and fluoxetine. Arzneim-Forsch/Drug Res 1999;49:289–296.

17. Schrader E, on behalf of the Study Group. Equivalence of St John's wort extract (ZE 117) and fluoxetine: a randomized, controlled study in mild-moderate depression. Int Clin Psychopharmacol 2000;15:61–68.

18. Brenner R, Azbel V, Madhusoodanan S, Pawlowska M. Comparison of an extract of Hypericum (LI 160) and sertraline in the treatment of depression: A double-blind, randomized pilot study. Clin Ther 2000;22:411–419.

19. Shelton RC, Keller MB, Gelenberg A, et al. Effectiveness of St John's wort in major depresssion. JAMA 2001;285:1978–1986.

20. Ernst E, Rand JI, Barnes J, Stevinson C. Adverse effects profile of the herbal antidepressant St. John's wort (Hypericum perforatum L.). Eur J Clin Pharmacol 1998;54:589–594.

21. Lane-Brown MM. Photosensitivity associated with herbal preparations of St John's wort (Hypericum perforatum). Med J Austral 2000;172:302(letter).

22. Brockmöller J, Reum T, Bauer S, et al. Hypericin and pseudohypericin: pharmacokinetics and effects on photosensitivity in humans. Pharmacopsychiatry 1997;30(Suppl):94–101.

23. Bove GM. Acute neuropathy after exposure to sun in a patient treated with St John's wort. Lancet 1998;352:1121–1122(letter).

24. Moses EL, Mallinger AG. St. John's wort: three cases of possible mania induction. J Clin Psychopharmacol 2000;20:115–117(letter).

25. O'Breasail AM, Argouarch S. Hypomania and St John's wort. Can J Psychiatry 1998;43:746–747(letter).

26. Nierenberg AA, Burt T, Matthews J, Weiss AP. Mania associated with St. John's wort. Biol Psychiatry 1999;46:1707–1708.

27. Piscitelli SC, Burstein AH, Chaitt D, et al. Indinavir concentrations and St. John's wort. Lancet 2000;355:547–548.

28. Johne A, Brockmöller J, Bauer S, et al. Pharmacokinetic interaction of digoxin with an herbal extract from St. John's wort (*Hypericum perforatum*). Clin Pharmacol Ther. 1999;66:338–345.

29. Roots I, Johne A, Schmider J, et al. Interaction of a herbal extract from St. John's wort with amitriptyline and its metabolites. Clin Pharmacol Therap 2000;67:159(Abstract PIII-69).

30. Breidenbach T, Hoffmann MW, Becker T, et al. Drug interaction of St John's wort with ciclosporin. Lancet 2000;355:1912(correspondence).

31. Ruschitzka F, Meier PJ, Turina M, et al. Acute heart transplant rejection due to Saint John's wort. Lancet 2000;355:548–549.

32. Yue Q-Y, Bergquist C, Gerden B. Safety of St John's wort (*Hypericum perforatum*). Lancet 2000;355:576–577 (correspondence).

33. Ernst E. Second thoughts about safety of St John's wort. Lancet 1999;354:2014–2016.

34. Moore LB, Goodwin B, Jones SA, et al. St. John's wort induces hepatic drug metabolism through activation of the pregnane X receptor. Proc Natl Acad Sci 2000;97:7500–7502.

35. Roby CA, Anderson GD, Kantor E, et al. St John's wort: effect on CYP3A4 activity. Clin Pharmacol Ther 2000;67:451–457.

36. Burstein AH, Horton RL, Dunn T, et al. Lack of effect of St John's wort on carbamazepine pharmacokinetics in healthy volunteers. Clin Pharmacol Ther 2000;68:605–612.

37. Lantz MS, Buchalter E, Giambanco V. St. John's wort and antidepressant drug interactions in the elderly. J Geriatr Psychiatry Neurol 1999;12:7–10.

38. Gordon JB. SSRIs and St. John's wort: possible toxicity? Am Fam Physician 1998;57;950, 953.

39. Irefin S, Sprung J. A possible cause of cardiovascular collapse during anesthesia: long-term use of St. John's wort. J Clin Anesth 2000;12:498–499.

40. Lee A, Minhas R, Ito S. Safety of St. John's wort during breast-feeding. Clin Pharmacol Ther 2000;67:130(Abstract PII-64).

41. Tyler VE. A guide to clinically tested herbal products in the U.S. market. Healthnotes Rev Complement Integ Med 2000;7:279–287.

SAM*e**

rating: 🐾 🐾

> - Possibly beneficial in mild-moderate depression and osteoarthritis; lack of quality evidence to support effectiveness
> - Potentially quicker onset of antidepressant effects compared to tricyclic antidepressants

S-adenosylmethionine is also known as ademetionine, SAM, or SAM*e*. The "*e*" in SAM*e* designates that SAM is endogenous. SAMe is a naturally occurring substance that functions as a methyl donor in methyl-transferase reactions for phospholipids, neurotransmitters, proteins, and deoxyribonucleic acid (DNA).

Uses: SAM*e* is mainly used for osteoarthritis and depression. It has been widely accepted in European countries, where it first became popular as a therapeutic agent in the 1980s. SAM*e* has also been employed to treat intrahepatic cholestasis of pregnancy, alcoholic liver cirrhosis, fibromyalgia, and migraine headaches, and for a variety of other conditions.[1-5]

Pharmacology: SAM*e* is formed by the amino acid methionine and adenosyltriphosphate (ATP); it is not an essential nutrient in humans. Endogenously, folic acid and vitamin B_{12} are required for its synthesis.[6] SAM*e* may offer chondroprotective properties by enhancing synthesis of proteoglycans in articular chondrocytes.[6] SAM*e* may also inhibit tumor necrosis factor-α (TNF-α) which is a pro-inflammatory cytokine that has been implicated in the pathogenesis of joint diseases and numerous other conditions.[6] SAM*e* inhibits platelet aggregation *in vitro* by increasing vascular production of prostacyclin (an endogenous prostanoid with anti-aggregant and vasodilator effects).[7]

SAM*e* is an ubiquitous methyl donor; in some animal studies it has been shown to increase the turnover and decrease neuronal levels of norepinephrine, serotonin, and dopamine.[8] In humans, contrasting research suggests that SAM*e* increases

---

* *Editor's Note:* Although not an herb, SAMe is a dietary supplement that is included because of its current popularity.

central serotonin levels, inhibiting the central reuptake of norepinephrine and dopamine.[9] SAMe has been reported to increase hepatic glutathione concentrations, and to serve as a methyl donator for other sulfur-containing amino acids which protect against oxidative stress and hepatotoxicity. SAMe supplementation may also prove useful in increasing folic acid production, thereby decreasing high homocysteine levels.[10]

Clinical Trials: While SAMe has been evaluated in limited clinical trials for a number of uses,[1-5] osteoarthritis and depression are the two primary indications that have been most studied using oral preparations.

• Osteoarthritis—Many randomized, controlled clinical trials have been conducted evaluating the effectiveness of SAMe for osteoarthritis.[11-19] These studies were all published in the 1980s, mainly in the proceedings of a SAMe osteoarthritis symposium. No new clinical trials have been published since then. All studies concluded that SAMe is effective in relieving the clinical symptoms associated with osteoarthritis. Improvements in pain relief, morning stiffness, walking distance, and active and passive range of motion were all observed. SAMe was considered to be equal in analgesic and anti-inflammatory efficacy to common nonsteroidal anti-inflammatory drugs (NSAIDs).[13,14,17-19]

However, these studies were poorly designed. For example, since SAMe is thought to increase proteoglycan synthesis in articular chondrocytes, the effects may take 1–2 months to be observed. The two double-blind, placebo-controlled trials lasted 3–4 weeks.[14,15] Furthermore, many of these comparative studies did not include a placebo control group, and they lacked adequate statistical power to detect differences between the SAMe and the NSAID groups.[17-19] One randomized, double-blind, placebo-controlled trial found SAMe was superior to placebo in relieving osteoathritis knee pain.[16] While this study is promising, the authors used an intravenous bolus dose of SAMe (which is not available to U.S. consumers) followed by oral doses.

• Depression—Many uncontrolled trials, placebo-controlled trials, and comparative trials with tricyclic antidepressants (TCAs) have been conducted.[20] A few studies have also evaluated the role of SAMe therapy in combination with other antidepressants.[20] These studies report modest improvements in depression; however, the findings were often contradictory and confounded by poor study design. The majority of these trials were small (less than 30 patients) and most involved SAMe as an intravenous formulation.

A meta-analysis of controlled trials using standardized criteria for diagnosis and clinical status found 13 studies that met inclusion criteria, five of which used oral SAMe.[21] A full clinical response was found in 38% of patients receiving SAMe compared to 22% of those receiving placebo. These results are lower than what is typically observed in antidepressant studies with active drugs. SAMe was equally effective as therapeutic doses of TCAs (e.g., imipramine, desipramine, amitriptyline) for major depression; a full response was found in 62% of SAMe-treated patients and 59% of TCA-treated patients.

The different mean response rates of SAMe compared to placebo (38%), and SAMe compared to TCAs (62%), indicate a large variation in patient response, which is not easily explained. Another important criticism of the comparative trials is the short study duration; many studies lasted only 2–3 weeks—too short a time to assess the effects of TCAs (which usually require 4–8 weeks before the full effect may be observed).

Adverse Effects: SAMe was generally well tolerated in the clinical trials. Side effects of the oral formulations, which were uncommon, included flatulence, nausea, vomiting, diarrhea, headache, and anxiety.[20] A few patients developed mania and hypomania after receiving SAMe,[22,23] which also occurs with pharmaceutical antidepressants.

Interactions: No serious drug interactions have been reported for SAMe. Since SAMe may increase central serotonin levels, it is possible that it can have additive effects when combined with other drugs that inhibit serotonin reuptake. There is one case report of a "serotonin syndrome" in a patient taking SAMe and clomipramine.[24] SAMe, however, has been combined with TCAs without any adverse consequences. Until more is known, patients should avoid combining SAMe with other antidepressants.

Cautions: SAMe should not be used in patients with a history of mania or bipolar disorder. The safety of the commercially available SAMe in pregnancy and lactation is unknown.

Preparations & Doses: To minimize gastrointestinal upset, oral SAMe is often initiated at 200 mg once or twice daily. For osteoarthritis, the dose may be increased every 1 or 2 weeks until a dose of 400–1600 mg daily is achieved. For depression, the typical initial dose used in the positive clinical trials was 1600 mg daily (in divided doses), or doses quickly increased up to this amount within 1 week; maintenance doses of 200 mg twice daily have been used. According to clinical trials, SAM*e* has an onset of action ranging from a few days to 2 weeks.[20]

SAM*e* has poor oral absorption and undergoes extensive first-pass metabolism by the liver.[25] Some of the clinical trials used intravenous or intramuscular routes of administration to avoid the high first-pass liver metabolism. Oral formulations are enteric coated to improve absorption. SAM*e* is synthesized from yeast fermentation and is not derived from human or animal sources. Large doses, such as 1600 mg/day, can be costly.

Summary Evaluation

While SAM*e* is well tolerated and may be mildly effective in both osteoarthritis and depression, significant study design flaws in the existing literature make it difficult to evaluate this agent. Patients should not expect major improvements. SAM*e* may be a useful alternative for those who do not want to use orthodox pharmaceuticals or who cannot tolerate prescribed drugs, but current clinical data regarding safety and efficacy with chronic use is preliminary and incomplete.

references

1. Floreani A, Paternoster D, Melis A, et al: S-adenosylmethionine versus ursodeoxycholic acid in the treatment of intrahepatic cholestasis of pregnancy: Preliminary results of a controlled trial. Eur J Obstet Gynecol Reprod Biol 67:109–113, 1996.
2. Frezza M, Surrenti C, Manzillo G, et al: Oral S-adenosylmethionine in the symptomatic treatment of intrahepatic cholestasis. A double-blind, placebo-controlled study. Gastroenterology 99:211–215, 1990.
3. Mato JM, Camara J, Fernandez de Paz J, et al: S-adenosylmethionine in alcoholic liver cirrhosis: A randomized, placebo-controlled, double-blind, multi-center clinical trial. J Hepatol 30:1081–1089, 1999.
4. Volkman H, Norregaard J, Jacobsen S, et al: Double-blind, placebo-controlled, cross-over study of intravenous S-adenosylmethionine in patients with fibromyalgia. Scand J Rheumatol 26:206–211, 1997.
5. Bottiglieri T, Hyland K, Reynolds EH: The clinical potential of ademethionine (S-adenosylmethionine) in neurological disorders. Drugs 48:137–152, 1994.
6. Harmand MF, Cilamitjana J, Maloche E, et al: Effects of S-adenosylmethionine on human articular chondrocyte differentiation: An in vitro study. Am J Med 83(suppl 5A):48–54, 1987.
7. Watson EH, Zhao Y, Chawla RK, et al: S-adenosylmethionine attenuates the lipopolysaccharide-induced expression of the gene for tumour necrosis factor alpha. Biochem J 342:21–25, 1999.

8. Fava M, Rosenbaum JF, MacLaughlin R, et al: Neuroendocrine effects of S-adenosyl-L-methionine, a novel putative antidepressant. J Psychiatr Res 24:177–184, 1990.

9. Baldessarini RJ: Neuropharmacology of S-adenosyl-L-methionine. Am J Med 83(suppl 5A):95–103, 1987.

10. Loehrer FMT, Angst CP, Haefeli WE, et al: Low whole blood S-adenylmethionine and correlation between 5-methyltetrahydrofolate and homocysteine in coronary artery disease. Arterioscler Thromb Vasc Biol 16:727–733, 1996.

11. Konig B: A long-term (2 years) clinical trial with S-adenosylmethionine for the treatment of osteoarthritis. Am J Med 83(suppl 5A):89–94, 1987.

12. Marcolongo R, Giordano N, Colombo B, et al: Double-blind multicentre study of the activity of S-adenosyl-methionine in hip and knee osteoarthritis. Curr Ther Res 37:82–94, 1985.

13. Maccagno A, Di Giorgio EE, Caston OL, et al: Double-blind controlled clinical trial of oral S-adenosylmethionine versus piroxicam in knee osteoarthritis. Am J Med 83(suppl 5A):72–77, 1987.

14. Caruso I, Pietrogrande V: Italian double-blind multicenter study comparing S-adenosylmethionine, naproxen, and placebo in the treatment of degenerative joint disease. Am J Med 83(suppl 5A):66–71, 1987.

15. Montrone F, Fumagalli M, Sarzi Puttini P, et al: Double-blind study of S-adenosyl-methionine versus placebo in hip and knee arthrosis. Clin Rheumatol 4:484–485, 1985.

16. Bradley JD, Flusser D, Katz BP, et al: A randomized, double blind, placebo-controlled trial of intravenous loading with S-adenosylmethionine (SAM) followed by oral SAM therapy in patients with knee osteoarthritis. J Rheumatol 21:905–911, 1994.

17. Müller-Fassbender H: Double-blind clinical trial of S-adenosylmethionine versus ibuprofen in the treatment of osteoarthritis. Am J Med 83(suppl 5A):81–83, 1987.

18. Vetter G: Double-blind comparative clinical trial with S-adenosylmethionine and indomethacin in the treatment of osteoarthritis. Am J Med 83(suppl 5A):78–80, 1987.

19. Domljan Z, Vrhovac B, Durrigl T, et al: A double-blind trial of ademetionine vs naproxen in activated gonarthrosis. Int J Clin Pharmacol Ther Toxicol 27:329–333, 1989.

20. Friedel HA, Goa KL, Benfield P: S-adenosyl-l-methionine: A review of its pharmacological properties and therapeutic potential in liver dysfunction and affective disorders in relation to its physiological role in cell metabolism. Drugs 38:389–416, 1989.

21. Bressa GM: S-adenosyl-l-methionine (SAMe) as antidepressant: Meta-analysis of clinical studies. Acta Neurol Scand Suppl 154:7–14, 1994.

22. Carney MWP, Chary TK, Bottiglieri T, et al: The switch mechanism and the bipolar/unipolar dichotomy. Br J Psychiatr 154:48–51, 1989.

23. Kagan BL, Sultzer DL, Rosenlicht N, et al: Oral S-adenosylmethionine in depression: A randomized, double-blind, placebo-controlled trial. Am J Psychiatr 147:591–595, 1990.

24. Iruela LM, Minguez L, Merino J et al: Toxic interaction of S-adenosylmethionine and clomipramine. Am J Psychol 150:522, 1993.

25. Stramentinoli G, Gualano M, Galli-Kienle M: Intestinal absorption of S-adenosyl-L-methionine. J Pharmacol Exp Ther 209:323–326, 1979.

Saw Palmetto (*Serenoa repens*)

rating: 🐾🐾🐾 +

> - Overall evidence supports benefit for the treatment of benign prostatic hypertrophy
> - Safe and well tolerated; no significant adverse effects or cautions

Saw palmetto is an American dwarf palm tree indigenous to the Eastern United States coastal region. The ripe fruit, or berry, is used medicinally.

Uses: Saw palmetto is commonly marketed and used to treat symptoms of benign prostatic hyperplasia (BPH). Standardized products are considered first-line therapy for BPH by doctors and patients in many European countries. Traditionally, the plant has also been used for a variety of urogenital and other conditions in both men and women, such as impotence and infertility, irritable bladder symptoms, and acute or chronic prostatitis.[1-3]

Pharmacology: Standardized saw palmetto products consist of an oily liposterolic extract of the saw palmetto berry, extracted with hexane, 90% ethanol, or liquid CO_2.[1-4] The extract contains a complex mixture of free fatty acids and their esters, with smaller quantities of aliphatic alcohols, sterols (such as beta-sitosterol), and other compounds.

The pharmacology and mechanism of action of saw palmetto have been extensively studied, but are still not fully elucidated. Initial *in vitro* and *in vivo* animal experiments found these extracts to have spasmolytic, anti-inflammatory, growth factor inhibitory, and anti-androgen properties.[3-7] Saw palmetto extracts (primarily the free fatty acid components) weakly inhibit 5-alpha reductase, potentially reducing the conversion of testosterone to dihydrotestosterone (DHT). Extracts were found to inhibit DHT binding to androgen receptors in prostate tissue. However, clinical investigations have not verified these potential anti-androgen effects in humans; saw palmetto does not affect serum levels of DHT at usual doses (unlike finasteride), nor does it significantly affect other serum hormone concentrations, prostate-specific antigen (PSA) levels, or prostate size.[8-11] Saw palmetto has alpha-receptor blocking activity *in vitro*,[12] but not *in vivo* at clinically therapeutic doses in humans.[13] It has recently been found to cause involution of prostatic epithelium,[11] and to reduce local DHT concentrations in the periurethral region of the prostate.[14] The most relevant mode of action is undetermined, and more than one mechanism may be involved.

Clinical Trials: Saw palmetto has been evaluated for effects on symptoms of BPH in many European randomized controlled trials (RCTs), and these trials have been extensively reviewed.[1-3,5,6,9,15] Although most studies were of short duration (1 to 3 months) and included small numbers of patients (20–80), both subjective symptoms and objective parameters (nocturia, post-void residual, and peak urine flows) generally improved relative to placebo. Benefits were reported within 1 month of starting treatment.[6] Studies are of varying quality; many trial results have been criticized due to smaller than usual effects seen in the placebo groups, lack of validated urologic symptom scales, and inadequate study methods or reporting of data.[6,7]

One high-quality, systematic review/meta-analysis of the worldwide literature found 18 RCTs of saw palmetto, alone or combined with other herbs, that met inclusion criteria.[9] Of 2939 patients, 1118 were involved in placebo-controlled trials, while the remainder were involved in trials vs. active controls (primarily two large studies with finasteride). Sixteen RCTs were double-blind (89%), and treatment allocation concealment was adequate in nine studies (50%). The mean study duration was 9 weeks (range, 4–48 weeks). The authors concluded that saw palmetto was statistically superior to placebo and similar to finasteride in improving urologic symptoms, nocturia, peak flow rates, and residual urine volumes.

The United States Pharmacopoeia evaluated 29 published studies of the herb's effect on BPH symptoms, and nine RCTs met sufficient quality criteria to permit objective analysis.[6] These included seven placebo-controlled trials, and two active control trials (finasteride and an alpha-blocker). Another meta-analysis evaluated the published clinical trial data on Permixon (a widely used European product), which included 11 RCTs.[15] Similar positive conclusions were reached in these two high-quality, systematic reviews/meta-analyses.

Saw palmetto was somewhat less effective than low doses of alpha-blockers, prazosin (4 mg/day) and alfuzosin (7.5 mg/day), in two European studies.[16,17] The prazosin study was not randomized or statistically analyzed, and the alfuzosin study lasted only 3 weeks.

The first published RCT of a U.S. supplement consisted of a 6-month double-blind trial of 44 men with symptomatic BPH.[11] Subjects took a saw palmetto herbal blend (NUTRALITE Saw Palmetto with Nettle Root; containing 106 mg saw palmetto lipoidal extract plus nettle root, pumpkin seed oil, lemon bioflavonoid extract, and vitamin A) or a placebo t.i.d. Using prostate MRI and ultrasound-guided biopsy, the saw palmetto product was found to be associated with involution of the prostatic epithelium, but without affecting prostate size. Testosterone, DHT, and PSA levels also were not affected. Clinical measurements such as symptom scores and flow rates were reduced in the herbal and placebo groups to a similar extent. The authors stated that these measures were secondary end points, and that the study was not adequately powered to detect slight changes.

Adverse Effects: There are no significant side effects. Mild gastrointestinal complaints comparable to placebo are generally reported in less than 2–4% of patients.[6,9,11] Unlike finasteride, saw palmetto does not cause erectile dysfunction.[8,9]

Interactions: There are no recognized drug interactions, and PSA levels are not affected.[8–11]

Cautions: There are no contraindications or other cautions with saw palmetto, although self-treatment of patients with unsuspected prostate cancer may delay medical therapy. Saw palmetto has not been studied in children and pregnant or nursing women,[6] but is not marketed for these populations.

Preparations & Doses: The oral dose of standard liposterolic extracts found beneficial in clinical studies is 160 mg b.i.d. Equivalent effects have been demonstrated when given as a single daily dose of 320 mg.[18,19] Although the most widely studied product (Permixon) is not currently marketed in the U.S., another European product found to be effective, Prostagutt (by Schwabe), is marketed under the brand name ProstActive (by Nature's Way). Commercial liposterolic extracts, similar to those marketed in European countries, are also available in the U.S., and are usually standardized to 85–95% combined fatty acids and sterols. Crushed berry products or whole extracts, equivalent to about 2–4 g/day of dried berries, should be equivalent to the standard liposterolic extract,[6,20] but have not been adequately studied.

Summary Evaluation

Saw palmetto extracts have been extensively studied in European countries, and found to be safe and effective in most RCTs. A single U.S. controlled trial that did not find clinical benefits may have been too small to detect a clinical effect. However, its results imply that benefits may be minimal, or that other products are more reliable. Nevertheless, based on the evidence to date, saw palmetto can be recommended as a safe herbal alternative or as an adjunct to standard medical therapy for patients with BPH. It has a shorter onset and is as effective as finasteride, but may not be as effective as alpha-blockers.

references

1. Chavez MJ, Chavez PI: Saw palmetto. Hosp Pharm 33:1335-1361, 1998.
2. Plosker GL, Brogden RN: *Serenoa repens* (Permixon): A review of its pharmacology and therapeutic efficacy in benign prostatic hyperplasia. Drugs & Aging 9:379–395, 1996.
3. Bombardelli E, Morazzoni P: *Serenoa repens* (Bartram) J.K. Small. Fitoterapia 68:99–113, 1997.
4. Barrett M: The pharmacology of saw palmetto in treatment of BPH. J Am Nutraceut Assoc 2(3):40–43, 2000.
5. Bone K: Saw palmetto—A critical review. Eur J Herbal Med 4:15–23, 1998.
6. U.S. Pharmacopoiea: Saw palmetto botanical monograph, 2000. http://www.usp.org/dietary/index.htm
7. Gerber GS: Saw palmetto for the treatment of men with lower urinary tract symptoms. J Urol 163:1408–1412, 2000.
8. Carraro JC, Raynaud JP, Koch G: Comparison of phytotherapy (Permixon) with finasteride in the treatment of benign prostatic hyperplasia: A randomized international study of 1098 patients. Prostate 29:231–242, 1996.
9. Wilt TJ, Ishani A, Stark G, et al: Saw palmetto extracts for treatment of benign prostatic hyperplasia: A systematic review. JAMA 280:1604–1609, 1998.
10. Gerber GS, Zagaja GP, Bales GT, et al: Saw palmetto (*Serenoa repens*) in men with lower urinary tract symptoms: Effects on urodynamic parameters and voiding symptoms. Urology 51:1003–1007, 1998.
11. Marks LS, Partin AW, Epstein JI, et al: Effects of a saw palmetto herbal blend in men with symptomatic benign prostatic hyperplasia. J Urol 163:1451–1456, 2000.
12. Goepel M, Hecker U, Krege S, et al: Saw palmetto extracts potently and noncompetitively inhibit human alpha-1 adrenoceptors in vitro. Prostate 38:208–215, 1999.
13. Goepel M, Dinh L, Mitchell A, et al: Do saw palmetto extracts block human alpha1-adrenoceptor subtypes in vivo? Prostate 46:226–232, 2001.
14. DiSilverio F, Monti S, Sciarra A, et al: Effects of long-term treatment with *Serenoa repens* (Permixon) on the concentrations and regional distribution of androgens and epidermal growth factor in benign prostatic hyperplasia. Prostate 37:77–83, 1998.

15. Boyle P, Robertson C, Lowe F, Roehrborn C: Meta-analysis of clinical trials of Permixon in the treatment of symptomatic benign prostatic hyperplasia. Urology 55:533–539, 2000.
16. Grasso M, Montesano A, Buonaguidi A, et al: Comparative effects of alfuzosin versus *Serenoa repens* in the treatment of symptomatic benign prostatic hyperplasia. Arch Esp de Urol 48:97–103, 1995.
17. Semino MA, Ortega JLL, Cobo EG, et al: Tratamiento sintomatico de la hipertrofia benigna de prostata. Estudio comparativo entre Prazosin y *Serenoa repens*. [Symptomatic treatment of benign prostate hypertrophy. Study comparing Prazosin with *Serenoa repens*.] Arch Esp de Urol 45:211–213, 1992 (English abstract).
18. Braeckman J, Bruhwyler J, Vanderkeckhove K, Geczy J: Efficacy and safety of the extract of *Serenoa repens* in the treatment of benign prostatic hyperplasia: Therapeutic equivalence between twice- and once-daily dosage forms. Phytother Res 11:558–563, 1997.
19. Stepanov VN, Siniakova LA, Sarrazin B, Raynaud JP: Efficacy and tolerability of the lipidosterolic extract of *Serenoa repens* (Permixon) in benign prostatic hyperplasia: A double-blind comparison of two dosage regimens. Adv Ther 16:231–241, 1999.
20. Mills S, Bone K: Principles and Practice of Phytotherapy: Modern Herbal Medicine. Edinburgh, Churchill Livingstone, 2000.

Siberian Ginseng
(*Eleutherococcus senticosus*)
rating: 🐾🐾

- Considered an adaptogen to help modulate stress and enhance mental and physical performance
- Claims primarily based on early research by Soviet scientists
- Beneficial effects on physical performance not validated by more recent trials
- Adverse effects poorly documented, but appear minimal

Eleutherococcus senticosus (syn. *Acanthopanax senticosus*) is in the same botanic family as the *Panax* ginsengs (Araliaceae), but is not a member of the *Panax* genus and is therefore not considered a true ginseng. *E. senticosus*, also known as Eleuthero, is commonly referred to as Siberian or Russian ginseng because it is indigenous to Eastern Russia. The root or root bark is used medicinally.

Uses: Siberian ginseng is claimed to have powerful adaptogenic and tonic properties that can modulate stress and improve mental and physical performance under a wide variety of stressful conditions. It was discovered by Soviet researchers who were searching for an alternative to Asian ginseng and other adaptogenic herbs.[1,2] Officially approved for use in Russia in 1962, Siberian ginseng became a popular commercial drink to help improve endurance.[3] In traditional Chinese medicine, this plant is considered a minor tonic (named ci wu jia). It has been employed for bronchitis, digestion, heart ailments, rheumatism, headaches, and insomnia, and to generally restore vigor and health.[2,4]

Pharmacology: The eleutherosides (A-G) are considered the most important constituents in the roots of Siberian ginseng. Unlike the ginsenosides of the Panax genus, however, the eleutherosides are a chemically diverse group of plant chemicals (lignans, sterols, phenylpropanoids, coumarins, and others), and are not unique to *E. senticosus*.[1,3,5]

Soviet researchers conducted numerous animal experiments with Siberian ginseng, and reported enhanced physical endurance and resistance to infection, radiation, cancer, toxins, and a variety of environmental extremes.[3,6,7] Anabolic, estrogenic, antiviral, hypotensive, and many other effects have also been demonstrated in animal models.[3,7] Conflicting reports in which extracts induced both hypoglycemia and hyperglycemia in animals, or enhanced both CNS sedation and stimulation, have been explained by the "adaptogenic" properties of the herb.[3] Alternatively, they may also be explained by different extracts or experimental conditions. Most of the earlier animal endurance studies were unblinded, which also raises the question of investigator bias; a more recent blinded study was negative.[8]

Limited pharmacologic data is available in humans. In a reportedly double-blind, placebo-controlled study, 10 ml t.i.d. of a German product for 4 weeks significantly increased lymphocytes by about 50% in 36 healthy volunteers.[9] In an unblinded, randomized, controlled study, 25 drops t.i.d. of an ethanolic root extract decreased glucose and cholesterol (total, LDL, and triglycerides), and increased neutrophil and lymphocyte activity in 50 healthy volunteers.[10]

Clinical Trials: Most of the original Russian clinical studies have been reviewed and summarized.[3,7] Initial research reported that athletes performed better; sportsmen had better endurance and concentration; and workers had fewer sick days when taking Siberian ginseng. In multiple studies that included over 2100 healthy subjects, Siberian ginseng was reported to demonstrate adaptogenic effects to help subjects withstand various adverse conditions and stressors (work load, noise, motion, heat, etc.), resulting in enhanced work performance. Studies in over 2200 unhealthy patients reported "benefits" in various diseases such as atherosclerosis and heart disease, acute pyelonephritis, diabetes, chronic bronchitis, hypertension and hypotension, trauma, neuroses, and cancer. However, outcome measures and actual clinical benefits are not well defined. Moreover, these studies were uncontrolled or unblinded, and would not meet today's standards for high-quality clinical research.

In more recent controlled trials, benefits for athletic endurance were initially reported in a single-blind, placebo-controlled study, and improvements in muscle strength demonstrated in a placebo-controlled trial with unclear blinding.[11,12] A Chinese study also reported an increased anaerobic threshold of power load and a decreased respiratory quotient (suggesting enhanced fat metabolism during exercise).[13] However, more rigorous double-blind studies have failed to verify these potential beneficial effects. A series of small controlled trials using treadmill or cycle ergometry found no ergonomic benefits for a brand of Siberian ginseng called Endurox.[14–16] Another well-designed trial of 20 runners found no ergonomic benefits with an ethanolic extract of eleutherosides B and E given daily for 6 weeks compared to placebo.[17] A well-designed, double-blind, crossover study found no measurable ergonomic or metabolic benefits in nine cyclists, randomly given placebo or 1200 mg Siberian ginseng daily for 7 days before two separate endurance cycling trials.[18]

Cognitive function (concentration and memory testing) was evaluated in a preliminary randomized, double-blind study of 24 adult volunteers who were given 1250 mg daily of Siberian ginseng, *Gingko biloba*, vitamins, or a placebo for 3 months. Results were published in abstract form only. Siberian ginseng did not objectively improve concentration compared to placebo, but it did improve results in a test for selective memory ($P < 0.02$).[19] In another randomized, double-blind study, Siberian ginseng significantly reduced the frequency, duration, and severity of herpes outbreaks. Questionnaires were distributed to 93 patients with herpes simplex infections, before and after a 6-month treatment with a standardized Eleutherococcus ethanolic extract (400 mg/day equivalent to 4 g dried root) or placebo. Improvements were reported in 75% of the ginseng group compared to 34% of the placebo group ($P < 0.0007$).[20]

Adverse Effects: Siberian ginseng is considered safe and nontoxic, although data is limited. No side effects were reported in any of the recent human trials, and there are no well-documented case reports of adverse effects. In the original Russian studies, adverse events were not reported in otherwise healthy subjects, although it was suggested that Siberian ginseng should not be used when blood pressures exceed 180/90.[3] In "unhealthy" patients, insomnia, arrhythmias, hypertension, headaches, irritability, and anxiety reactions were occasionally reported.[3] Caution is thus advised for patients with cardiac disease, hypertension, psychiatric diseases, or when using caffeine or other stimulants, although these potential side effects are not well established.

Interactions & Cautions: In two separate case reports, adulterated or mislabeled eleutherococcus preparations (most likely with *Periploca sepium*, which contains cardioactive glycosides) were associated with androgenization in a newborn[21,22] and with an increased digoxin level absent toxicity.[23] Safety of Siberian ginseng is unknown in women who are pregnant or breast feeding.

Preparations & Doses: Multiple products are on the U.S. market, from dried herb preparations to a variety of extracts. In the original Russian studies, doses were usually taken for up to 4–8 weeks at a time, interrupted by 2- to 3-week ginseng-free intervals;[3] however, there is no data to support these regimens. Common doses of encapsulated extracts currently on the market include one to three 100–400 mg capsules given 2–3 times daily, roughly equivalent to 1–4 g/day or more of a dried root product.[1]

Summary Evaluation

Siberian ginseng is commonly used as an adaptogen to help modulate responses to stressors and to enhance mental and physical stamina and endurance. These claims are primarily based on animal studies and early clinical investigations by Soviet researchers. Siberian ginseng does not enhance physical endurance based on more recent, well-designed clinical trials. Limited studies suggest that Siberian ginseng may enhance WBC activity, reduce cholesterol and glucose, enhance memory, and benefit patients with herpes simplex infections, but these studies require confirmation and, in general, the efficacy of Siberian ginseng is not established beyond a reasonable doubt for any indication. Based on limited data, Siberian ginseng appears safe, with no well-documented adverse effects.

---

references

1. Davydov M, Krikorian AD. *Eleuthorococcus senticosus* (Rupr. & Maxim.) Maxim. (Araliaceae) as an adaptogen: A closer look. J Ethnopharmacol 72:345–393, 2000.
2. Mills S, Bone K. Principles and Practice of Phytotherapy: Modern Herbal Medicine. Edinburgh, Churchill Livingstone, 2000.
3. Farnsworth NR, Kinghorn AD, Soejarto DD, Waller DP. Siberian ginseng (*Eleutherococcus senticosus*): Current status as an adaptogen. In Wagner H, Hikino H, Farnsworth NR (eds): Economic and Medicinal Plant Research. Vol 1. Orlando, FL, Academic Press, 1985, pp 155–215.
4. Blumenthal M, Goldberg A, Brinckmann J (eds). Herbal Medicine: Expanded Commission E Monographs. Newton, MA, Integrative Medicine Communications, 2000.

5. Baranov AI. Medicinal uses of ginseng and related plants in the Soviet Union: Recent trends in the Soviet literature. J Ethnopharmacol 6:339–353, 1982.

6. Brekhman II, Kikrillov OI. Effect of Eleutherococcus on alarm-phase of stress. Life Sci 8(I):113–121, 1969.

7. Fulder S. The drug that builds Russians. New Scientist 87:576–579, 1980.

8. Lewis WH, Zenger VE, Lynch RG. No adaptogen response of mice to ginseng and eleutherococcus infusions. J Ethnopharmacol 8:209–214, 1983.

9. Bohn B, Nebe CT, Birr C. Flow-cytometric studies with *Eleutherococcus senticosus* extract as an immunomodulatory agent. Arzneim-Forsch 37:1193–1196, 1987.

10. Szolomicki J, Samochowiec L, Wojcicki J, Drozdizik M. The influence of active components of *Eleutherococcus senticosus* on cellular defence and physical fitness in man. Phytother Res 14:30–35, 2000.

11. Asano K, Takahashi T, Miyashita M, et al. Effect of *Eleutherococcus senticosus* extract on human physical working capacity. Planta Med Jun(3):175–177, 1986.

12. McNaughton L, Egan G, Caelli G. A comparison of Chinese and Russian ginseng as ergogenic aids to improve various facets of physical fitness. Int Clin Nutr Rev 9:32–35, 1989.

13. Wu YN, Wang XQ, Zhao YF, et al. Effect of ciwujia (*Radix Acanthopanax senticosis*) preparation on human stamina. [Chinese; English abstract] J Hyg Res 25:57–61, 1996.

14. Smeltzer KD, Gretebeck RJ. Effect of *Radix Acanthopanax senticosus* on submaximal running performance. (Abstract) Med Sci Sports Exerc 30(Suppl.):S278, 1998.

15. Dustman K, Plowman SA, McCarthy K, et al. The effects of Endurox on the physiological responses to stair-stepping exercise. (Abstract) Med Sci Sports Exerc 30(Suppl.):S323, 1998.

16. Cheuvront SN, Moffatt RJ, Biggerstaff KD, et al. Effect of Endurox on various metabolic responses to exercise. (Abstract) Med Sci Sports Exerc 30(Suppl.): S323, 1998.

17. Dowling EA, Redondo DR, Branch J, et al. Effect of *Eleutherococcus senticosus* on submaximal and maximal exercise performance. Med Sci Sports Exercise 28:482–489, 1996.

18. Eschbach LC, Webster MJ, Boyd JC, et al. The effect of Siberian ginseng (*Eleutherococcus senticosus*) on substrate utilization and performance during prolonged cycling. Int J Sport Nutr Exercise Metab 10:444–451, 2000.

19. Winther K, Ranlov C, Rein E, Mehlsen J. Russian root (Siberian ginseng) improves cognitive functions in middle-aged people, whereas Ginkgo biloba seems effective only in the elderly. (Abstract) J Neurological Sci 150(Suppl.):S90, 1997.

20. Williams M. Immuno-protection against herpes simplex type II infection by eleutherococcus root extract. Int J Altern Complem Med 13:9–12, 1995.

21. Koren G, Randor S, Martin S, Danneman D. Maternal ginseng use associated with neonatal androgenization. JAMA 264:2866, 1990.

22. Awang DVC. Maternal use of ginseng and neonatal androgenization. JAMA 266:363, 1991.

23. McRae S. Elevated serum digoxin levels in a patient taking digoxin and siberian ginseng. Can Med Assoc J 155:293–295, 1996.

Slippery Elm (*Ulmus rubra*)

rating: 🐝

- Traditional demulcent remedy for respiratory, intestinal, and skin diseases
- No clinical trials performed

This American herbal remedy is traditionally obtained from the bark of the red elm tree, *Ulmus rubra* (also known as *Ulmus ulva*). The inner bark is required, and this may result in the death of the tree; thus, different species of elm bark are sometimes found in current preparations.

Uses: Today, the product is used mainly in lozenges and teas to treat pharyngitis. It is also employed for bronchitis, colitis, digestive disorders, peptic ulcer, gout, rheumatism, cystitis, and skin inflammation.[1] Slippery elm was used by traditional native Americans to treat wounds and as a poultice or salve for skin diseases, including bruises and burns.[1] The herb is also one of several herbal ingredients found in the popular alternative anti-cancer remedies Essiac and Flor-Essence.[2]

Pharmacology: A hygroscopic, mucilaginous material is extracted from the bark; it swells considerably when water is added.[3] Tannins, phytosterols, sesquiterpenes, sugars, starch, and other minor constituents are present.[1,3–5] The mucilage soothes the skin and mucous membranes.

Clinical Trials: No clinical trials have been conducted. A pilot study is planned to see if a controlled trial can be carried out on the multi-herb anti-cancer formulation, Flor-Essence.[2]

Adverse Effects: None, other than occasional allergic skin reactions.[1]

Interactions: No drug interactions are recognized.

Cautions: Slippery elm has a reputation as an abortifacient; this effect results from its deliberate use to dilate the cervical canal.[6]

Preparations & Doses: Slippery elm products are available in tablets, capsules, lozenges, liquid extracts, and powders.[7,8] It can also be prepared as an infusion or as a poultice. The usual dose is 200 mg given a few times a day. Alternatively, 4–6 g of powdered bark can be added to 100–500 ml heated water to make a mucilaginous drink. When 1 g is added to 40 ml cold water, a jelly forms within 1 hour.[8] The powder can be added to milk, and was formerly used as a food supplement.[1,6]

―――――――――― **Summary Evaluation** ――――――――――

Slippery elm is like marshmallow candy and other soft, bland, demulcent herbal products, such as plantain, coltsfoot, and comfrey. Although no specific benefits have been demonstrated, it is still favored in preparations such as throat pastilles for coughs or sore throat and for soothing various gastrointestinal symptoms.

references

1. Kemper KJ: Slippery elm. Accessed January 12, 2001 at Longwood Herbal Taskforce: Herb and Supplement Monographs, http://www.mcp.edu/herbal/default.htm
2. Richardson MA, Sanders T, Tamayo C, et al: Flor-Essence herbal tonic use in North America: A profile of general consumers and cancer patients. HerbalGram 50:40–46, 2000.
3. Mills S, Bone K: Principles and Practice of Phytotherapy: Modern Herbal Medicine. Edinburgh, Churchill Livingstone, 2000.
4. Brown D (ed): The Herb Society of America. Encyclopedia of Herbs and Their Uses. New York, DK Publishing, 1995.
5. Newall CA, Anderson LA, Phillipson JD: Herbal Medicines: A Guide for Health-Care Professionals. London, The Pharmaceutical Press, 1996.
6. Peirce A: The American Pharmaceutical Association Practical Guide to Natural Medicines. New York, William Morris and Company, 1999.
7. Blumenthal M, Busse WR, Goldberg A, et al (eds): The Complete German Commission E Monographs: Therapeutic Guide to Herbal Medicines (English translation). Austin, TX, American Botanical Council, 1998.
8. British Herbal Medicine Association: British Herbal Pharmacopoeia, 4th ed. Biddles, Ltd, Guildford, UK, 1996.

Tea Tree Oil (*Melaleuca alternifolia*)
rating: 🐾🐾

- Used for mild fungal and other topical infections
- *In vitro* antibacterial and antifungal activity well documented, but *in vivo* and clinical activity less well characterized
- Not for internal use

Tea tree oil, or melaleuca oil, is an essential oil from the leaves of *Melaleuca alternifolia*, a tree native to Australia.

Uses: Tea tree oil is primarily used as a topical anti-infective. It is found in facial care products to treat or prevent acne, mouthwashes and toothpaste, and skin and nail care products to treat or prevent fungal infections.

Pharmacology: Components of the essential oil are numerous; the primary antimicrobial constituents are terpinen-4-ol, 1-8-cineole, and alpha-terpineol. Antimicrobial activity has been demonstrated *in vitro* against various aerobic (e.g., *Staphylococcus aureus*, *Escherichia coli*, *Propionibacterium acnes*, *Pseudomonas aeruginosa*) and anaerobic bacteria.[1] *In vitro* antifungal activity is established for *Candida*, *Trichophyton*, and other species.[2-4] Minimum inhibitory concentrations (MICs) and/or microbicidal concentrations for most organisms range from 0.25% to 8%. *S. aureus* and most gram-negative bacteria have much lower MICs (0.25–0.5%) than the common resident skin flora.[5] In addition, *in vitro* testing of *Gardnerella vaginalis*, *Bacteroides*, and other gram-positive anaerobic cocci commonly associated with bacterial vaginosis indicates MIC_{90} of less than or equal to 0.5%.[6]

Clinical Trials:

- Fungal Infections—Uncontrolled trials and case series have reported benefits for various fungal skin and nail infections.[7-9] However, minimal benefits for tinea infections were demonstrated in two double-blind, randomized, controlled trials. For the treatment of *Tinea pedis*, one trial compared topical tolnaftate 1%, tea tree oil 10%, and placebo in 121 patients. Mycological cure was demonstrated in 85%, 30%, and 21% of patients, respectively. Effective therapy, defined as achievement of both mycological cure (negative culture results) and improvement by > 2 points on a 0–4 numeric symptom scale, was demonstrated in 46%, 22%, and 9% of patients.[10]

For the treatment of toe onychomycosis, a trial of 117 patients comparing clotrimazole 1% solution and 100% tea tree oil found no significant differences in mycological cure rate between the groups (clotrimazole 11%, tea tree oil 18%). Approximately 60% of patients in both groups had resolution of symptoms at the end of the 6-month treatment period.[11] However, topical clotrimazole is a poor therapy for onychomycosis, and tea tree oil did not prove superior.

In an uncontrolled trial of 13 AIDS patients with fluconazole-resistant oral candidiasis, 15 ml of a commercially available melaleuca oral solution (concentration unknown) was "swished and expelled" four times daily for 2–4 weeks. Of the 12 patients evaluated, two showed mycological cure, and six had improvement of symptoms at 4 weeks. One patient had worsening symptoms, and three were unchanged.[12]

• Other Uses—For the treatment of mild to moderate acne, one randomized, single-blinded trial compared 5% tea tree oil gel to 5% benzoyl peroxide (BZP) in 124 patients for 3 months. Both treatments significantly decreased the mean number of inflamed lesions, although there was a significant difference between groups in favor of BZP. Both treatments also significantly decreased the mean number of non-inflamed lesions (open and closed comedones), with no difference between the groups. Side effects of dryness, scaling, and pruritis occurred in 79% of BZP patients versus 44% of tea tree oil patients.[13]

A crossover trial of eight patients compared development of dental plaque after 4-day use of 0.1% chlorhexidine, water as placebo, or 0.34% tea tree oil solution.[14] No difference was found between tea tree oil and placebo; however, the tea tree oil concentration was well below the MIC required for many common oral bacteria.

There is one published case report of successful treatment of bacterial vaginosis with tea tree oil vaginal pessaries.[15] Although tea tree oil is often used for this purpose, and *in vitro* activity has been documented against most bacterial vaginosis organisms, no clinical trials have been conducted.

Adverse Effects: Contact dermatitis from tea tree oil, tea tree oil products, and tea tree foliage is well documented.[16–18] Reported adverse events of irritation from low-concentration products used in trials are < 10%.[7,10,13]

Interactions: Tea tree oil used in conjunction with other topical medications containing surfactants may affect antimicrobial activity.

Cautions: Tea tree oil should not be taken internally. High-percentage oil products should be kept away from children; ingestion of < 10 ml of 100% oil has resulted in central nervous system effects such as drowsiness and ataxia in toddlers.[19,20] Because large topical doses used on animals have demonstrated similar side effects,[21] topical use in infants and small children should be limited to small areas. Poisoning has been associated with respiratory depression, coma, abdominal pain, diarrhea, and death.[22] Also, the 100% essential oil can be irritating to mucous membranes. Tea tree oil should not be used for treatment of ear infections; one animal study demonstrated ototoxicity with topical application to the middle ear.[23]

Consumers should be aware that oil from other Melaleuca species is sometimes sold. These oils do not contain the same antimicrobial constituents and cannot be substituted for *Melaleuca alternifolia* oil. Use in pregnant or lactating women is contraindicated due to the lack of information regarding transdermal absorption.

Preparations & Doses: Products in published studies or reports have varied considerably in concentrations and preparations. These include 100% oil, 10% oil, 8% ointment, 5% cream, and 1% lozenge preparations. The concentration of tea tree oil necessary to optimize antimicrobial activity while minimizing the incidence of dermal irritation is unknown. MICs for most organisms as determined *in vitro* are quite low, but interference from surfactants, as well as other organic materials that may be present in products, increases the MICs for some organisms.[24] Products with concentrations of at least 10% may be needed to ensure that MICs are exceeded.

Summary Evaluation

The *in vitro* antibacterial and antifungal activities of tea tree oil lend support to theories that skin and nail care topical products may be of some benefit in prevention of infections. Benefits of varying degree have been demonstrated in controlled clinical trials for the treatment of tinea pedis and acne. Because side effects appear mild and typical dermatophyte infections are generally not serious, it is not unreasonable for patients who wish to use an herbal alternative to try tea tree oil for the treatment of mild fungal skin infections. However, the existing evidence does not support this recommendation; the clinical trials have many limitations and lack consistent results.

references

1. Concha JM, Moore LS, Holloway WJ: Antifungal activity of *Melaleuca alternifolia* (tea-tree) oil against various pathogenic organisms. J Am Podiatr Med Assoc 88:489–492, 1998.
2. Hammer KA, Carson CF, Riley TV: In-vitro activity of essential oils, in particular *Melaleuca alternifolia* (tea tree) oil and tea tree oil products, against *Candida* spp. J Antimicrob Chemother 42:591–595, 1998.
3. Nenoff P, Haustein U-F, Brandt W: Antifungal activity of the essential oil of *Melaleuca alternifolia* (tea tree oil) against pathogenic fungi in vitro. Skin Pharmacol 9:388–394, 1996.
4. Hammer KA, Carson CF, Riley TV: *Melaleuca alternifolia* (tea tree) oil inhibits germ tube formation by *Candida albicans*. Med Mycology 38:355–362, 2000.
5. Hammer KA, Carson CF, Riley TV: Susceptibility of transient and commensal skin flora to the essential oil of *Melaleuca alternifolia* (tea tree oil). Am J Infect Control 24:186–189, 1996.
6. Hammer KA, Carson CF, Riley TV: In vitro susceptibilities of Lactobacilli and organisms associated with bacterial vaginosis to *Melaleuca alternifolia* (tea tree) oil. Antimicrob Agents Chemother 43:196, 1999.
7. Walker M: Clinical investigation of Australian *Melaleuca alternifolia* oil for a variety of common foot problems. Current Podiatry 21(4):7,8,12–15, 1972.
8. Belaiche P: Traitment des infections cutanées par l'huile essentielle de *Melaleuca alternifolia*. [Treatment of skin infections with the essential oil of *Melaleuca alternifolia*.] [abstract]. Phytotherapy 15:15–17, 1985.
9. Shemesh A, Mayo WL: Australian tea tree oil: A natural antiseptic and fungicidal agent. Australia J Pharmacy 72:802–803, 1991.
10. Tong MM, Altman PM, Barnetson RStC: Tea tree oil in the treatment of tinea pedis. Australasian J Dermatol 33:145–149, 1992.
11. Buck D, Nidorf DM, Addino JG: Comparison of two topical preparations for the treatment of onychomycosis: *Melaleuca alternifolia* (tea tree) oil and clotrimazole. J Fam Practice 38:601–605, 1994.
12. Jandourek A, Vaishampayan JK, Vazquez JA: Efficacy of melaleuca oral solution for the treatment of fluconazole refractory oral candidiasis in AIDS patients. AIDS 12:1033–1037, 1998.
13. Bassett IB, Pannowitz DL, Barnetson RStC: A comparative study of tea-tree oil versus benzoylperoxide in the treatment of acne. Med J Australia 153:455–458, 1990.
14. Arweiler NB, Donos N, Netuschil L, Reich E: Clinical and antibacterial effect of tea tree oil - a pilot study. Clin Oral Invest 4:70–73, 2000.
15. Blackwell AL: Tea tree oil and anaerobic (bacterial) vaginosis. Lancet 337:300, 1991.

16. Osborne F, Chandler F: Australian tea tree oil. Canadian Pharm J 131(2):42–46, 1998.
17. Bushan M, Beck MH: Allergic contact dermatitis from tea tree oil in a wart paint. Contact Derm 36:117–118, 1997.
18. DeGroot AC: Airborne allergic contact dermatitis from tea tree oil. Contact Derm 35:304–305, 1996.
19. Del Beccaro MA: Melaleuca oil poisoning in a 17-month-old. Vet Hum Toxicol 37:557–558, 1995.
20. Jacobs MR, Hornfeldt CS: Melaleuca oil poisoning. J Toxicol Clin Toxicol 32:461–464, 1994.
21. Villar D, Knight MJ, Hansen SR, Buck WB:. Toxicity of melaleuca oil and related essential oils applied topically on dogs and cats. Vet Hum Toxicol 36:139–142, 1994.
22. Seawright A: Tea tree oil poisoning [comment]. Med J Australia 159:831, 1993.
23. Zhang SY, Robertson D: A study of tea tree oil ototoxicity. Audiol Neuro-Otol 5(2):64–68, 2000.
24. Hammer KA, Carson CF, Riley TV: Influence of organic matter, cations and surfactants on the antimicrobial activity of *Melaleuca alternifolia* (tea tree) oil in vitro. J Applied Microbiol 86:446–452, 1999.

Turmeric (*Curcuma longa*)

rating: 🐾 🐾 +

- This Indian herb is used traditionally as a flavor, dye, and digestive aid.
- Anti-inflammatory, anti-arthritis, anti-cancer, and antioxidant effects are currently gaining attention; controlled trials do not adequately show clinical benefits.
- A major constituent, curcumin, is also used as a phytomedicine.

Turmeric is the root (or rhizome) of the Asian plant, *Curcuma longa* or *C. domestica* (red valerian, haldi, jiang huang). When the roots are ground up, they yield a yellowish powder that resembles saffron; it is sometimes referred to as Indian saffron. Turmeric is used as a curry component and as a spice in Indian cooking, and can be used as a dye. Turmeric and its major component, curcumin, are both used as phytomedicines.

Uses: Turmeric has been traditionally recognized in India as a flavorful, colorful condiment, and as an Ayurvedic medicine to improve appetite, act as a carminative, and treat gallstones and other biliary problems, as well as dyspepsia.[1,2] It is a traditional remedy in India, China, and other Southeast Asian countries to treat asthma and colds, and is applied as an ointment, paste, or poultice for scabies, boils, bruises, insect bites, and other skin lesions. Turmeric is given orally for many other conditions, including menstrual problems, pain, epilepsy, respiratory tract infections, bleeding, diarrhea, jaundice, and rheumatic disorders.[3] More recently, it has gained a reputation as an anti-inflammatory agent, a treatment for hypercholesterolemia, an antioxidant, and a cancer preventative, and is claimed to prevent cardiovascular and other degenerative changes of aging. Claims also are made for its value in allergy, AIDS, cataracts, and other diseases. Curcumin is added to foods such as butter and margarine to prevent oxidation and to improve the color.

Pharmacology: More than 100 components have been isolated from turmeric.[4] The main medical component of the root is a volatile oil, containing turmerone, and other coloring agents, called curcuminoids. Curcumin (diferuloylmethane) is the major constituent, usually found in a concentration of < 6%.[5] Turmeric shares some compounds, such as zingiberene, with ginger, to which it is related.

Turmeric components have been shown in animal studies to inhibit leukotriene biosynthesis and to inhibit cyclo-oxygenase and arachidonic acid release; antiplatelet aggregation, and fibrinogen-lowering properties have also been demonstrated.[1,5] It has been suggested (without adequate evidence, however) that turmeric acts like a COX-2 inhibitor in the treatment of arthritis.[6] Curcumin and other turmeric components, such as borneol, curcumene, and azulene, have been shown in animal studies to have anti-inflammatory properties,[7] and to have protective effects for hepatocytes against toxins, hepatitis C virus, and HIV.[3,4] Other hepatic benefits of turmeric have been described, including inhibition of cytochrome P450 and glutathione 2-transferase; aflatoxin damage in ducklings has been reversed by curcumin.[8] Turmeric has free-radical scavenging and other antioxidant properties that result in a reduction of lipid peroxidation and the breakdown of polyunsaturated fatty acids.[9]

Curcumin may be a stimulator of apoptosis of osteoclasts, as well as prostate, gastric, and colon cancer cells in vitro.[10–12] Turmeric or curcumin has shown antiproliferative effects against human breast tumor cells in vitro,[13] and can inhibit prostate cancer angiogenesis.[11] Curcumin has antimutagenic, anti-HIV, and immune-enhancing effects in laboratory studies.[5,14–16]

Turmeric is regarded as a choleretic based on animal studies that demonstrate increased bile flow.[2,5] However, the clinical value of stimulating bile in humans is not well defined, especially as it is unlikely to exceed the normal digestive flow that accompanies the eating of a fatty or spicy meal. An ultrasound study in 10 healthy volunteers who were administered an oral dose of 20 mg curcumin found a 10–30% contraction of the gallbladder that lasted significantly longer than placebo; this was still considered to be significantly less than that caused by a normal meal (> 50% contraction).[17]

Although it is claimed that curcumin has about 65% bioavailability after oral administration,[18] this is contested by other studies that showed very poor absorption.[14,19] Many of the reported benefits seen with animal studies depend upon the turmeric extract being given by the intravenous route.[19] In the stomach and bowel, orally ingested turmeric may inhibit nitrosamine formation[5]; this compound may have a role in the development of colonic cancer.

Clinical Trials: Clinical trials have been primarily published in local journals from Asian countries. There have been no clinical studies on turmeric or curcumin from Europe or North America.

• Inflammation and Arthritis—In a randomized, double-blind, crossover trial from India, of 6-month duration and conducted on 42 patients with osteoarthrits, Articulin-F, an herbal mixture containing turmeric (plus ashwagandha, frankincense, and zinc) improved pain and disability scores compared to placebo.[20] Although the results were statistically significant, the individual effect of turmeric was not evaluated and the dose of turmeric (300 mg/day) was relatively small. A "preliminary" double-blind RCT on 18 patients with rheumatoid arthritis suggested curcumin 400 mg t.i.d. was as effective as phenylbutazone 100 mg t.i.d.; however, upon analyses of the results, phenylbutazone appeared more effective, and there was no adequate placebo control.[21]

Another RCT on the anti-inflammatory effects of curcumin in a dose of 400 mg t.i.d. involved 40 men who underwent surgical repair of a hernia or hydrocele.[22] The study was double-blinded and controlled with both phenylbutazone 100 mg t.i.d. and a placebo. Reductions in the intensity of postoperative inflammation after 6 days for curcumin and phenylbutazone (84.2% and 86%, respectively) were both reported as superior to placebo (61.8%). However, the results for curcumin from days 1–5 were no better than placebo, whereas phenylbutazone appeared superior.

• Dyspepsia and Ulcer Disease—In a double-blind RCT from Thailand on 116 patients with dyspepsia (which was not clearly defined in Western terms), 86% subjectively improved with turmeric 500 mg q.i.d. versus 53% on placebo after 1 week. However, patient satisfactory ratings for the two agents were identical.[23] A non-controlled Thai study of 25 patients with duodenal or gastric ulcers found that 600 mg of turmeric administered five times daily was associated with an ulcer healing rate of 48% after 4 weeks, and 76% after 12 weeks.[24] Controlled trials, however, have not confirmed any clinical benefits for ulcer disease. A well-designed Vietnamese double-blind study of 130 patients found that turmeric, at a dose of 2 g t.i.d., was no more effective than placebo for the symptoms and healing rate of duodenal ulcers after 8 weeks of treatment.[25] Similar negative findings were found in an open RCT of 50 patients with benign gastric ulcers confirmed endoscopically; a typical liquid antacid formulation was significantly superior to 250 mg q.i.d. of turmeric in inducing ulcer healing at both 6 weeks (65.2% vs. 33.3%) and 12 weeks (94.1% vs. 70.6%).[26]

• Other Indications—An open study on patients with chronic anterior uveitis evaluated 53 patients, with 21 lost to follow-up. Eighteen patients with a weak reaction to purified protein derivative (PPD) received 375 mg t.i.d. of turmeric alone for 12 weeks, versus 12 patients with a strong PPD reaction who received turmeric combined with antitubercular drugs for 1 year. The 18 patients receiving turmeric alone all improved within the initial 12 weeks, compared to 86% of the combined treatment group. After 3 years of follow-up, there was a higher recurrence rate in the turmeric group (55%) than the combination treatment group (36%), with similar rates of vision loss. The authors suggest that turmeric may be beneficial in treating chronic anterior uveitis, but the results of this non-blinded and poorly controlled study are difficult to interpret.[27]

Small uncontrolled studies in India and China have reported potential effects of turmeric or curcumin in lowering serum cholesterol.[28,29] In an open study of 45 patients that assessed cholesterol as a secondary endpoint over 4 weeks, triglycerides were reduced, but total cholesterol was unaffected.[24] An uncontrolled pilot study in India involving 814 patients reported that a paste of turmeric combined with neem was beneficial to treat scabies.[30]

Adverse Effects: Encapsulated turmeric or curcumin administered in the clinical trials was well tolerated; side effects were generally similar to placebo. In one trial of patients with duodenal ulcers, a burning sensation was reported twice as often in the turmeric group than in the placebo group (13% and 7%, respectively).[23] There are rare cases of allergic contact dermatitis reported.[18]

Interactions: Turmeric has antiplatelet effects *in vitro*, which could have an additive effect with anticoagulants or antiplatelet drugs.[5] However, antiplatelet effects have not been demonstrated *in vivo*, and no adverse effects or interactions have been reported in the clinical trials or from individual cases.

Cautions: The safety of the herb (especially the turmeric extract, curcumin) in pregnancy and during breast feeding has not been determined. Its choleretic effect may, in theory, cause an increase in symptoms in patients with gallbladder or biliary disease,[1] but this has not been reported in humans, and the effect is unlikely.

Preparations & Doses: Turmeric is used in foods, and is readily available as powders or capsules. Various extracts containing curcumin are available in liquid form or in proprietary mixtures. In the clinical trials, turmeric root or powder preparations were administered in a dose of 1–6 g/day, typically divided three times daily, whereas doses of about 400 mg t.i.d. of curcumin were used. Quality turmeric products are allegedly standardized to contain not less than 3% curcumin, and not less than 3% volatile oils.[2] Much larger amounts of curcumin can be administered than turmeric; the usual dose of 1200 mg/day of curcumin is equal to about 40 g/day of turmeric (containing 3% curcumin). A heaping teaspoon of powdered turmeric is about 4 g.[5]

--------------------- **Summary Evaluation** ---------------------

Turmeric is a valued spicy condiment that has been traditionally used to improve digestion and to treat dyspepsia and inflammatory disorders. Turmeric and its major component, curcumin, are also promoted as antioxidants; cancer, HIV, and hypercholesterolemia treatments; and cardiovascular disease preventatives. However, controlled clinical trials are either lacking for these indications or have not shown convincingly positive results. A clinical benefit has not been demonstrated for peptic ulcer disease, and one study was inconclusive for dyspepsia. Controlled trials for arthritis and inflammation also do not adequately demonstrate beneficial effects. Other uses have not been evaluated in controlled clinical trials.

references

1. Leung A, Foster S. Encyclopedia of Common Natural Ingredients Used in Food, Drugs, and Cosmetics, 2nd ed. New York, John Wiley & Sons, 1996.

2. Blumenthal M, Goldberg A, Brinckmann J (eds). Herbal Medicine. Expanded Commission E Monographs. Newton, MA, Integrative Medicine Communications, 2000.

3. Rhizoma Curcurmae Longae. WHO Monographs on Selected Medicinal Plants, Vol 1. Geneva, World Health Organization, 1999, pp 115–124.

4. Wichtl W. *Curcuma* (Turmeric): Biological activity and active compounds. In Lawson LD, Bauer R (eds): Phytomedicines of Europe. Chemistry and Biological Activity. Washington, DC, 1998, pp 133–139.

5. Mills S, Bone K. Principles and Practice of Phytotherapy. Modern Herbal Medicine. Edinburgh, Churchill Livingstone, 2000.

6. Duke JA. Clippings from my COX box. J Medicinal Food 1998/99:1(4): 293–298.

7. Beckwith JV. Herbal medications and nutraceuticals used to treat rheumatoid or osteoarthrits. In Miller LG, Murray WJ (eds): Herbal Medicinals. A Clinician's Guide. New York, The Haworth Press, Inc, 1998, pp 95–113.

8. Hamilton WR, Stohs SJ. Hepatic effects of herbal remedies. In Miller LG, Murray WJ (eds): Herbal Medicinals. A Clinician's Guide. New York, The Haworth Press, Inc, 1998, pp 37–63.

9. Quiles JL, Aguilera C, Mesa MD, et al. An ethanolic-aqueous extract of *Curcuma longa* decreases the suseptibility of liver microsomes and mitochondria to lipid peroxidation in atherosclerotic rabbits. Biofactors 1998; 8:51–57.

10. Ozaki K, Kawata Y, Amano S, Hanazawa S. Stimulating effects of curcumin on osteoclast apoptosis. Biochem Pharmacol 2000; 59:1577–1581.

11. Dorai T, Cao YC, Dorai B, et al. Therapeutic potential of curcumin in human prostate cancer. III Curcumin inhibits proliferation, induces apoptosis, and inhibits angiogenesis of LNCaP prostate cells in vivo. Prostate 2001;47:293–303.

12. Moragoda L, Jaszewski R, Magnondar AP. Curcumin induced modulation of cell cycle and apoptosis in gastric and colon cancer cells. Anticancer Res 2001;21(2A):873–878.

13. Mehta K, Pantazis P, McQueen T, Aggarwal BB. Antiproliferative effect of curcumin (diferuloyl/methane) against human breast tumor cell lines. Anticancer Drugs 1997; 8:470–481.

14. Sharma RA, McLelland HR, Hill KA, et al. Pharmacodynamic and pharmacokinetic study of oral curcumin extract in patients with colorectal cancer. Clin Cancer Res 2001;7:1894–1900.

15. Mazumder A, Raghavan K, Weinstein J, et al. Inhibition of human immunodeficiency virus type I-integrase by curcumin. Biochem Pharmacol 1995; 49:1165–1170.

16. Hosein SR. Curcumin and the immune system. Treatment update 104. Community AIDS Treatment Information Exchange, Canada, Vol 11, no. 10, 2000. Accessed July 29, 2001 at http://www.aegis.com/pubs/catie/2000/cate 10406.html

17. Rasyid A, Lelo A. The effect of curcumin and placebo on human gall-gladder function: An ultrasound study. Aliment Pharmacol Ther 1999;13:245–249.

18. Grant KL, Schneider CD. Alternative therapies: Turmeric. Am J Health-Syst Pharm 2000;57:1121–1122.

19. Ammon HP, Wahl MA. Pharmacology of *Curcuma longa*. Planta Med 1991; 57:1–7.

20. Kulkarni RR, Patki PS, Jog VP, et al. Treatment of osteoarthritis with a herbomineral formulation: A double-blind, placebo-controlled, cross-over study. J Ethnopharmacol 1991;33:91–95.

21. Deodhar SD, Sethi R, Srimal RC. Preliminary study on antirheumatic activity of curcumin (diferuloyl methane). Indian J Med Res 1980;71:632–634.

22. Satoskar RR, Shah SJ, Shenoy SG. Evaluation of anti-inflammatory property of curcumin (diferuloyl methane) in patients with post-operative inflammation. Int J Clin Pharmacol Ther Toxicol 1986;24:651–654.

23. Thamlikitkul V, Dechatiwongse T, Chantrakul C, et al. Randomized double blind study of *Curcuma domestica* Val. for dyspepsia. J Med Assoc Thai 1989;72:613–619.

24. Prucksunand C, Indrasukhsri B, Leetchochawalit M, Hungspreugs K. Phase II clinical trial on effect of the long turmeric (*Curcuma longa* Linn) on healing of peptic ulcer. Southeast Asian J Trop Med Public Health 2001;32:208–215.

25. Van Dau N, Ngoc Ham Y, HuyKhac D, et al. The effects of a traditional drug, turmeric (*Curcuma longa*), and placebo on the healing of duodenal ulcer. Phytomedicine 1998;5:29–34.

26. Kositchaiwat C, Kositchaiwat S, Havanondha J. *Curcuma longa* Linn. in the treatment of gastric ulcer compared to liquid antacid: a controlled trial. J Med Assoc Thai 1993;76:601–605.

27. Lal B, Kapoor AK, Asthana OP, et al. Efficacy of curcumin in the management of chronic anterior uveitis. Phytother Res 1999;13:318–322.

28. Soni KB, Kuttan R. Effect of oral curcumin administration on serum peroxides and cholesterol levels in human volunteers. Indian J Physiol Pharmacol 1992;36:273–275.

29. Chang H-M, But PP-H. Pharmacology and Applications of Chinese Materia Medica. Vol. 2. Singapore, World Scientific, 1986, pp 936–939.

30. Charles V, Charles SX. The use and efficacy of *Azadirachta indica* Adr ("neem") and *Curcuma longa* ("turmeric") in scabies: A pilot study. Trop Geogr Med 1992;44:178–181.

Uva Ursi (*Arctostaphylos uva-ursi*)

rating: 🐾🐾 –

- Traditionally used as a urinary antiseptic and diuretic
- A single clinical trial has reported benefits for prevention of UTIs.
- Appears safe for intermittent short-term use; excessive amounts should be avoided.

Uva ursi, also called bearberry, refers to the plant *Arctostaphylos uva-ursi*, the leaves of which are used in herbal medicine.

Uses: Uva ursi has long been used as a urinary antiseptic for mild urinary tract infections (UTIs) or inflammation, and as an herbal diuretic. The herb is a common ingredient in a number of "bladder and kidney" teas and products, which are popular in European countries. Uva ursi also has been employed for centuries as an astringent or hemostatic for diarrhea and hemorrhages, probably due to its high tannin content.[1–5]

Pharmacology: Key constituents of the leaf include hydroquinone glycosides (4–15%) such as arbutin, polyphenols such as tannins (10–20%), flavonoids, and triterpenes.[1,2,5] Arbutin is most likely hydrolyzed to hydroquinone in the gastrointestinal tract, which is eliminated in the urine in small amounts.[5,6] Uva ursi extracts, arbutin, and hydroquinone all have antimicrobial activity.[3,5] In a series of European experiments, hydroquinone was found to be the most active constituent of uva ursi, which has antimicrobial activity *in vitro* against typical urinary pathogens in an alkaline urine environment (pH of 8), but not in an acidic urine (pH of 6).[2,5] In rats with experimentally induced pyelonephritis, 25 mg/kg doses of a uva ursi extract were reported to have significant antibacterial and nephroprotective activity.[5]

Uva ursi's diuretic potential has not been scientifically evaluated in humans. Conflicting studies in animals have found diuretic activity when given by intraperitoneal injection; no activity when given orally; and anti-diuretic activity in one study.[7–9]

In other animal experiments, both uva ursi extracts and arbutin enhanced the anti-inflammatory effects of steroids administered topically or systemically.[10,11] Uva ursi fed to diabetic mice improved certain diabetic symptoms, but did not affect insulin or glucose concentrations.[12] Hydroquinone is also used in pharmaceutical drug products to reduce hyperpigmentation.

Clinical Trials: Monopreparations of uva ursi have not been evaluated in clinical trials. However, a combination herbal product (UVA-E) was evaluated in one randomized, double-blind, placebo-controlled trial for UTIs.[13] This extract product (containing uva ursi as an antiseptic and dandelion as a mild diuretic) or a placebo was given to 57 healthy women with recurrent cystitis. Treatment for 1 month significantly reduced recurrence during the 1-year follow-up period, with no cystitis in the herbal group (0 of 30) versus 23% recurrence in the placebo group (5 of 27; P < 0.05). Another combination herbal preparation (containing uva ursi, hops, and peppermint) was used to treat patients suffering from frequent and painful urination.[3] Of 915 patients treated for 6 weeks, success was reported in 70%; however, this study was not controlled. No studies have evaluated uva ursi's potential diuretic effects in humans.

Adverse Effects: There are no reported side effects from uva ursi products. The high tannin content (10–20%) may cause GI upset, and oxidation of hydroquinone may turn the urine a green-brown color.[1-3,5]

Interactions: The high tannin content of the herb could precipitate alkaloid drugs, and bind iron or other metal ions.[5] Foods or drugs that produce an acidic urine could presumably reduce the urinary antimicrobial effects of uva ursi, while alkanization of the urine would enhance this effect.

Cautions: Hydroquinone is toxic in large doses. Severe toxicity has been reported from ingesting 1 g, and death from 5 g.[3,14] However, large doses of the herb have reportedly been consumed without adverse effects, probably because hydroquinone is primarily available as arbutin; the concentration of hydroquinone ingested in usual doses is not thought to be toxic.[3] Nevertheless, hydroquinone has poorly documented hepatotoxic, mutagenic, and carcinogenic potential.[2-4] Coupled with hydroquinone's known toxic effects in large doses, and uva ursi's high tannin content, these concerns have persuaded herbal authorities to recommend limiting uva ursi's duration of therapy to 1–2 weeks at a time.[2–5] For similar reasons, the herb is best avoided in pregnancy and lactation, and in children.

Preparations & Doses: Two to three g of an oral dried-leaf preparation (containing roughly 100–200 mg of arbutin) are usually taken 3–4 times daily.[1,3,5] The combination product used in the positive clinical trial, UVA-E (Medic Herb AB, Sweden), was dosed as 3 tablets t.i.d., but the quantities of uva ursi and dandelion extracts were not reported.[13] Teas, fluid extracts, and tinctures are also used, and cold water extraction of the leaves should reduce the level of irritating tannins.

--------------- **Summary Evaluation** ---------------

Uva ursi has a long history of use as a urinary antiseptic and diuretic. Beneficial anti-infective effects are suggested based on *in vitro* antimicrobial activity (in alkaline urine only), animal studies, and a single positive clinical trial of a combination herbal product. These studies are promising, but should be considered preliminary. Diuretic properties have not been studied, and are mainly claimed on the basis of traditional usage. Excessive or prolonged use of uva ursi should be avoided due to the potential toxicities of hydroquinone.

references

1. Blumenthal M, Goldberg A, Brinckmann J (eds): Herbal Medicine: Expanded Commission E Monographs. Newton, MA, Integrative Medicine Communications, 2000.
2. European Scientific Cooperative on Phytotherapy: Uvae ursi folium: Bearberry leaf. Monographs on the Medicinal Uses of Plant Drugs. Exeter, UK, ESCOP, July 1997.
3. Newall CA, Anderson LA, Phillipson JD: Herbal Medicines: A Guide for Health-Care Professionals. London, The Pharmaceutical Press, 1996.
4. Schulz V, Hänsel R, Tyler VE: Rational Phytotherapy: A Physicians' Guide to Herbal Medicine, 4th ed. New York, Springer, 2001.
5. Mills S, Bone K: Principles and Practice of Phytotherapy: Modern Herbal Medicine. Edinburgh, UK, Churchill Livingstone, 2000.
6. Deisenger PJ, Hill TS, English JC: Human exposure to naturally occurring hydroquinone. J Toxicol Environ Health 47:31–46, 1996.
7. Beaux D, Fleurentin J, Mortier F: Effect of extracts of *Orthosiphon stamineus* Benth, *Hieracium pilosella* L., *Sambucus nigra* L. and *Arctostaphylos uva-ursi* (L.) Spreng. in rats. Phytother Res 13:222–225, 1999.
8. Grases F, Melero G, Costa-Bauza A, et al: Urolithiasis and phytotherapy. Int Urol Nephrol 26:507–511, 1994.
9. Borkowski VB. Diuretische wirkung einiger flavondrogen. Planta Med 8:95–104, 1960. [English abstract]

10. Matsuda H, Tanaka T, Kubo M: [Pharmacological studies on leaf of *Arctostaphylos uva-ursi* (L.) Spreng. III. Combined effect of arbutin and indomethacin on immuno-inflammation]. Yakugaku Zasshi 111:253–258, 1991. [English abstract]

11. Matsuda H, Nadamura S, Tanaka T, Kubo M: [Pharmacological studies on leaf of *Arctostaphylos uva-ursi* (L.) Spreng. V. Effect of water extract from *Arctostaphylos uva-ursi* (L.) Spreng. (bearberrry leaf) on the antiallergic and anti-inflammatory activities of dexamethasone ointment]. Yakugaku Zasshi 112:673–677, 1992. [English abstract]

12. Swanston-Flatt SD, Day C, Bailey CJ, Flatt PR: Evaluation of traditional plant treatments for diabetes: Studies in streptozotocin diabetic mice. Acta Diabetolog Latina 26:51–55, 1989.

13. Larsson B, Jonasson A, Fianu S: Prophylactic effect of UVA-E in women with recurrent cystitis: A preliminary report. Curr Therap Res 53:441–443, 1993.

14. Windholz M (ed): The Merck Index, 9th ed. Rahway, New Jersey, Merck & Co., Inc, 1976.

Valerian (*Valeriana officinalis*)
rating: 🐾 🐾

> - Commonly used for insomnia, but not conclusively demonstrated to be effective
> - Well tolerated with low abuse potential in usual therapeutic doses

The *Valeriana* genus contains hundreds of species; *V. officinalis* is commonly used in Europe and North America. The root or rhizome is used medicinally. It has a distinct and disagreeable odor when dried.

Uses: Valerian is considered to be a mild sedative-hypnotic herb, primarily promoted for insomnia in the U.S. It is a popular hypnotic and daytime sedative in many European countries. Traditionally, valerian has been used as a gastrointestinal antispasmodic and for a wide variety of physical conditions associated with anxiety, stress, and nervous complaints.[1-4]

Pharmacology: Numerous constituents have been identified, many of which have pharmacologic properties. The volatile oil, consisting of monoterpenes and sesquiterpenes such as valerenic acid, is one of the more biologically active components found in valerian root.[2-4] Valepotriates, such as valtrate and isovaleric acid, are pharmacologically active but very unstable, and are unlikely to be in finished products or absorbed systemically.[1] Alkaloids, amino acids, and other compounds may also contribute to activity, but no single constituent has been shown to account for all of valerian's effects.[2,3] Inhibitory GABA receptors are stimulated in the CNS by valerian extract, but the precise action is unknown and may involve more than one mechanism.[2,3]

There is a large body of pharmacologic literature from animal and *in vitro* studies; the details have been extensively reviewed.[1-7] In summary, extracts and isolated chemical constituents of valerian root have sedative, tranquilizing, and anticonvulsant properties in animal models. Barbiturate-induced sleep is enhanced, and peripherally acting antispasmodic effects have also been demonstrated. Outcomes vary considerably based on the individual extracted fractions, and doses used in the animal studies are often orders of magnitude greater than those recommended for humans.

Clinical Trials: A systematic review of the worldwide literature identified nine randomized, double-blind, placebo-controlled trials, conducted in Europe, of valerian mono-preparations.[8] Overall interpretation of the results of these trials was difficult because of the inconsistent methodologic quality and study designs, and variable results.[8] Based on questionnaires, polysomnography evaluations, or crude wrist meters, clinical improvements in sleep onset and/or sleep quality were observed in five trials, while effects were equivalent to placebo in four trials. Favorable EEG changes resulting from valerian were demonstrated in two of four studies. While two high-quality trials contained more than 100 patients (both with positive results),[9,10] most studies were much smaller, containing 8–14 patients each.[8] Clinical effects were usually observed within 1–2 days in shorter or acute-dose trials, but beneficial effects on sleep quality became statistically significant only after 4 weeks of treatment in one of the larger and better quality trials with 121 patients.[10]

Valerian has been compared with low doses of benzodiazepines in two double-blind trials. A combination valerian/hops product had no significant hypnotic effect compared to placebo in 20 healthy adults, but did have effects comparable to triazolam 0.125 mg in a post-hoc subset of "poor sleepers."[11] In a 4-week trial, sleep quality improved similarly in 75 patients given a valerian mono-preparation or 10 mg of oxazepam, compared to baseline. A higher number of patients in the oxazepam group (70%) rated the effects positive as compared to valerian (55%), but this was not reported to be statistically different.[12]

Valerian's efficacy was not confirmed in a more recent well-designed and well-conducted European study, which compared one night versus 14 nights of therapy.[13] Sixteen patients with insomnia, in a randomized, double-blind, placebo-controlled crossover trial with a 13-day washout period, were evaluated with objective polysomnographic recordings (measuring sleep efficiency, sleep latency, and sleep stages) as well as structured questionnaires (measuring subjective sleep latency, sleep quality, and morning feeling). After a single nighttime dose of valerian given as 600 mg of LI-156 (Sedonium), no significant effects were observed on any parameter. Even after 14 days of treatment, no subjective or objective parameters were affected by valerian, except slow-wave sleep latency, which was reduced compared to placebo. In the subjective questionnaire, a slight tendency toward reduced subjective sleep-onset latency was observed, which was not verified by objective measurements.

Although this study was small and thus not powered to detect slight effects, the rigorous study design compared to previous randomized controlled trials gives it added weight. Possible conclusions are that valerian has minimal or no objective benefits; dosing should last longer than 2 weeks; or the particular product used in this study is not as effective as others that had favorable findings.

Adverse Effects: Side effects were similar to placebo in the controlled trials.[5,8] In contrast to benzodiazepines, valerian does not appear to cause a hangover effect or adversely affect reaction time, alertness, or concentration the following day[14,15] although slight impairment of vigilance was found 1–2 hours after administration in one study.[15] Dependence and withdrawal reactions have not been observed with usual doses, but these responses have not been adequately evaluated.

In case reports, hepatotoxicity has been associated with herbal products that contain valerian, but most of these reports involve combinations with known or suspected hepatotoxic herbs.[5,16] One patient taking excessive doses of a U.S. valerian product (530 mg to 2 g per dose, 5 times daily for many years) developed high-output cardiac failure and delirium after discontinuing the herbal medicine while undergoing an open lung biopsy under general anesthesia. His condition slowly reversed with midazolam, raising the possibility of a valerian "withdrawal reaction" from excessive chronic dosing.[17] Valerian appears to be relatively safe in acute overdose cases. A suicide attempt by an 18-year-old college student who ingested 40–50 valerian capsules resulted in non-life-threatening effects such as fatigue, lightheadedness, body pains, and tremor, which all resolved within 24 hours.[18]

Interactions: There are no documented drug interactions. Valerian did not increase impairment due to alcohol according to one European placebo-controlled trial.[3] However, it is prudent to warn patients not to mix excessive doses of valerian with CNS-depressant drugs.

Cautions: Valerian byproducts are cytotoxic and mutagenic *in vitro*. It is doubtful that these effects are relevant for humans, however, as the most cytotoxic products (valepotriates) are very unstable and may not be present in marketed products; furthermore, they deteriorate rapidly in the intestines and are poorly absorbed.[3–5,19] In addition, chronic high doses of valepotriates in animals did not produce tumors, and oral administration did not produce teratogenic effects.[4] However, there is a lack of clinical data for pregnant and nursing women, and therefore valerian is not recommended for these subjects.[4]

Preparations & Doses: Traditionally, 2–3 g/day of dried root or rhizome (usually as an infusion or extract) is taken as needed 2–3 times per day as a sedative, or before bedtime for insomnia.[1,4] The dose for insomnia used in the controlled clinical trials ranged from 400 to 900 mg of an aqueous or ethanolic root extract, roughly equivalent to 1.5–3 g of dried herb, given 1/2 to 1 hour before bedtime.[8] The only product evaluated in these trials that is currently distributed in the U.S. is Sedonium (Lichtwer Pharma); it was not effective in a recent trial.[13] American products vary widely and are not uniform in content. Some contain whole herb, while others contain a variety of different proprietary extracts. Some valerian products are standardized to valerenic acid, which is a useful marker compound for *V. officinalis* as it is not found in other species.[3,4]

Summary Evaluation

Valerian root has traditionally been used as a mild sedative-hypnotic, but evidence from randomized, controlled trials is inconclusive. Valerian is well tolerated and with low abuse potential in usual therapeutic doses. It is not unreasonable for patients to try valerian root as a mild sedative or hypnotic, especially for those who want a non-addictive alternative to drugs such as benzodiazepines. However, valerian's efficacy has not been demonstrated beyond a reasonable doubt, especially with short-term use.

---

references

1. European Scientific Cooperative on Phytotherapy: Valerianae radix: Valerian root. Monographs on the Medicinal Uses of Plant Drugs. Exeter, UK, ESCOP, July 1997.
2. Houghton PJ: The scientific basis for the reputed activity of valerian. J Pharm Pharmacol 51:505–512, 1999.
3. Upton R (ed): Valerian root. American Herbal Pharmacopoeia and Therapeutic Compendium. Santa Cruz, CA, American Herbal Pharmacopeia, April 1999.

4. World Health Organization: WHO monographs on selected medicinal plants. Vol. 1. Geneva, WHO, 1999.

5. Bos R, Woerdenbag HJ, De Smet PAGM, Scheffer JJC: Valeriana species. In De Smet PAGM (ed): Adverse Effects of Herbal Drugs. Vol. 3. Berlin, Springer, 1997, pp 165–180.

6. Schulz V, Hänsel R, Tyler VE: Rational Phytotherapy: A Physicians' Guide to Herbal Medicine, 4th ed. New York, Springer, 2001.

7. Morazzoni P, Bombardelli E: *Valeriana officinalis:* traditional use and recent evaluation of activity. Fitoterapia 66:99–112, 1995.

8. Stevinson C, Ernst E: Valerian for insomnia: A systematic review of randomized clinical trials. Sleep Med 1:91–99, 2000.

9. Leathwood PD, Chauffard F, Heck E, Munoz-Box R: Aqueous extract of valerian root (*Valeriana officinalis* L.) improves sleep quality in man. Pharmacol Biochem Behav 17:65–71, 1982.

10. Vorbach EU, Görtelmeyer R, Brüning J: Therapie von insonmien. Wirksamkeit und vertraglichkeit eines baldrianpraparats. Psychopharmakotherapie 3:109–115, 1996 [English translation].

11. Dressing, Riemann D, Löw H, et al: Insomnia: Are valerian/balm combinations of equal value to benzodiazepine? Therapiewoche 42:726–736, 1992.

12. Dorn M: [Baldrian versus oxazepam: Efficacy and tolerability in non-organic and non-psychiatric insomniacs-A randomised, double-blind, clinical, comparative study]. Forsch Komplementärmed Klass Naturheilkd 7:79–84, 2000. Reviewed in Reichert R: Valerian root compares favorably to oxazepam in the treatment of insomnia. Healthnotes Rev Complem Integrat Med 7:295–296, 2000.

13. Donath F, Quispe S, Diefenbach K, et al: Critical evaluation of the effect of valerian extract on sleep structure and sleep quality. Pharmacopsychiatry 33:47–53, 2000.

14. Kuhlmann J, Berger W, Podzuweit H, Schmidt U: The influence of valerian treatment on "reaction time, alertness and concentration" in volunteers. Pharmacopsychiatry 32:235–241, 1999.

15. Gerhard U, Linnenbrink N, Georghiadou C, Hobi V: Vigilanzmindernde effekte zweier pflanzlicher schlafmittel [Effects of two plant-based sleep remedies on vigilance]. Schweiz Rund Med (PRAXIS) 85:473–481, 1996. [English summary]

16. Shaw D, Leon C, Kolev S, Murray V: Traditional remedies and food supplements: A 5-year toxicological study (1991-1995). Drug Safety 17:342–356, 1997.

17. Garges HP, Varia I, Doraiswamy PM: Cardiac complications and delirium associated with valerian root withdrawal. JAMA 280:1566–1567, 1998.

18. Willey LB, Mady SP, Cobaugh DJ, Wax PM: Valerian overdose: A case report. Vet Human Toxicol 37:364–365, 1995.

19. Bos R, Hendriks H, Scheffer JJC, Woerdenbag HJ: Cytotoxic potential of valerian constituents and valerian tinctures. Phytomed 5:219–225, 1998.

Willow (*Salix alba*)

rating: 🐾 🐾

> - Contains salicin, which is metabolized to salicylic acid
> - Effective mild analgesic at appropriate dosage
> - Caution in patients with contraindications to salicylates

There are over 300 species of willow trees found mainly in Europe and North America. The species of medical interest include *Salix alba* (white willow), *S. nigra* (black willow), and *S. purpurea* (purple willow); however, *S. daphnoides* and *S. fragilis* along with *S. purpurea* provide the greatest yield of salicylate precursors. The willow is the source of acetylsalicylic acid (aspirin); indeed, this well-known drug is generically named for its phytomedicinal source.

Uses: In ancient Greece, willow bark was used for gout and for febrile and painful disorders.[1,2] In 1763 the Reverend Edward Stone of Oxfordshire reported on its value in treating fevers.[3] Subsequently, salicylic acid was prepared from salicin in willow bark, and eventually aspirin was synthesized in 1853. Salicylic acid is also obtained from the meadowsweet, *Spira ulmaria*; aspirin was named after this plant.[5] Used for a variety of traditional indications in the past (including gastritis, gonorrhea, and as an aphrodisiac and sedative), willow bark is now mainly used to treat rheumatic disorders, and is a common alternative to aspirin as an analgesic and antipyretic. Recently, willow bark has been introduced into weight loss preparations.

Pharmacology: Willow bark contains 1.5–11% phenolic glycosides, including salicortin and its hydrolysis product salicin, as well as variable quantities of salicylic acid esters and their derivatives.[1,6,7] Other constituents include proanthocyanidins, catechins, and flavonoids (e.g., isoquercitin). Tannins are present in a concentration as high as 20%.

Salicin and salicortin are prodrugs which are split by intestinal flora into glucose and saligenin (salicyl alcohol), and both of these are well absorbed; saligenin is oxidized in the blood and liver to salicylic acid.[2] Since these chemical conversions take time, the effect of willow bark is slower in onset than that of aspirin. Furthermore, the amount of active drug in the popular *S. alba* is much lower than in other willows.[1,2] Thus, relatively low blood levels of active salicylates are obtained after oral use of crude willow herb preparations. Only concentrated willow bark extracts can provide sufficient active drug to reach blood levels of clinical value, since 80 g or more of a typical crude willow bark preparation would be needed to obtain 794 mg of salicin, which is the equivalent of 500 mg of aspirin.[2,5]

A study of 10 healthy volunteers given 1.4 g of a specific willow bark product reported a maximum salicylic acid serum level of 9.8 μm/L. This level is equivalent to what is attained with an oral dose of 40 mg of acetylsalicylic acid.[5] Such a result suggests that other agents in willow bark may account for its anti-inflammatory effect.

Clinical Trials: In spite of its long use, only a few controlled trials have been conducted with willow bark to support it as an analgesic or antipyretic. Collectively, these studies suggest that appropriate extracts may be beneficial for milder painful conditions. A recently published, randomized, double-blinded, and placebo-controlled study of 191 patients with chronic low back pain showed a positive dose-dependent effect, with pain relief within 1 week in patients taking 1400 mg of willow bark extract (containing 240 mg salicin) per day.[8] A 2-month, randomized, non-crossover study in 82 patients with chronic arthritis pain showed a small but statistically significant improvement in symptoms with a low-dosage combination willow bark formulation (Reumalex; containing 100 mg white willow bark extract, guaiacum, black cohosh, sarsaparilla, and poplar bark) compared to placebo.[9] An unpublished study is commented on in two reviews in which 78 inpatients in a German hospital were treated for 2 weeks for osteoarthritis of the hip or knee.[5,10] This was a double-blind, placebo-controlled trial that used a daily dose of 1360 mg of coated tablets of willow bark extract, equivalent to 240 mg salicin. The pain index significantly improved on the herbal preparation compared to placebo ($P < 0.05$).[5] A preceding pilot study had also shown the superiority of willow extract over placebo.[10]

Adverse Effects: In general, willow bark has been reported to be very well tolerated, with adverse effects—such as nausea, skin rashes, and wheezing—in less than 4% of patients.[10] Typical doses of salicin do not irritate the stomach, and recommended doses of willow bark extracts contain small amounts of salicylate; willow bark is therefore far less likely to cause gastric damage, bleeding, and allergic reactions than aspirin.[1] The high tannin content, rather than the salicylate components, is more likely to cause gastric disturbance. However, large doses of willow bark may have effects similar to those of aspirin.

Interactions: Salicin does not inhibit platelet aggregation, and is thus safer than aspirin with respect to interference with coagulation and interaction with anticoagulant medications. The use of willow in combination with other anti-inflammatory agents may theoretically increase the risk of gastric irritation, although this has not been described.[1]

Cautions: Willow bark should not be used in asthmatic subjects or other patients who develop allergic respiratory problems or rashes from salicylates, and a cautious approach should be adopted in patients who have had gastric complications or bleeding with aspirin. Although it is likely to be safe, it is advisable not to give it to children at risk of Reye's syndrome. The general precautions for aspirin should be taken when using willow products, although the bleeding risks are less with willow. Its safety has not been evaluated in pregnancy and in breast-feeding mothers.[11]

Preparations & Doses: Willow bark is available from various sources, which differ in their proportion of active components. Solid products and extracts, including alcoholic preparations and teas, are available, and are often incorporated in multiple-herb preparations.[12] Topical products are also in use. The recommended adult daily dose by mouth is usually 60–120 mg of the salicin component, but 240 mg/day may be more reasonable based on controlled trials.[8,10,11] The usual dose of dried willow bark is 1.5–3 g given three to five times a day.[2] Willow bark extract may contain as much as 17% salicin, but the amount is closer to 1% in some specimens[11]; thus correlation of bark dosages with salicin doses is unreliable. Standardized products with the amount of salicin listed on the label are recommended.

Summary Evaluation

Willow bark, which contains the analgesic salicin, is safer than aspirin, but effective dosing may be difficult to attain, and many experts are dubious about its value.[5,12] Nevertheless, products are promoted for use in treating fever, pain, and inflammatory joint disease. Several controlled trials have demonstrated benefits for extract products in the treatment of rheumatic and musculoskeletal pain. There is no established basis for incorporating willow bark in composite products for weight control or in "diaphoretic" teas. Its value in topical therapy has not been established. Although some authorities believe that willow bark is purely of historic interest, the evidence of recent studies suggests that this may be a premature judgment.

references

1. Highfield ES, Kemper KJ: White willowbark. The Longwood Herbal Task Force. Accessed January 14, 2001 at http://www.mcp.edu/herbal/default.htm
2. Blumenthal M, Goldberg A, Brinckmann J (eds): Herbal Medicine: Expanded Commission E Monographs. Newton, MA, Integrative Medicine Communications, 2000.
3. Mann RD: Modern Drug Use. An Enquiry on Historical Principles. Lancaster, England, MTP Press Limited, 1984.
4. Sneader W: Drug Discovery: The Evolution of Modern Medicines. New York, John Wiley & Sons, 1985.
5. Schulz V, Hänsel R, Tyler VE: Rational Phytotherapy: A Physician's Guide to Herbal Medicine, 4th ed. Berlin, Springer, 2001.
6. Newall CA, Anderson LA, Phillipson JD: Herbal Medicines. A Guide for Health-Care Professionals. London, The Pharmaceutical Press, 1996.
7. Willow bark. The Review of Natural Products. St. Louis, MO, Facts and Comparisons, March 2000.
8. Chrubasik S, Eisenberg E, Balan E, et al: Treatment of low back pain in exacerbations with willow bark extract: A randomized double-blind study. Am J Med 109:9–14, 2000.
9. Mills SY, Jacoby RK, Chacksfield M, Willoughby M: Effect of a proprietary herbal medicine on the relief of chronic arthritis pain: A double-blind study. Br J Rheumatol 35:874–878, 1996.
10. Ernst E, Chrubasik S: Phyto-anti-inflammatories. A systematic review of randomized, placebo-controlled, double-blind trials. Rheum Clin North Am 26:13–27, 2000.
11. Salicis cortex. Willow bark. ESCOP Monographs on the Medicinal Uses of Plant Drugs. European Scientific Cooperative on Phytotherapy. Facsimile 4, July 1997.
12. Willow bark (Adapted from the Complete German Commission E Monographs). Accessed March 13, 2001 at http://www.onhealth.webmd.com/alternative/resource/herbs

Wormwood (*Artemisia* spp.)

ratings: Common wormwood 🐾 —

       Chinese wormwood extract 🐾 🐾 🐾

> - Common wormwood, often used as a "bitter" herb, has not been well studied.
> - Pure wormwood oil is poisonous when ingested.
> - Chinese wormwood extracts (artemisinin compounds) are useful antimalarial agents.

Wormwood is a common name for specific plants of the *Artemisia* genus, which includes over 350 species worldwide. Two species used commonly in herbal medicine include *A. absinthium* (common wormwood) and *A. annua* (Chinese wormwood, or "qing hao").

Uses: Preparations of wormwood have been used as medicine for thousands of years. Common wormwood (*A. absinthium*) has traditionally been employed to eliminate parasitic worms and as an aromatic "bitter" to promote intestinal secretory activity for treating anorexia, dyspepsia, and "biliary dyskinesia."[1,2] Absinthe, an alcoholic beverage made from *A. absinthium* extract, was extremely popular in turn-of-the-century France.[3,4] Its mild hallucinogenic properties led to the belief that it stimulated "creative" and intellectual powers. Numerous artists, including Van Gogh, celebrated these effects; however, its use was ultimately banned because of purported CNS toxicity.

Chinese wormwood (*A. annua*) has been used for thousands of years by Chinese practitioners for the treatment of fever and related conditions, including malaria. In the 1970s, Chinese researchers isolated an active constituent of the herb, artemisinin (qinghaosu), and found that it had parasiticidal activity against both chloroquine-sensitive and chloroquine-resistant strains of *Plasmodium falciparum*. Artemisinin and several semi-synthetic derivatives are now used in Southeast Asia and Africa, especially for severe *P. falciparum* and multi-resistant malaria.[5]

Pharmacology: Common wormwood contains a number of biochemical compounds that have physiological effects. Absinthin and artabsin are believed responsible for the bitter properties of the herb. Several studies of bitter oral wormwood extracts have demonstrated increased gastric and biliary secretion in both animals and humans.[1,6] The essential oil contains the terpenoid thujone, which in toxic doses can cause autonomic excitability and convulsions.[2,4] Thujone is believed to be the ingredient in absinthe that is responsible for CNS toxicity. The structure of thujone is related to camphor and tetrahydrocannabinol, the active component in marijuana, which may account for some of the hallucinatory effects attributed to its use. Santonin, a sesquiterpene lactone isolated from *A. absinthium*, can paralyze helminthic worms, which are then unable to maintain their position within the bowel lumen.[7] Other constituents of wormwood, including flavonoids, phenolic compounds, and coumarins, have *in vitro* antimicrobial, anti-tumor, hepatoprotective, anti-inflammatory, and insecticidal activity.[8]

Extracts of Chinese wormwood also contain a number of volatile oils, including camphor, thujone, cineole, caryophyllene and artemisia ketone.[9] The sesquiterpene lactone artemisinin (qinghaosu) has antimalarial activity both in animals and *in vitro*. Artemisinin and an active metabolite, dihydroartemisinin, have a rapid action, and parasite clearance times are much shorter than with other antimalarial drugs.[5]

Clinical Trials:

• Common Wormwood—Despite the long history of use as an antihelminthic, there are no controlled trials of the crude herb for use in humans. Santonin, isolated from *A. absinthium*, was reportedly used effectively for roundworm (Ascaris) infections in the early 20th century; it is no longer used due to significant neurotoxic and other adverse effects.[7] The "bitter" activity of wormwood, applied by herbalists as a digestive stimulant for a variety of gastrointestinal complaints, has not been evaluated in controlled clinical trials for any medical disorder.

• Chinese Wormwood—Artemisinin and its derivatives from *A. annua* have demonstrated effective antimalarial activity in large randomized controlled trials from several countries with endemic malaria.[5] Falciparum malaria has been treated with great efficacy (generally 80–100%) and minimal side effects. Even patients with cerebral malaria, considered to be the most dangerous form of the disease, are generally cured, with mortality rates less than 10–20%, which is at least equivalent to standard antimalarial treatment. Two systematic reviews/meta-analyses found artemisinin agents to be at least as effective as quinine for the treatment of severe malaria (16 randomized trials), and similar to standard drug regimens for treating uncomplicated malaria (41 randomized trials) in non-blinded studies.[10,11] Despite the rapid clearance of parasitemia and malaria symptoms with artemisinin compounds, there is a relatively high malaria recrudescence rate following treatment; this has been reduced by more prolonged courses or by combining therapy with longer-acting antimalarial drugs.[5]

Adverse Effects: Dilute aqueous extracts of common wormwood have few acute side effects other than a bitter taste, which often limits consumption. More concentrated forms, especially pure wormwood oil that contains significant amounts of thujone, have severe toxicity.[6] In one case report, a 31-year-old man mistakenly ingested 10 ml of wormwood oil sold as topical "aromatherapy"; he developed seizures, rhabdomyolysis, and acute renal failure.[12] Abnormalities of hearing and vision, seizures, and brain damage are associated with chronic drinking of absinthe ("absinthism"), although it is unknown to what extent the alcohol content of absinthe contributes to these toxicities.[4]

Artemisinin compounds from Chinese wormwood are generally well tolerated, with the incidence of side effects (primarily gastrointestinal) being equivalent to or lower than that of comparable antimalarial regimens.[5,10,11] Of concern is that neurotoxicity has been demonstrated with high doses of artemisinin agents in animal models.[13] There is one case report of chronic cerebellar dysfunction in a patient who self-administered a 5-day course of an oral artemisinin agent for *P. falciparum* malaria.[14] Rare reports of neurotoxicity, and a potential neurotoxic risk with chronic use, prohibit use of these compounds for malaria prophylaxis in the absence of additional safety data.[5,15]

Interactions: Thujone in *A. absinthium* is a porphyrogenic terpenoid, and may exacerbate bouts of porphyria in patients with this disease.[4]

Cautions: Ingestion of pure wormwood oil from *A. absinthium* is absolutely contraindicated, and may be life threatening. Common wormwood should also be avoided in pregnant and breast-feeding women due to the concern over the toxic potential of thujone.[6] There are no specific contraindications to the use of antimalarial artemisinin compounds in pregnant or lactating women, but there is little data in these populations.[5]

Preparations & Doses: Common wormwood is prepared from the aerial parts of the flowering plant, and may be administered in tablets, teas, tinctures, and other extracts. Usual doses range from 5–10 drops of a dilute tincture (as an aromatic "bitter") to 1–1.5 g of crude herb brewed as a tea or decoction up to three times daily.[1,6] The volatile oil is used topically and for aromatherapy.

Artemisinin derivatives from Chinese wormwood are available in a number of different forms in countries outside the U.S.[5] Artemisinin extracted from the plant can be administered orally. Semi-synthetic derivatives with better water or oil solubility have been developed for intravenous, intramuscular, or rectal use (e.g., artemether, arteether, artesunate, artelenic acid). While dosing regimens vary widely, most successful trials have treated patients for 5–7 days.

--- **Summary Evaluation** ---

Common wormwood may have some efficacy as an anti-helminthic, although its clinical effectiveness has not been adequately evaluated. It may also increase gastrointestinal secretions (the "bitter" property of the herb), accounting for its use in mild gastrointestinal disorders; however, its clinical utility has not been studied and is not well defined in conventional allopathic medicine. The potential neurotoxic effects associated with thujone give this herb a low benefit-to-risk ratio.

In contrast, artemisinin compounds derived from Chinese wormwood appear to be a genuine advance in the therapy of malaria. These products may play a particularly important role in areas that have high rates of chloroquine-resistant *P. falciparum*.

references

1. Mills S, Bone K: Principles and Practice of Phytotherapy: Modern Herbal Medicine. Edinburgh, Churchill Livingstone, 2000.
2. Schulz V, Hänsel R, Tyler VE: Rational Phytotherapy: A Physicians' Guide to Herbal Medicine, 4th ed. New York, Springer, 2001.
3. Arnold WN: Absinthe. Scientific American 260:112–117, 1989.
4. Strang J, Arnold WN, Peters T: Absinthe: What's your poison? BMJ 319:1590–1592, 1999.
5. Van Agtmael MA, Eggelte TA, van Boxtel CJ: Artemisinin drugs in the treatment of malaria: From medicinal herb to registered medication. Trends Pharmacol Sci 20:199–205, 1999.
6. Absinthii herba: Wormwood. Monographs on the Medicinal Uses of Plant Drugs. European Scientific Cooperative on Phytotherapy, July 1997.

7. Woerdenbag HJ, Van Uden W, Pras N: *Artemisia cina.* In De Smet PAGM (ed): Adverse Effects of Herbal Drugs. Vol. 3. Berlin, Springer, 1997, pp 15–22.
8. Tan RX, Zheng WF, Tang HQ: Biologically active substances from the genus *Artemisia.* Planta Med 64:295–302, 1998.
9. Chang H-M, But PP-H (eds): Pharmacology and Applications of Chinese Materia Medica. Vol. 1, Singapore, World Scientific Publishing, 1986.
10. McIntosh HM, Olliaro P: Artemisinin derivatives for treating severe malaria (Cochrane Review). In The Cochrane Library, Issue 4. Oxford, Update Software, 2000.
11. McIntosh HM, Olliaro P: Artemisinin derivatives for treating uncomplicated malaria (Cochrane Review). In The Cochrane Library, Issue 4. Oxford, Update Software, 2000.
12. Weisbord SD, Soule JB, Kimmel PL: Poison online-Acute renal failure caused by oil of wormwood purchased through the internet. N Engl J Med 337:825–827, 1997.
13. Brewer TG, et al: Neurotoxicity in animals due to arteether and artemether. Trans Roy Soc Trop Med Hyg 88(Suppl. 1):S33–S36, 1994.
14. Miller LG, Panosian CB: Ataxia and slurred speech after artesunate treatment for falciparum malaria. (Letter) N Engl J Med 336:1328, 1997.
15. Hoffman S: Artemether in severe malaria—Still too many deaths. N Engl J Med 335:124–125, 1996.

Yarrow (*Achillea millefolium*)
rating: 🐝

> - Reputed to have a variety of uses, especially as an anti-inflammatory and astringent
> - Few clinical trials; effects not substantiated
> - Appears safe and well tolerated; data limited

Yarrow is a common name for many similar species and subspecies of Achillea; *Achillea millefolium* (common yarrow) is also referred to as Achillea, milfoil, and soldier's woundwort. It is a member of the Asteraceae family. The plant is named after Achilles, who was fabled to have used yarrow to treat wounds and staunch bleeding. The stems, leaves and flower are used medicinally.

Uses: Yarrow is reputed to have a host of beneficial effects in many cultures.[1-4] It is variably described as a diaphoretic, antipyretic, astringent, analgesic, anti-inflammatory, spasmolytic, and diuretic. Traditional indications include fevers, colds, digestive disorders, hemorrhoids, menstrual cramps, menorrhagia, and urogenital problems, and it is also used for wounds, bruises, sprains, and rashes. In the U.S., yarrow is approved as a flavoring in alcoholic beverages when the product is thujone-free.[3]

Pharmacology: Many organic constituents have been isolated from yarrow, including fatty acids, flavonoids, tannins, coumarins, alkaloids, and a volatile oil.[2-5] The oil contains sesquiterpene lactones, terpineol, camphor, thujone and many other constituents. Extracts contain variable amounts of the anti-inflammatory azulene or chamazulene; these may be found only in subspecies of *A. millefolium* that do not include common yarrow.[3,4,6] Azulene, chamazulene, and the flavonoids have demonstrated anti-inflammatory activity, while the flavonoids have the greatest antispasmodic activity in animal studies.[3-5] Yarrow extracts are reported to have antipyretic, sedative, antispasmodic, diuretic, hypoglycemic, and hypotensive actions in animal models, and antibacterial and antifungal activity *in vitro*.[3-5] Intravenous injection of an alkaloid constituent (achilleine) decreased bleeding time by 32% in rabbits,[7] potentially supporting its use as a hemostatic agent by herbalists.

Clinical Trials: There are few clinical trials of yarrow, and none using the herb as a monopreparation. In 34 patients with acute viral hepatitis, a combination herbal product from India (Liv-52) that included yarrow and seven other herbs reduced clinical symptoms and bilirubin levels faster than placebo in a double-blind, randomized trial over 6 weeks.[8] In a more recent randomized, controlled trial, an herbal mixture of yarrow, juniper, and nettle used as a mouthwash on 45 subjects with moderate gingivitis failed to affect plaque growth and gingival health compared to a placebo.[9]

Adverse Effects: Yarrow is considered to be well tolerated, with no known side effects.[1,4]

Interactions: Based on animal studies, large doses of yarrow may theoretically potentiate sedatives and antihypertensives, or counteract anticoagulants.[3] These properties have not been studied or reported in humans, and clinical effects are unlikely.

Cautions: Allergic subjects may develop contact dermatitis and systemic allergic manifestations, and patients with known sensitivity to Asteraceae plants (e.g., chrysanthemum, daisy, chamomile) may be more susceptible.[3,10] A minor component of the volatile oil is thujone, which is a toxic chemical in large amounts. The small concentration found in the herb is unlikely to cause toxicity; however, thujone is reputed to be an abortifacient and to affect the menstrual cycle.[3] Yarrow's safety in pregnancy and during breast feeding have not been established.

Preparation & Doses: Leaves, stems, and flower tops are employed in a variety of preparations, including decoctions, infusions, and tinctures. There is no standardized dose or formulation. A typical oral dose is 1–2 g dry herb or its equivalent, three times daily.[1,3] In the U.S., the herb is available in oral capsule form, or in a variety of liquid extract products.

Summary Evaluation

Clinical studies are few; thus, there is insufficient data to make evidence-based recommendations for the use of yarrow monopreparations. Yarrow extract may have some clinical benefit as a topical astringent or anti-inflammatory agent, but this use is based on anecdotal experience or tradition, and has not been substantiated in clinical studies. The alleged benefits of oral dosing for hepatitis and other disorders also have not been validated by controlled trials using monopreparations. Yarrow is likely to be safe and well tolerated for most patients (except those allergic to the plant), based on a long history of traditional use.

---

references

1. Blumenthal M, Goldberg A, Brinckmann J (eds). Herbal Medicine: Expanded Commission E Monographs. Newton, MA, Integrative Medicine Communications, 2000.

2. Hedley C. Yarrow—a monograph: *Achillea millefolium* L. Eur J Herbal Med 2:14–18, 1996.

3. Newall CA, Andersen LA, Phillipson JD. Herbal Medicines. A Guide for Health-Care Professionals. London, The Pharmaceutical Press, 1996.

4. Chandler RF, Hooper SN, Harvey MJ. Ethnobotany and phytochemistry of yarrow, *Achillea millefolium*, Compositae. Econ Botany 36:203–223, 1982.

5. Yarrow. The Review of Natural Products. St. Louis, MO, Facts and Comparisons, 1998.

6. Zeylstra H. Just yarrow? Br J Phytother 4:184-189, 1997.

7. Miller FM, Chow LM. Alkaloids of *Achillea millefolium* L. I. Isolation and characterization of achilleine. J Am Chem Soc 76:1353–1354, 1954.

8. Sama SK, Krishnamurthy L, Ramachandran K, Lal K. Efficacy of an indigenous compound preparation (Liv-52) in acute viral hepatitis: A double-blind study. Indian J Med Res 64:738–742, 1976.

9. Van der Weijden GA, Timmer C, Timmerman MF, et al. The effect of herbal extracts in an experimental mouthrinse on established plaque and gingivitis. J Clin Periodontol 25:399–403, 1998.

10. Hausen BM. A 6-year experience with Compositae mix. Am J Contact Dermat 7:94–99, 1996.

Yohimbe (*Pausinystalia yohimbe*)

rating: 🐾🐾 −

> - Commonly used for erectile dysfunction or sexual potency; results of controlled clinical trials inconsistent
> - Adverse effects mild with usual doses, but dose dependent
> - Many drug and disease interactions

Yohim<u>be</u> is the crude herbal product derived from the dried bark of *Pausinystalia yohimbe*, a West African evergreen tree. Yohim<u>bine</u> is the active chemical isolated from yohimbe, also found in smaller concentrations in the root of *Rauwolfia*.

Uses: Yohimbe bark was originally used in Africa as an aphrodisiac and to restore erections in impotent men.[1] Crude yohimbe and the isolated chemical yohimbine are similarly used in Western countries to increase sexual desire and for erectile dysfunction. These products are also used in male "performance" supplements, and for fatigue, orthostatic hypotension, obesity, and clonidine overdose.

Pharmacology: The bark of *P. yohimbe* contains up to 6% mixed indole alkaloids, of which yohimbine is the principal active constituent.[1] Structurally related to reserpine, yohimbine has been well characterized as a selective alpha$_2$ adrenergic receptor antagonist.[2,3] Yohimbine readily enters the central nervous system (CNS), where it increases sympathetic outflow, potentiating the release of norepinephrine from sympathetic nerve terminals. These effects activate alpha and beta receptors in the heart and peripheral vasculature, with a consequent rise in heart rate and blood pressure.[2] These actions are opposite to those of clonidine, an alpha$_2$ receptor *agonist*, which *decreases* sympathetic outflow. At high concentrations, yohimbine also inhibits monoamine oxidase (MAO) and acetylcholinesterase enzymes, and has other pharmacologic properties.[3]

Yohimbine successfully stimulates sexual behavior in animal models.[4,5] The most likely mechanisms include a direct CNS effect, and/or a peripheral effect on alpha$_2$ adrenergic receptors in penile tissue that relaxes smooth muscle in the corpus cavernosum.[6,7]

Clinical Trials: Yohimbe, the crude herb, has not been studied clinically. However, yohimbine has been studied in many randomized, controlled trials, and a systematic review and meta-analysis evaluated the placebo-controlled trials published through early 1997.[8] Only moderate- to high-quality studies were included, and seven trials met criteria for yohimbine monotherapy. These trials contained 11 to 100 patients each, lasted from 4 to 10 weeks, and included patients with both organic and psychogenic impotence. The usual dose was 5–10 mg t.i.d. Outcome measures were not uniform among the studies, and included questionnaires of self-reported treatment success, objective rating scales, and penile tumescence monitoring.

All studies found that yohimbine was more effective than placebo; this reached statistical significance in five of the seven trials. Statistically significant results were found less often for patients with identified organic etiologies. A meta-analysis of the studies also favored the drug over placebo, with a calculated overall odds ratio of 3.85 (95% confidence interval 6.67–2.22). Positive responders varied from 34% to 73% with yohimbine, and from 4% to 45% with placebo.

Despite these overall positive findings, three subsequent chronic trials of good quality found negative results. In one randomized, double-blind, placebo-controlled crossover study, 36 mg/day of yohimbine had identical findings to placebo in 29 patients with mixed-type impotence.[9] In an unrandomized placebo-controlled trial, a large dose of 100 mg/day also had similar activity to placebo in 22 patients with organic erectile dysfunction.[10] Lastly, a randomized, controlled crossover study of 5.4 mg t.i.d. (combined with isoxsuprine or pentoxifylline) found none of 20 patients with vasculogenic erectile dysfunction to have a complete therapeutic response. In addition, no improvement was seen in arterial flow velocity or resistance indexes by penile duplex ultrasonography.[11]

Yohimbine has been reported to have some success in controlled studies for treating autonomic orthostatic hypotension[3,12]; as an antidote for clonidine overdose[13,14]; to reverse symptoms of dry mouth by increasing salivary flow[15]; and to decrease symptoms of opiate withdrawal.[16]

Adverse Effects: In most of the clinical trials using usual doses of 5–10 mg t.i.d., adverse effects were observed in about 10–30% of patients, but were considered to be minor and well tolerated. These primarily included anxiety, headache, dizziness, nausea, tachycardia, and hypertension.[8] In a clinical trial using an excessively large dose of 100 mg q.d., adverse effects were identified in 80% of patients compared to 20% of placebo controls. The most frequently reported side effects for yohimbine were increased urinary frequency (32%), tachycardia (27%), and anxiety (18%).[10]

Yohimbine should be avoided in patients with hypertension; it has been associated with increased blood pressure in these patients, and with a case of hypertensive crisis.[3,17,18] Based on its pharmacologic effects, yohimbine should also be avoided in patients with angina, claudication, or other cardiovascular diseases. Anxiety or an exacerbation of symptoms is more likely to occur in patients with psychiatric disorders such as panic attacks, post-traumatic stress disorder, and bipolar-affective disease.[19–21]

Yohimbine has also been associated with isolated case reports of bronchospasm,[22] agranulocytosis,[23] and a lupus-like syndrome with renal failure[24]; product contamination is also a possible cause of these disparate reports. Overdoses with several hundred milligrams have resulted in cardiovascular, gastrointestinal, and nervous system toxicities, with clinical outcomes ranging from benign to fatal.[3,25]

Interactions: Yohimbine antagonizes the antihypertensive properties of central alpha$_2$ agonists such as clonidine and guanabenz, and the effects of yohimbine can similarly be reduced.[3] Yohimbine may cause exaggerated cardiovascular and anxiety responses in patients concurrently taking psychiatric medications, especially tricyclic antidepressants that inhibit norepinephrine reuptake.[3] These effects are not expected with selective serotonin reuptake inhibitors.[3,26] Some authors have advised that yohimbine should not be used concurrently with sympathomimetic drugs or tyramine-containing foods, based on the herb's potential MAO inhibitor effects.[1] These concerns are probably not warranted at usual therapeutic doses, and no interactions have been reported.[3] However, it would be advisable to avoid yohimbine with other sympathomimetic drugs (including caffeine and other stimulants) due to the potential for enhanced cardiovascular and CNS toxicity.

Cautions: Due to lack of data and the potential for cardiovascular or CNS effects, yohimbine should generally be avoided in pregnant and breast-feeding women.[3]

Preparations & Doses: Yohimbine and yohimbe are widely available herbal medicines as monopreparations or combined with many other herbs and supplements. The usual oral dose of yohimbine for erectile dysfunction is 5–10 mg t.i.d. Yohimbine is also available as an FDA-approved prescription drug (5.4-mg tablet as the HCl salt), marketed as a "sympatholytic and mydriatic," although actual pharmacologic effects may be quite different.

Summary Evaluation

Yohimbine is widely used for erectile dysfunction and sexual potency. The results of randomized controlled clinical trials are generally positive, especially for nonorganic etiologies, but study results are inconsistent and do not demonstrate efficacy beyond a reasonable doubt. Benefits, if any, appear to be mild; yohimbine is not expected to be as effective as sildenafil or other well-characterized pharmacologic therapies for erectile dysfunction. Side effects of usual doses of yohimbine appear to be well tolerated in selected patients in controlled studies, but adverse effects are dose-dependent. There are also many potential and reported drug and disease interactions.

references

1. Blumenthal M, Goldberg A, Brinckmann J (eds): Herbal Medicine: Expanded Commission E Monographs. Newton, MA, Integrative Medicine Communications, 2000.
2. Hoffman BB, Lefkowitz RJ: Catecholamines, sympathomimetic drugs, and adrenergic receptor antagonists. In Hardman JG, Limbird LE (eds): Goodman & Gilman's The Pharmacological Basis of Therapeutics, 9th ed. New York, McGraw-Hill, 1996, pp 199–248.
3. De Smet PAGM: Yohimbe alkaloids—General discussion. In De Smet PAGM (ed): Adverse Effects of Herbal Drugs. Vol. 3. Berlin, Springer, 1997, pp 181–205.
4. Clark JT, Smith ER, Davidson JM: Evidence for the modulation of sexual behavior by alpha-adrenoceptors in male rats. Neuroendocrinol 41:36–43, 1985.
5. Sala M, Braida D, Leone MP: Central effect of yohimbine on sexual behaviour in the rat. Physiol Behav 47:165–173, 1990.
6. Morales A: Yohimbine in erectile dysfunction: The facts. Int J Impotence Res 12 (Suppl 1):S70–S74, 2000.
7. Maggi M, Filippi S, Ledda F, et al: Erectile dysfunction: From biochemical pharmacology to advances in medical therapy. Eur J Endocrin 143:143–154, 2000.
8. Ernst E, Pittler MH: Yohimbine for erectile dysfunction: A systematic review and meta-analysis of randomized clinical trials. J Urology 159:433–436, 1998.
9. Kunelius P, Häkkinen J, Lukkarinen O: Is high-dose yohimbine hydrochloride effective in the treatment of mixed type impotence? Urology 49:441–444, 1997.

10. Telöken C, Rhoden EL, Sogari P, et al: Therapeutic effects of high-dose yohimbine hydrochloride on organic erectile dysfunction. J Urol 159:122–124, 1998.

11. Knoll LD, Benson RC Jr, Bihartz DL, et al: A randomized crossover study using yohimbine and isoxsuprine versus pentoxifylline in the management of vasculogenic impotence. J Urol 155:144–146, 1996.

12. Lacomblez L, Bensimon G, Isnard F, et al: Effect of yohimbine on blood pressure in patients with depression and orthostatic hypotension induced by clomipramine. Clin Pharmacol Ther 45:241–251, 1989.

13. Roberge RJ, McGuire SP, Krenzelok EP: Yohimbine as an antidote for clonidine overdose. Am J Emerg Med 14:678–680, 1996.

14. Shannon M: Yohimbine. Ped Emerg Care 16:49–50, 2000.

15. Bagheri H, Schmitt L, Berlan M, Montastruc JL: A comparative study of the effects of yohimbine and anetholtrithione on salivary secretion in depressed patients treated with psychotropic drugs. Eur J Clin Pharmacol 52:339–342, 1997.

16. Hameedi FA, Woods SW, Rosen MI, et al: Dose-dependent effects of yohimbine on methadone maintained patients. Am J Drug Alcohol Abuse 23:327–333, 1997.

17. Musso NR, Vergassola C, Pende A, Lotti G: Yohimbine effects on blood pressure and plasma catecholamines in human hypertension. Am J Hyperten 8:565–571, 1995.

18. Ruck B, Shih RD, Marcus SM: Hypertensive crisis from herbal treatment of impotence (correspondence). Am J Emerg Med 17:317–318, 1999.

19. Southwick SM, Morgan CA, Charney DS, High JR: Yohimbine use in a natural setting: Effects on posttraumatic stress disorder. Biol Psychiatry 46:442–444, 1999.

20. Gurguis GN, Vitton BJ, Uhde TW: Behavioral, sympathetic, and adrenocortical responses to yohimbine in panic disorder patients and normal controls. Psychiatr Res 71:27–39, 1997.

21. Price LH, Charney DS, Heninger GR: Three cases of manic symptoms following yohimbine administration. Am J Psychiatry 141:1267–1268, 1984.

22. Landis E, Shore E: Yohimbine-induced bronchospasm. Chest 96:1424, 1989.

23. Siddiqui MA, More-O'Ferrall D, Hammod RS, et al: Agranulocytosis associated with yohimbine use. Arch Int Med 156:1235–1238, 1996.

24. Sandler B, Aronson P: Yohimbine-induced cutaneous drug eruption, progressive renal failure, and lupus-like syndrome. Urology 41:343–345, 1993.

25. Friesen K, Palatnick W, Tenenbein M: Benign course after massive ingestion of yohimbine. J Emerg Med 11:287–288, 1993.

26. Ashton AK, Hamer R, Rosen RC: Serotonin reuptake inhibitor-induced sexual dysfunction and its treatment: A large-scale retrospective study of 596 psychiatric outpatients. J Sex Marital Ther 23:165–175, 1997.

Yucca (*Yucca* spp.)

rating: 🐾 🐾

> - Usually employed for purported anti-inflammatory properties
> - Evidence not convincing for any indication
> - Appears to be safe and well tolerated

Yucca plants include a number of different trees and shrubs found in arid portions of North and Central America. Common species include *Yucca aloifolia* (Spanish bayonet), *Y. brevifolia* (Joshua tree), *Y. filamentosa* (Adam's needle), *Y. glauca* (soapweed), and many others. All parts of the plant, as well as many different species, are used.

Uses: As a dietary supplement in the U.S., yucca is commonly marketed as an anti-inflammatory herb, primarily for the treatment of arthritis symptoms. There are also claims that yucca may help reduce blood pressure and cholesterol levels. Traditionally, yucca has been used by different cultures for a wide variety of medical conditions, including gout, gall bladder problems, diabetes, genitourinary disorders, indigestion, and constipation, and also has been used as a diuretic and topically for inflammation or general skin cleansing.[1–5] Native Americans have created soap, shampoo, rope, and textiles from yucca plants. Plant constituents are also used commercially as foaming agents and flavorings.

Pharmacology: Yucca plants contain steroidal saponins such as sarsasapogenin and tigogenin.[1,6] Saponins are widely used for their detergent and foaming properties, and have also been studied in animals for their potential anticholesterol, anti-inflammatory, and anticarcinogenic activities.[7,8] Yucca leaf protein can interfere *in vitro* with the protein synthesis of cells infected by herpes simplex virus and cytomegalovirus.[9] Flowers of certain yucca species contain polysaccharides with tumor-inhibiting effects in mice.[10,11]

Clinical Trials: Yucca has been evaluated in two controlled trials from the 1970s by the same principal investigator; both studies have significant methodologic flaws.

In one supposedly randomized, double-blind, placebo-controlled study, adults with osteoarthritis or rheumatoid arthritis took

2–8 tablets daily of a saponin extract (amount unknown) from an unidentified desert yucca plant. Of 165 patients enrolled, 149 replied to a questionnaire after 1 week to 15 months of treatment. Subjective benefits were found in the yucca group in 49–77% of patients based on different types of questions, while only 21.5% of the placebo group indicated improvement. Although the results are suggestive of benefit, study weaknesses and poorly described methodology severely limit the value of the study. Only 17 of 51 placebo patients answered the questionnaire (other results were abstracted from charts); questionnaire results were incompletely reported for the placebo group; and randomization was flawed (at one site, all the patients received yucca tablets). In addition, duration of treatment and follow-up was highly variable, and compliance was not measured.[12]

In the second study, of similar design, 2 tablets of yucca extract or placebo were given with each meal to 212 arthritic patients for up to 16 months to study the effects on cholesterol, triglycerides, and blood pressure. The investigators claimed that yucca reduced all three parameters compared to placebo. However, the study had similar design and methodologic weaknesses to those of the previous study. In addition, the data descriptions are confusing; there is no statistical analysis; and study "blinding" was faulty (the office nurses, who dispensed the tablets, were aware of which patients were in each group).[13]

Adverse Effects: In general, saponins may cause dose-dependent gastrointestinal distress, especially in raw plant form.[2,8,14] In one of the controlled clinical trials using yucca tablets, mild and transient complaints were reported in about 9% of patients, and unfavorable gastrointestinal effects were reported in 4%.[12] Native Americans and others have used the yucca plant as food for centuries without known adverse effects.

Interactions: No interactions are recognized.

Cautions: Safety in pregnant and breast-feeding women has not been established. Injected directly into the bloodstream, saponins can cause hemolysis.[1,8]

Preparations & Doses: Precise doses have not been established. In the clinical studies that used a yucca saponin extract, 2 tablets were taken three times daily, usually with or after meals. The amount of yucca or saponin in each tablet, and other ingredients in the extract, were not described.[12,13] Traditionally, herbalists have made decoctions by boiling the roots or young shoots in water.[2]

Summary Evaluation

Yucca is most commonly used for the inflammatory symptoms of arthritis. The one controlled study that claimed benefits for this condition was severely flawed. Similarly, effects on lipids and blood pressure are poorly characterized. Yucca appears to be safe and well tolerated, but there is no convincing evidence that it is effective in treating any medical disorder.

references

1. Yucca. Lawrence Review of Natural Products. St. Louis, MO, Facts and Comparisons, March 1994.
2. Moore M: Medicinal Plants of the Desert and Canyon West. Santa Fe, NM, Museum of New Mexico Press, 1989.
3. Morton JF: Atlas of Medicinal Plants of Middle America. Springfield, Ill, Thomas Books, 1981.
4. Foster SF, Duke JA: A Field Guide to Medicinal Plants: Eastern and Central North America. Boston, Houghton Mifflin Co, 1990.
5. Heinerman J: Aloe Vera, Jojoba, and Yucca: The Amazing Health Benefits They Can Give You. New Canaan, Connecticut, Keats Publishing, 1982.
6. Mahato SB, Ganguly AN, Sahu NP: Steroid saponins. Phytochem 21:959–978, 1982.
7. Hostettmann K, Marston A: Saponins. New York, Cambridge University Press, 1995.
8. Mills S, Bone K: Principles and Practice of Phytotherapy: Modern Herbal Medicine. Edinburgh, Churchill Livingstone, 2000.
9. Hayashi K, Nishino H, Niwayama S, et al: Yucca leaf protein stops the protein synthesis in HSV-infected cells and inhibits virus replication. Antiviral Res 17:323–333, 1992.
10. Sokoloff B: The oncostatic and oncolytic factors present in certain plants. Oncology 22:49–60, 1968.
11. Ali MS, Shapma GC, Asplund RO, et al: Isolation of antitumor polysaccharide fractions from *Yucca glauca* Nutt. (Lilliaceae). Growth 42:213–223, 1978.
12. Bingham R, Bellew BA, Bellew JG: Yucca plant saponin in the management of arthritis. J Applied Nutrition 27:45–51, 1975.
13. Bingham R, Harris DH, Laga T: Yucca plant saponin in the treatment of hypertension and hypercholesterolemia. J Applied Nutrition. 30:127–136, 1978.
14. Tilford GL: Edible and Medicinal Plants of the West. Missoula, Montana, Mountain Press Publishing, 1997.

Herbal Medicines Categorized By Levels of Evidence and Indications

A. Categorized By Benefit and Safety Ratings

🐞 🐞 🐞 = Convincing Evidence of Clinical Benefit Demonstrated in Multiple Randomized, Controlled Trials

Safety Rating	Herb	Best-Studied Indication or Use
[+]	Ginger	Nausea, motion sickness
[+]	Glucosamine*	Osteoarthritis pain
[+]	Horse chestnut seed extract	Chronic venous insufficiency
[+]	Saw palmetto	Benign prostatic hypertrophy
	Chinese wormwood (artemisinin)	Malaria
	Chondroitin*	Osteoarthritis pain
	Echinacea	Acute viral upper respiratory infections
	Hawthorn	Heart failure
	Vitex (chaste berry)	Premenstrual syndrome/cyclic mastalgia
[–]	Kava	Anxiety
[–]	Peppermint oil	Irritable bowel syndrome, dyspepsia
[–]	St. John's wort	Depression

* Although not herbal medicines, these dietary supplements are evaluated in the herbal summary sections of this book.

♣ ♣ = Clinical Benefit Suggested By Controlled Clinical Trials, But Study Results Conflicting or Evidence Inadequate and Inconclusive

Safety Rating	Herb	Best-Studied Indication or Use
[+]	Aloe vera gel	Abrasions and dermatologic conditions
[+]	Chamomile	Skin inflammation, dyspepsia
[+]	Cranberry	Urinary tract infection prophylaxis
[+]	Fenugreek	Diabetes, hyperlipidemia
[+]	Milk thistle	Hepatitis/liver disease
[+]	Nettle	Arthritis, allergic rhinitis, benign prostatic hypertrophy
[+]	Pygeum	Benign prostatic hypertrophy
[+]	Turmeric	Inflammation
	Bilberry	Ophthalmic and peripheral vascular disorders
	Black cohosh	Menopausal symptoms
	Black currant oil	Dermatitis, arthritis, other inflammatory conditions
	Borage oil	Dermatitis, arthritis, other inflammatory conditions
	Capsicum peppers	Arthritis/pain syndromes
	Coenzyme Q10*	Heart disease, hypertension
	Devil's claw	Pain and inflammation
	Elderberry	Upper respiratory illnesses
	Evening primrose oil	Eczema, PMS, arthritis, diabetic neuropathy
	Feverfew	Migraine headache prophylaxis
	Garlic	Hyperlipidemia, hypertension, cardiovascular disease
	Ginkgo	Dementia, intermittent claudication
	Ginseng, American	Hyperglycemia
	Ginseng, Asian	Physical or cognitive performance
	Ginseng, Siberian	Physical or cognitive performance
	Gotu kola	Chronic venous insufficiency

(Table continued on next page.)

🐾 🐾 = Clinical Benefit Suggested By Controlled Clinical Trials, But Study Results Conflicting or Evidence Inadequate and Inconclusive (*Continued*)

Safety Rating	Herb	Best-Studied Indication or Use
	Ivy leaf	Bronchopulmonary disease
	Lemon balm	Herpes simplex infection, anxiety/insomnia
	Melatonin*	Insomnia, jet lag
	Papaya	Inflammation, wounds
	Red clover	Menopausal symptoms
	SAMe*	Osteoarthritis, depression
	Tea tree oil	Dermatophyte infections
	Uva ursi	Urinary antiseptic
	Valerian	Insomnia
	Willow bark	Pain and inflammation
	Yucca	Arthritis symptoms
[–]	Ephedra	Performance enhancer, weight loss
[–]	Licorice	Viral hepatitis, peptic ulcer disease
[–]	PC-SPES	Prostate cancer
[–]	Yohimbe	Erectile dysfunction

* Although not herbal medicines, these dietary supplements are evaluated in the herbal summary sections of this book.

🜂 = Minimal To No Evidence of Benefit
in the Clinical Literature

Safety Rating	Herb	Common Use(s)
	Ashwagandha	General tonic, stress, arthritis, anemia
	Astragalus	Infections, "immune-stimulant"
	Cat's claw	Arthritis, GI disorders, "immune-stimulant"
	Dong quai	Menopausal symptoms, women's health
	Goldenseal	Infections, dyspepsia, "immune-stimulant"
	Horehound	Expectorant, antitussive
	MSM*	Arthritis, pain syndromes
	Mullein	Expectorant, antitussive
	Passion flower	Sedative-hypnotic, anxiolytic
	Slippery elm	Cough, sore throat
	Yarrow	Anti-inflammatory, astringent, wounds
[–]	Coltsfoot	Antitussive
[–]	Comfrey	Expectorant, antitussive, topical anti-inflammatory
[–]	Lobelia	Asthma, cough
[–]	Pokeroot	Inflammatory and infectious disorders
[–]	Wormwood	Herbal "bitter", parasites

* Although not herbal medicines, these dietary supplements are evaluated in the herbal summary sections of this book.

B. Categorized By Best-Studied Indications

Indications/Uses	Benefit Rating/Level of Evidence	
	🐾🐾🐾 Rating	🐾🐾 Rating
Cardiovascular		
Chronic venous insufficiency	horse chestnut (+)	bilberry, gotu kola
Heart disease	hawthorn	Co-Q10*, garlic
Hypercholesterolemia		evening primrose oil, fenugreek (+), garlic
Hypertension		Co-Q10*, garlic
Peripheral arterial disease		bilberry, garlic, ginkgo
Dermatologic		
Abrasions, wounds		aloe gel (+), chamomile (+), papaya
Dermatitis, eczema		aloe gel (+), black currant oil, borage oil, topical chamomile (+), evening primrose oil
Dermatophyte infections		tea tree oil
Herpes simplex infections		aloe gel (+), lemon balm, Siberian ginseng
Endocrine		
Diabetes/hyperglycemia		American ginseng, fenugreek (+)
Gastrointestinal		
Dyspepsia, irritable bowel syndrome, colic	peppermint oil (−)	chamomile (+)
Hepatitis/liver disease		milk thistle (+), licorice (−)
Nausea/motion sickness	ginger (+)	
Peptic ulcer disease	licorice (−)	
Genitourinary		
Benign prostatic hypertrophy	saw palmetto (+)	nettle (+), pygeum (+)
Erectile dysfunction		yohimbe (−)
Prostate cancer		PC-SPES (−)
Urinary tract infection		cranberry (+), uva ursi
Psychiatric		
Anxiety	kava (−)	lemon balm
Dementia/cognitive performance		Asian ginseng, ginkgo, gotu kola, Siberian ginseng

(Table continued on next page.)

Indications/Uses	Benefit Rating/Level of Evidence	
	♣♣♣ Rating	♣♣ Rating
Psychiatric *(cont.)*		
Depression	St. John's wort (−)	SAMe*
Insomnia		lemon balm, melatonin*, valerian
Respiratory		
Allergic rhinitis		nettle (+)
Asthma/bronchitis/ expectorant		ephedra (−), elderberry, ivy
Upper respiratory infection	echinacea	
Rheumatologic/Neurologic		
Arthritis/pain syndromes	chondroitin*, glucosamine (+)*	black currant oil, borage oil, capsicum, devil's claw, evening primrose oil, nettle (+), papaya, SAMe*, turmeric (+), willow, yucca
Headaches, migraine		feverfew
Headaches, tension		topical peppermint oil (−)
Neuralgias/neuropathies		black currant oil, borage oil, topical capsicum, evening primrose oil
Women's Health		
Dysmenorrhea		bilberry
Menopausal symptoms		black cohosh, red clover
Premenstrual syndrome/ cyclical mastalgia	vitex (chaste berry)	evening primrose oil
Miscellaneous		
Malaria	Chinese wormwood (artemisinin)	
Physical performance enhancer		Asian ginseng, ephedra (−), Siberian ginseng
Vision/eye disorders		bilberry, ginkgo
Weight loss		ephedra (−)

* Although not herbal medicines, these dietary supplements are evaluated in the herbal summary sections of this book.

III: Special Topics

Chinese Herbs

Chinese herbal medicine is based on ancient experience, philosophy, and poetic thinking. Many Chinese "diseases" are related to non-Western concepts, making it difficult to translate original terminology or the underlying "science" into English. The Chinese pharmacopeias of ancient times, which are still used as guides in current herbal therapy, identified diseases in picturesque terms, and ascribed cosmic and philosophic explanations for the herbs' effects on disease. Confucian political theory influenced the formulation of multiple herb prescriptions, resulting in the structural hierarchy of a prime (king or ruler) herb, supported by minister herbs, whose effectiveness is enhanced and balanced by adjutant (military assistant) and emissary (secret agent) herbs.

Herbal studies from China and other Asian countries that practice Traditional Chinese Medicine (TCM) do not always conform to established Western procedures of objective, unbiased pharmacotherapeutic evaluations.[1] Thus, for the most part, an analysis of such investigations has not been attempted in preparing this book, and only a few of the most popular Chinese herbal medicines are included in the herbal summaries. There are many difficulties in evaluating the role of, and problems using, individual Chinese herbs (see table).

Uses of Chinese Herbs
In the typical practice of TCM, herbal recipes contain numerous components. The formulations are often based on important

Problems With the Use of Chinese Herbs

- Different spellings of the English names of herbs cause confusion and errors.
- Specific herbs that have been written about over many centuries may have numerous variants, depending on location of origin and source of gathering.
- Individual Chinese references sometimes give totally different accounts of the qualities of herbs and their recommended uses.
- Many Chinese herbs are used in multi-herb combination formulations (often with animal parts), making it extremely difficult to determine the role of individual components.
- There are few well-designed, randomized, controlled trials of Asian herbal preparations; only in the last few years have Western study methodologies been introduced.
- A prescription by a Chinese herbalist is often adapted to the basic constitution and psychology of the patient.
- Traditional Chinese medical diagnoses are made on the basis of pulse and tongue examination; thus, many illnesses are not interpretable in Western terms.
- Some Chinese herbs are used for unmeasurable effects (such as increasing longevity).
- Possible contamination or adulteration of Chinese herbs with drug products or potential toxins is a major concern.

pharmacopeias, or the various *Pen-ts'ao*. The most famous of these was the Pen-ts'ao Kang Mu of the great 16th century physician Li shi-chen.[2] The most potent herbs offer the prime (king) effect, whereas others amplify, modify, harmonize, and balance this action so as to ensure gentle, natural restoration of normal bodily function. Since each herb consists of numerous chemicals, the resulting pharmacologic potpourri can be quite complex. Although it is possible that various active chemicals potentiate one another, this is difficult to assess. Nevertheless, some proprietary drugs appear to be effective. An example is Zemaphyte, which is based on licorice: several good, controlled trials have shown it to be useful in atopic eczema,[3,4] and further investigations are merited.

Many popular asthma drug mixtures, such as Ge Jie Anti-Asthma Pill, Crocodile Bile Pill, and Minor Blue Dragon Mixture,[5,6] are based on ephedra, which has some value as an allopathic bronchodilator drug. A critical analysis of the literature revealed 17 randomized, controlled clinical trials of herbal medicines for asthma. These studies suggested that, of the Chinese herbs, gingko, ephedra, and possibly some Chinese herbal mixtures and Japanese traditional mixtures (such as Saibuko-to) were of clinical benefit.[7]

A red yeast (*Monascus purpureus*), which produces a natural cholesterol-lowering agent that inhibits HMG-CoA reductase, has been shown to be effective in high-quality studies on hypercholesterolemic patients.[8] The agent, a monacholin, is marketed under the name Cholestin (chemically identical to lovastatin). Other newly rediscovered herbs may offer benefits, such as *Cordyceps sinensis* (for asthma),[9] reishi mushrooms (for various problems, including allergy), and *Tripterygium wilfordii* (for rheumatic diseases).[10]

Mixtures of herbs (sometimes with animal and mineral components) are used in many Asiatic countries where TCM made inroads in the past. The Jamu system in Indonesia is largely based on mixtures of herbs acting as specific tonics for various types of impaired organ-system function. In Japan, Kampo medicine is popular, and several combinations such as Saibuko-to have been shown to have clinical or laboratory anti-inflammatory effects.[7,11]

Many of the popular Chinese herbs are credited with a variety of indications by herbalists and marketers, and there is often a striking lack of agreement as to the appropriate uses or specific benefits of these herbs (see table, next page). It must be concluded that many of the claims are based on imagination and hope, since there is rarely any convincing evidence in favor of the more important indications. Chinese herbs cannot be recommended for use in major disorders such as cancer, AIDS or other major infections, serious diseases such as multiple sclerosis, and any urgent or emergent condition such as heart failure. It is evident that patients are investing in hope when they purchase Chinese herbs for such indications from catalogues, the internet, or herbal outlet stores.

Dangers of Chinese Herbs

Some Chinese herbal mixtures can be dangerous.[12] For example, a popular slimming preparation that was supposed to be based on the herb han fang ji (*Stephania tetranda*) was contaminated, possibly with the herb guang fang ji (*Aristolochia fangchi*).[13] The latter herb contains aristolochic acid, which is nephrotoxic. Cases were reported of rapidly progressive interstitial nephritis resulting in renal fibrosis and chronic renal failure. In addition, the preparation appears to have caused urinary tract malignancies in some patients.[13] In Taiwan in 1995, an herbal weight-control

Selected Traditional Chinese Herbal Medicines *

Latin Name	Chinese Name(s)	English Name(s)	Characteristic Constituent(s)	Indications/Purported Effects
Acanthopanax senticosa	ci wu jia	Siberian ginseng	eleutherosides	immune booster, anti-cancer, fat reducer, laxative, tonic
Aconitum carmichaelii	chuan wu tou	aconite, monkshood	aconitine	cardiotonic, analgesic, diarrhea, anti-inflammatory
Adenophora tetraphylla	nan sha sheng	ladybell	stigmasterol	antitussive, expectorant
Angelica sinensis	dong quai, tang-kuei	Chinese angelica	ligustilide	menopause, gynecologic problems, anti-inflammatory, allergies
Artemesia annua	quing hao	sweet Annie	artemisinin	malaria, lupus, diarrhea
Asarum sieboldi	hsi hsin	azamaru, wild ginger	asarinine	analgesic, expectorant, colds
Astragalus membranaceous	huang qi	milk vetch	astragalosides	infections, fatigue, adaptogen, AIDS, immunostimulant
Atractylodes chinensis	cang zhu	thistle	atractylol	digestive disorders, stimulant, analgesic
Bupleurum falcatum	chai hu	hare's ear	saikosaponins	liver diseases, gynecological problems, autoimmune diseases, infections
Camellia sinensis	chai	tea	polyphenols, theophylline	digestive, stimulant, antioxidant
Chysanthemum morifolium	ji hua	chysanthemum	stachydrine	antipyretic, conjunctivitis
Cimifuga foetida	sheng ma	bugbane	cimifugin	headache, fever, bronchitis, tonsillitis, infections
Cinnamomum cassia	gui zhi	Chinese cinnamon	cinnamaldehyde	diaphoretic, GI disorders, carminative, antiseptic
Codonopsis pilosula	dang shen	poor-man's ginseng	tangshenosides	tonic, diabetes, hypertension
Coptis sinensis	huang lian	mishmi bitter, goldthread	coptisine	antipyretic, diarrhea

(Table continued on next page.)

Latin Name	Chinese Name(s)	English Name(s)	Characteristic Constituent(s)	Indications/Purported Effects
Cordyceps sinensis	dong chong-xia cao	summer-herb, winter-worm	cordycepin	tonic, hyper-cholesterolemia, cough, asthma, antioxidant, kidneys
Corydalis ambigua	yan hu suo	corydalis	tetrahydro-palmatine	analgesic, hypnotic, dysmenorrhea
Datura metel	yang jin hua	loco weed	hyoscyamine	bronchospasm, colic
Dioscorea opposila	shan yao	yam	glutamine	tonic, diabetes, digestive
Ephedra sinica	ma huang	ephedra	ephedrine	asthma, cough, sinusitis, diuretic
Eriobotrya japonica	pi pa ye	loquat	amygdaline	expectorant, antitussive
Fritillaria verticillata	bei mu	fritillary	fritillin	antitussive, expectorant
Ganoderma lucidum	ling chi	reishi mushroom	ganoderic acids	bronchitis, anti-cancer, anti-allergy, immunostimulant
Ginkgo biloba	bai guo	maidenhair tree	ginkgolides	dementia, circulation, asthma
Glehnia littoralis	sha shen	glehnia		cough, expectorant
Glycyrrhiza uralensis	gan cao	licorice	glycyrrhizin	harmonizer, hepatitis, eczema, cough
Gynostemma pentaphyllum	jiao gu lan	sweet tea vine, southern ginseng	gypenosides	adaptogen, sedative, tonic, hypertension
Huperzia serrata	qian ceng ta	Chinese club moss	huperzine A	antioxidant, dementia
Ligusticum wallichii	chuan xiong	cinidium	ligustilide	colds, rheumatism, allergies, ischemia
Ligustrum lucidum	nu zheng zi	glossy privet	ligustrin	immune function, infection
Lonicera japonica	jin yin hua	honeysuckle	saponins	antipyretic, pharyngitis, diarrhea
Lycium chinense	guo ji zi	wolfberry	β-carotene, terpenoids	tonic, eye problems, anti-obesity
Magnolia liliflora	xin yi	magnolia	citral	decongestant, sinusitis

(Table continued on next page.)

Latin Name	Chinese Name(s)	English Name(s)	Characteristic Constituent(s)	Indications/Purported Effects
Momordica charantia	ku gua zi	bitter melon, balsam pear	charantin	diabetes, antimicrobial, AIDS
Momordica grosvernorii	lo han kuo	monk fruit	mogrosides	antitussive, digestant, sweetener
Morus alba	sang ye	mulberry	carotene	expectorant, colds
Ophiopogon japonicus	chiu'tzu ts'ao	onion grass	mucilage	bronchitis, laryngitis, cough
Paeonia lactiflora	bai shao	peony	paeoniflorin	dysmenorrhea, spasms
Panax ginseng	ren shen	ginseng	ginsenosides	tonic, adaptogen, diabetes, heart disease, cancer
Panax notoginseng	tian qi, tien chan	tienchi ginseng	ginsenosides	bleeding disorders, heart disease
Perilla frutescens	zi su zi	beefsteak plant	perilla aldehyde	colds, cough, fever
Phellodendron chinense	huang bai	cork-tree, philodendron	isoquinolines	diarrhea, vaginitis, anti-inflammatory
Picrorrhiza kurroa	hu huang lian	kutki	kutkin	antipyretic, asthma, vitiligo
Pinellia ternata	ban xia	pinellia	coniine	expectorant, sedative
Platycodon grandiflora	jie geng	balloon flower	playcodigen	bronchitis, tonsillitis, parasites
Polygala tenuifolia	yuan zhi	Chinese senega	tenuifolin	expectorant, sedative
Polygonum multiflorum	fo-ti, he shou wu	knotweed, cornbind, fleece flower	anthraquinones	neurasthenia, antimicrobial, atherosclerosis, cathartic
Poria cocos	fu ling, fushen	Indian bread, hoelen	pectin	expectorant, diuretic, sedative
Prunus persica	tao ren	peach	emulsin	menstrual problems, analgesic
Pueraria lobata	geh gen	kudzu vine	asparagin	antipyretic, alcoholism
Pulsatilla chinensis	bai tou weng	anemone, pasque flower	anemonin	antipyretic, amebic dysentery, analgesic

(Table continued on next page.)

Selected Traditional Chinese Herbal Medicines* *(Continued)*

Latin Name	Chinese Name(s)	English Name(s)	Characteristic Constituent(s)	Indications/Purported Effects
Rehmania glutinosa	di huang	Chinese foxglove	jionosides	allergies, bleeding disorders, rheumatism
Rheum palmatum	da huang	rhubarb	anthraquinones	laxative, antipyretic
Salvia miltiorrhiza	dan shen	red root sage	tanshinones	circulatory diseases, hepatitis, menstrual disorders
Schisandra chinensis	wu wei zi	magnolia vine	schizandrins	liver disease, cough, adaptogen, antioxidant
Scutellaria baicalensis	huang qin	scute, skullcap	baicalin	allergy, anti-inflammatory, bronchitis, enteritis, hypertension
Sophora japonica	huai hua	pagoda tree	sophoretin	bleeding disorders, hypertension, fever
Stemona tuberosa	bai bu	spring drug-root	stemonine	antitussive, analgestic, parasites
Syzgium aromaticum (Eugenia caryophyllata)	ding xiang	clove	eugenol	antiemetic, local anesthetic, antiseptic
Tricosanthes kirilowii	gua lou, tin hua fen	Chinese cucumber	tricosanthin	cancer, AIDS, angina
Tripterygium wilfordii	lei gong teng	thunder god vine	triptolides	arthritis, anti-inflammatory, immunosuppressor
Zizyphus vulgaris	da zao	Chinese date, jujube	zizyphic acid	fatigue, hypertension

* This table has been compiled from many sources. It is not an evidence-based list; information on indications and effects is not definitive and is intended primarily as a selected guide to familiarize health professionals with the array of traditional Chinese herbal medicines that are used by patients.

References consulted in constructing this table:

Websites

www.acupuncture.com/Herbology/Toxic.htm
www.advancedherbals.co.uk/herbs
www.dragonherbs.com/herbs
www.healthwell.com/healthnotes/herb
www.holisticonline.com/Herbal-Med
www.newcenturynutrition.com/cgi-bin/singleherbs
www.rain-tree.com
www.rxlist.com/cgi/alt
www.thorne.com/altmedrev/fulltext/china3-5.html (Sinclair S. Chinese herbs: A clinical review of Astragalus, Ligusticum, and Schizandra.)

(Table continued on next page.)

Books

1. Bone K. Clinical Applications of Ayurvedic and Chinese Herbs. Monographs for the Western Herbal Practitioner. Warwick, Australia, Phytotherapy Press, 1996.
2. Brown D. The Herb Society of America Encyclopedia of Herbs & Their Uses. New York, DK Publishing, 1995.
3. Chevalier A. The Encyclopedia of Medicinal Plants. New York, DK Publishing, 1996.
4. Ebling D. The Chinese Herbalist's Handbook. Santa Fe, NM, InWord Press, 1996.
5. Huang KC. The Pharmacology of Chinese Herbs, 2nd ed. Boca Raton, FL, CRC Press, 1999.
6. Leung AY, Foster S. Encyclopedia of Common Natural Ingredients Used in Food, Drugs, and Cosmetics, 2nd ed. New York, John Wiley & Sons, Inc, 1996.
7. Ross IA. Medicinal Plants of the World. Towata, NJ, Humana Press, 1999.
8. Mills S, Bone K. Principles and Practice of Phytotherapy. Modern Herbal Medicines. Edinburgh, Churchill Livingstone, 2000.
9. Reid D. A Handbook of Chinese Healing Herbs. Boston, Shambhala, 1995.
10. Reid DP. Chinese Herbal Medicine. Wellingborough, UK, Thorsons Publishing Group, 1987.
11. The Revolutionary Health Committee of Hunan Province. A Barefoot Doctor's Manual. Mayne Isle & Seattle, Cloudburst Press, 1997.
12. Yan X, Zhou, Xie G (Edited by Milne GWA). Traditional Chinese Medicines. Aldershot, England, Ashgate Publishing, 1999.
13. Ziment I. Alternative therapies in asthma. In: Gershwin ME, Albertson TE (eds): Bronchial Asthma. Principles of Diagnoses and Treatment, 4th ed. Towota, NJ, Humana Press, 2001, pp 255-278.

preparation was found to result in severe bronchiolitis obliterans in some patients. The apparent cause was the leaves of the herb, *Sauropus androgynous*.[14] Another example of toxicity attributed to an herbal mixture was the development of hepatitis in patients taking jin bu huan, an anodyne tablet. There are many other well-analyzed reports of toxicity caused by Chinese herbs.[12]

Furthermore, the potency of the active component in some herbal mixtures could cause serious inadvertent side effects. For example, PC-SPES, a commercial mixture of eight herbs (chysanthemum, isatis, licorice, reishi, *Panax pseudoginseng*, *Rabdosia rubescens*, saw palmetto, and skullcap), is used for treating prostate cancer. It has been shown to have potent estrogenic activity, resulting in pulmonary embolism in some patients.[15] In addition, many proprietary Chinese medicines have been found to be contaminated or adulterated with heavy metals, pesticides, and pharmaceutical drug products (e.g., steroids, benzodiazepines).[12,16]

Conclusions

Although there may be many useful traditional Chinese herbal preparations, future evaluations must be of much higher quality so that better evidence-based decisions can be made about clinical value and use.[1,17] A greater effort will be required to determine which chemical components account for specific pharmacologic effects of Chinese herbs,[18] and to establish whether any are dangerous. Nevertheless, whatever future developments occur, traditional Chinese herbs will continue to be used and to satisfy increasing numbers of people throughout the world.

references

1. Critchley JAJH, Zhang Y, Suthisisang CC, et al. Alternative therapies and medical science: Designing clinical trials of alternative/complementary medicines—Is evidence-based traditional Chinese medicine attainable? J Clin Pharmacol 40:462–467, 2000.
2. Cheung SC, Kwan PS, Kong YC. An Introduction to *Pen-Ts'ao* Study. Hong Kong, The Chinese University of Hong Kong. Shatin, NT, 1984.
3. Sheehan MP, Rustin MH, Atherton DJ, et al. Efficacy of a traditional Chinese herbal therapy in adult atopic dermatitis. Lancet 340:13–17, 1992.
4. Armstrong NC, Ernst E. The treatment of eczema with Chinese herbs: A systematic review of randomized clinical trials. Br J Clin Pharmacol 48:262–264, 1999.
5. But P, Chang C. Chinese herbal medicine in the treatment of asthma and allergies. Clin Rev Allergy Immunol 14:253–269, 1996.
6. Bielory L, Lupoli, K. Herbal interventions in asthma and allergy. J Asthma 36:1–65, 1999.
7. Huntley A, Ernst E. Herbal medicines for asthma: A systematic review. Thorax 55:925–929, 2000.
8. Heber D, Yip I, Ashley JM, et al. Cholesterol-lowering effects of a proprietary Chinese red-yeast-rice dietary supplement. Am J Clin Nutr 69:231–236, 1999.
9. Zhu J-S, Halpern GM, Jones K. The scientific rediscovery of an ancient Chinese herbal medicine: *Cordyceps sinensis*. J Altern Comp Med 3:289–303,429–456, 1998.
10. Tao X, Lipsky PE. The Chinese anti-inflammatory and immunosuppressive herbal remedy, *Tripterygium wilfordii* Hook F. Rheum Dis Clin N Am 26:29–50, 2000.
11. Ziment I. How your patients may be using herbalism to treat their asthma. J Respir Dis 19:1070–1081, 1998.
12. Tomlinson B, Chan TYK, Chan JCN, et al. Toxicity of complementary therapies: An Eastern perspective. J Clin Pharmacol 40:451-456, 2000.
13. Nortier JL, Martinez MC, Schmeiser HH, et al. Urothelial carcinoma associated with the use of a Chinese herb (*Aristolochia fangchi*). N Engl J Med 342:1686-1692, 2000.
14. Lai R-S, Chiang AA, Wu M-T, et al. Outbreak of bronchioltis obliterans associated with consumption of *Sauropus androgynus* in Taiwan. Lancet 348:83-85, 1996.
15. DiPaola RS, Zhang H, Lambert GH, et al. Clinical and biologic activity of an estrogenic herbal combination (PC-SPES) in prostate cancer. N Engl J Med 339:785–791, 1998.
16. Ko RJ. Adulterants in Asian patent medicines. N Engl J Med 339:847, 1998.
17. Tang J-L, Zhan S-Y, Ernst E. Review of randomized controlled trial of traditional Chinese Medicine. BMJ 319:160–161, 1999.
18. Ziment I. The management of common respiratory diseases by traditional Chinese drugs. Orient Heal Arts Internat Bull 13:133–140, 1988.

Ayurvedic Herbs

Several indigenous systems of traditional medical practice flourish in India. The best recognized one is Ayurveda, the "knowledge of life," which combines diet, exercise, spiritual activities, and herbal medicines in a holistic healing system. Ayurveda's major healing principles involve cleansing to remove toxins and balancing influences on the body so as to ensure a prolonged life. The Ayurvedic practitioner gives careful attention to the particular constitution of the patient and designs therapies that are individualized to balance the three basic energy forces, the tridosha; these correspond roughly to the Chinese major opposing forces, yin and yang. As is the case with Traditional Chinese Medicine, Ayurvedic herbal therapies combine experience with philosophy, and Western concepts of pharmacology have only recently been employed in evaluating their effectiveness.

Ayurveda arose from the Hindu texts of ancient herbalists. The best known were the Caraka Samhita and the Sushruta Samhita, which were written in Sanskrit. The three doshas (the tridosha) are *vata* (wind), *pitta* (fire), and *kapha* (phlegm). They emphasize the importance of respiratory disease in ancient societies. Imbalances of these basic elements and the underlying life forces (*prana*) cause disease. Disorders of function are further subdivided, with the seven *dhatus* or basic constituents each having individual vulnerability (i.e., plasma, marrow, blood, muscle, fat, bone, semen or ova). An important concept in Ayurveda is to promote rejuvenation, or rasayana, in part by eliminating noxious *malas* or *ama* that result from disturbance of metabolism (*agni*), which consumes the basic elementary substances (*mahabhutas*). These basic terms are often used by Ayurvedic practitioners in analyzing health disturbances and in prescribing herbal medicines designed to correct the specific impairment.

The use of herbs in traditional Indian medical systems is based on experience, philosophy, and crude beliefs such as the "Doctrine of Signatures," which was coincidentally favored by Paracelsus in Europe. Over 2000 drugs have been described in Ayurveda, and numerous popular and individually recommended formulations are favored. Traditional formulations often contain mineral and metallurgical components in addition to botanical products.

Many traditional herbal therapies in Ayurvedic practice are used as nonspecific aids to health which are thought to work by improving the body's ability to fight disease. Others are considered of value in enhancing physical and mental performance or in retarding aging. This unproved last claim is purely fanciful. In more recent Ayurvedic texts, specific indications are emphasized based on modern concepts of disease and symptoms, and numerous herbs are recommended for asthma, bronchitis, gastrointestinal disturbances, infections, and rheumatic disorders. Most investigations that are carried out in India are difficult to evaluate since the scientific methods are not as rigorous as those of Western medicine. Studies are often uncontrolled, unblinded, and lacking adequate statistical analysis. Moreover, many reports are based on isolated studies that are not further evaluated; thus, their credibility is rarely challenged or confirmed.

As is the case with Chinese herbs, a number of Indian herbs are becoming fashionable in the West, although the evidence in their favor is meager. Tea (both green and black) from India as well as China is receiving surprisingly vigorous support from promoters who claim, on the basis of limited and controversial epidemiologic evidence, that the polyphenols, flavonoids, and tannins of this beverage can be of value in protecting the heart and brain and in preventing cancer. Similar claims are made for turmeric, the yellow component of curry powder, which is also alleged to have anti-inflammatory properties. It is noteworthy that Indian herbs long used for asthma (including those that contain atropine and other anticholinergic drugs, theophylline, and numerous expectorants and antitussives) have not maintained their importance in the current era of asthma management.

In general, Ayurvedic herbs have made only small inroads in the West. In contrast, Chinese herbs were introduced into North America by groups of Chinese immigrants a century or more ago. Chinese herbal practice has been sanctioned by "grandfathering" and the U.S. FDA allows these herbs to be prescribed by Chinese herbalists in U.S. communities. Ayurvedic herbs have not held a traditional status in North America, and regulatory agencies are less likely to permit large-scale importation. However, numerous Ayurvedic herbs are available through health magazines and on the internet, and patients are able to self-medicate themselves with these products. Fortunately, most Ayurvedic herbs are benign, although adulteration or contamination can be a major problem with products obtained from less reliable purveyors.

Ayurvedic herbs include many spices, which are well known as condiments, although their therapeutic effects are less well recognized (see table below). Many Ayurvedic herbs are popular in the West (see table, page 400), but few of the claims have been validated in well-designed clinical trials. Most are based on traditional and empiric usage, quasi-scientific studies, or folkloric anecdotes. Many of the herbs are marketed in mixtures, making it extremely difficult to define the actions of individual ingredients and their potential synergy.

In general, one should be wary of lesser-known Ayurvedic herbs and maintain a healthy skepticism about herbs or mixtures that promise extraordinary benefits. As is the case with Chinese medicines, there is insufficient evidence to justify the use of any of these products in the treatment of serious diseases such as cancer or AIDS. It is evident that many purveyors appeal to desperate or poorly informed buyers, who are then exploited by extravagant promises.

Major Indian Spices Used In Herbal Medicine*

Spice	Indian Name	Latin Name	Alleged Properties or Indications**
Ajowan	Ajvini, Ajwain	*Trachyspermum ammi*	antispasmodic, antimicrobial
Allspice	Kattukkaruva	*Pimenta dioca*	tonic, purgative, analgesic
Aniseed	Vilayati saunf	*Pimpinella anisum*	carminative, expectorant
Asafetida	Hing	*Ferula asafoetida*	flatulence, cough
Basil	Tulsi	*Ocimum sanctum*	colds, kidney disease, diarrhea, tonic
Caraway	Shia jira	*Carum carvi*	colic, antihelminth, scabies
Cardamon	Elaichi	*Elattaria cardamomum*	digestive, aphrodisiac
Chile peppers	Marich, Katuvira	*Capsicum annuum,* etc.	analgesic, counter-irritant, colds
Cinnamon (and Cassia)	Dalchini	*Cinnamomum zeylanicum*, etc.	gastrointestinal disorders, antiseptic
Cloves	Laung	*Syzgium aromaticum*	dental analgesic, dyspepsia
Coriander (and Cilantro)	Dhania	*Coriandrum sativum*	antibacterial, anti-inflammatory
Cumin	Safaid jeera	*Cuminum cyminum*	anticancer, antimicrobial
Curry leaves	Meetha neem	*Murraya koenigii*	tonic, vomiting, carminative

(Table continued on next page.)

Major Indian Spices Used In Herbal Medicine* *(Continued)*

Spice	Indian Name	Latin Name	Alleged Properties or Indications**
Dill	Surva	*Anethum graveolens*	flatulence, hiccups, colic
Fennel	Saunf, Shata-pushpa	*Foeniculum vulgare*	carminative, diuretic
Fenugreek	Methi	*Trigonella foenum-graecum*	digestive, diabetes, hypercholesterolemia
Garlic	Lasuna	*Allium sativum*	high cholesterol, hypertension, colds
Ginger	Adrak, Shunthi	*Zingiber officinale*	colds, anti-emetic, stimulant
Lemongrass	Bhustrina, Gandhatrina	*Andropogon citratus*	diuretic, tonic, colic, fever
Licorice	Jethimadh, Mulethi	*Glycyrrhiza glabra*	pharyngitis, peptic ulcers
Marjoram	Mirzamjosh	*Majorana hortensis*	indigestion, colic
Mint	Podina	*Mentha piperita*	antispasmodic, sinusitis
Mustard	Banarsi rai	*Sinapsis alba*	emetic, counter-irritant
Nigella (Black cumin)	Kalonji	*Nigella sativa*	carminative, indigestion
Nutmeg (and Mace)	Jatipatra, Javitri	*Myristica fragrans*	hallucinogen, counter-irritant
Onion	Piyaz	*Allium cepa*	anti-cancer, colds
Parsley	Ajmood	*Petroselinum crispum*	gas, digestive, breath smell, diuretic
Pepper (black)	Kali mirch, Krishna	*Piper nigrum*	expectorant, antimicrobial
Rosemary	Rusmary	*Rosmarinus officinalis*	anti-cancer
Saffron	Kesar	*Crocus sativus*	rheumatism, neuralgia
Sage	Salvia	*Salvia officinalis*	gastroenteritis, antiseptic
Sesame	Gingli	*Sesamum indicum*	laxative, demulcent
Star anise	Anasphal	*Illicium verum*	digestive, rheumatism
Tamarind	Imli	*Tamarindus indicus*	digestive, antipyretic, astringent
Thyme	Banajwain	*Thymus vulgaris*	antiseptic, expectorant
Turmeric	Haldi, Halad	*Curcuma domestica*	digestive, arthritis, high cholesterol

* This table has been compiled from several sources. It is not an evidence-based list, and information on alleged properties or indications is not definitive. It is intended primarily as a selected guide to familiarize health professionals with the array of traditional Indian spices that may be used by patients.

** Different accounts often show significant disagreements. The alleged values listed here offer a partial summary of suggested properties of, or indications for, these spices.

Based on: www.ang.kfunigraz.ac.at/ (Gernot Katzer's Spice Pages)
www.theepicenter.com/ (Encyclopedia of spices)
www.thehimalayadrugco.com

Selected Ayurvedic Herbs Popular in the West*

Latin Name	Selected Indian Name(s)**	English Name(s)	Main Constituent(s)	Major Properties or Indications
Abies webbiana	Gobra sala, Talisa	silver fir	alpha-pinene	expectorant, tonic, carminative
Acorus calamus	Vacha, Bach, Vayambu	sweetflag	asarones	expectorant, sedative, antispasmodic, worms
Adhatoda vasica	Vasaka, Amalaka	malabar nut tree	vasicine	asthma, expectorant, bleeding gums
Aegle marmelos	Bilva, Shivaphala	bael tree	marmelosin	diarrhea, colitis, worms
Albizzia lebbek	Pit Shirish Shrisha	mimosa	glycosides, saponins	atopic diseases, diarrhea, cholesterol
Alpinia galanga	Kulinjan, Rasna	galangal(e)	galangol	aphrodisiac, bronchitis, rheumatism
Andrographis paniculata	Kirata, Kalmehi	king of bitters	andrographolides	infections, liver disease, cardiovascular disease
Areca catechu	Supari Puga, Gubak, Tambool, Kramuka	betelnut	arecoline	stimulant, breath sweetener
Asparagus racemosus	Shatavari	asparagus	asparasaponins	immunostimulant, antispasmodic, lactagogue
Azadiracta indica	Neem, Arishta, Nimba	Indian lilac, neem tree	azadiratin	antibacterial, skin diseases, tonic
Bacopa monniera	Brahmi, Jalnaveri	thyme leaved gratiola	bacosides	epilepsy, dementia, diuretic
Boerhaavia diffusa	Punarnava, Tazhutama	hogweed	boeravinones	diuretic, expectorant, tonic
Boswellia serrata	Salai guggal, Sallaki	frankincense	boswellic acid	anti-inflammatory, arthritis
Centella asiatica	Gotu kola, Madukaparni	Indian pennywort	flavonoids	memory, tonic, adaptogen
Coleus forskohlii	Makandi, Garmalu	coleus	forskolin (colforsin)	asthma, heart disease, glaucoma
Commiphora mukul	Guggul	Indian myrrh, bdellium	guggulsterone	hypercholesterolemia, arthritis
Convolvulus pluricalis	Shankapushpi	aloeweed, bindweed	convolvine	tranquilizer, insomnia, memory
Crataeva nurvala	Vasuna	three leaved caper	lupeol	urinary tract disease
Datura metel	D'hatura	jimson weed	scopolamine	asthma, spasms, eye disease
Emblica officinalis	Amalaki, Amla, Dhatri	Indian gooseberry, emblic myrobalan	phyllemblin	tonic, antimicrobial, expectorant, hypercholesterolemia

(Table continued on next page.)

Selected Ayurvedic Herbs Popular in the West* *(Continued)*

Latin Name	Selected Indian Name(s)**	English Name(s)	Main Constituent(s)	Major Properties or Indications
Gymnema sylvestre	Gurmar, Meshashringi	small Indian ipecac	gymnemic acids	diabetes, cholesterol
Hemidesmus indicus	Anatamula	Indian sarsaparilla	coumarins	skin diseases, tonic, arthritis
Inula racemosa	Pushkar-moola	"elecampane"	alantolactone	bronchitis, angina
Momordica charantia	Karela	bitter gourd	momordicine	diabetes, adaptogen
Phyllanthus amarus	Bahupatra	feather foil	phyllanthin	viral hepatitis, pain, diabetes
Picrorrhiza kurroa	Kutaki, Katuka	picrorrhiza	kutkoside	infections, hepatitis, immunostimulant
Piper longum	Pippali, Biplo, Pipli	long pepper	piperine, piplartine	expectorant, digestive, tonic
Rauwolfia serpentina	Sarpagandha, Vijaysar	snakeroot, kino tree	reserpine	hypertension, tranquilizer
Terminalia arjuna	Arjuna	arjun tree	arjungenin	cardioprotective, diuretic
Terminalia chebula	Haritaki	chebulic myrobalan	chebulagic acid	expectorant, digestive, laxative
Tinospora cordifolia	Guduchi, Gurcha	heart leaf	tinosporaside	arthritis, hepatitis, tonic, immune modifer
Tribulus terrestris	Gokshura	small caltrops	harmine	genitourinary disorders, analgesic
Tylophora asthmatica	Anthra-pachaka	Indian ipecac	tylophorine	asthma, diarrhea, autoimmunity
Withania somnifera	Ashwagandha, Dunal	winter cherry	withanolides	adaptogen, tonic, debility

* This table has been compiled from several sources. It is not an evidence-based list, and information on properties and indications is not definitive. It is intended primarily as a selected guide to familiarize health professionals with the array of traditional Ayurvedic herbal medicines that are used by patients.
** Numerous different names are used; this is a selection of more common names.
Websites consulted in constructing this table: www.ayurveda.com (The Ayurvedic Institute, Albuquerque, NM); www.niam.com (The National Institute of Ayurvedic Medicine); www.thehimalayadrugco.com; www.oilbath.com

references

Journals

Chopra A. Ayurvedic medicine and arthritis. Rheum Dis Clin North Am 26:133–144, 2000.

Ernst E, Chrubasik S. Phyto-anti-inflammatories. Rheum Dis Clin North Am 26:13–27, 2000.

Kapoor LD. Ayur-Vedic medicine of India. J Herbs Spices Medic Plants 1(4):37–219, 1993.

Thatte UM, Dahanukar SA. Immunotherapeutic modification of experimental infections by Indian medicinal plants. Phytother Res 3:43–49, 1989.

Ziment I. Historic overview of mucoactive drugs. In Braga PC, Allegra (eds): Drugs in Bronchial Mucology. New York, Raven Press, 1989, pp 1–34.

Ziment I. Eastern "alternative" medicine: What you need to know. J Respir Dis 19:630–644, 1998.

Ziment I. How patients may be using herbalism to treat their asthma. J Respir Dis 19:1070–1081, 1998.

Books

Bone K. Clinical Applications of Ayurvedic and Chinese Herbs. Monographs for the Western Herbal Practitioner. Warwick, Australia, Phytotherapy Press, 1996.

Chevalier A. The Encyclopedia of Medicinal Plants. New York, DK Publishing, 1996.

Dastur JF. Everybody's Guide to Ayurvedic Medicine. Bombay, DB Taraporevala Sons & Co., 1960.

Lad DV. Ayurvedic medicine. In Jonas WB, Levin JS (eds): Essentials of Complementary and Alternative Medicine. Philadelphia, Lippincott Williams & Wilkins, 1999, pp 200–215.

Pruthi JS. Spices and Condiments. New Delhi, National Book Trust, 1976.

Rosengarten F. The Book of Spices. New York, Pyramid Books, 1973.

Mexican Herbs

A large number of Mexican herbs are available at ethnic markets and botanicas in the U.S. In general, these herbs are similar to the popular herbal remedies that are widely available in Mexico. Many Mexican herbs are the same as those used in the Southwestern United States, and their popular indications are generally similar in both countries.

The average Mexican or other user who purchases such herbs relies on family and cultural tradition to provide guidance in their use. Mexican healers, such as curanderos, are more knowledgeable about their use, but they rely on experience and word of mouth rather than on standard textbooks. In comparison with Chinese and Indian herbal resources, there are surprisingly few scientific publications on Mexican drugs in English; similarly, although there are several useful websites, relatively few provide credible scientific data on their uses. Thus, Mexican herbs represent a very visible but largely unseen and generally ignored element of health care in the U.S.

The typical traditional herbal remedy from Mexican plant sources has a long, complex, and often confusing history. Similar plants are given different local names in the various regions of the country, whereas quite different plants may be given the same names in different areas. Some plants have several official and vernacular names, and the exact identification of a plant and a corresponding herb may undergo changes through confusion or misinterpretation.

As an example, the term gordolobo, which is usually applied to the flower of *Verbascum thapsis* (mullein), is also given to some species of *Gnaphthalum*. Moreover, a more dangerous herb of the *Senecio* species is sometimes used under the name gordolobo, and this can lead to poisoning. Comparable confusion exists with *Artemesia* and *Aristolochia* plants: different variants and entirely different species may share the same name.

Other areas of confusion are created by similar plants being identified variously and interchangeably, as occurs with plants called manzanilla, maguey, century plant, agave, or aloe. Different accounts may confuse their traditional properties.

The indications for most Mexican herbs are generally unsubstantiated. A surprising number of very different plants are used for similar purposes, for example as expectorants or laxatives, or for treating gastrointestinal disorders, insomnia, or nervousness. Sometimes, the same herb is recommended for opposing disorders, such as constipation and diarrhea, with no guidelines as to how to make the specific choice. There is a similar confusion between so-called immunostimulants and immunosuppresants, and it is not unusual for herbs to be labeled as stimulants or tonics while being recommended as sedatives.

The situation is similar to that for aromatherapy and all indigenous folk medicine systems; equal confusion can occur with Indian and Chinese herbs. However, Mexican herbal recommendations come from a more empiric background. Asiatic herbal medical practices have evolved in highly sophisticated fashions over the course of several thousand years.

Many Mexican herbs are also used as teas or soups, in a manner comparable to the way American and European herbs (such as mint and ginger) are packaged as herbal beverages and promoted for pleasure as much as for their medical benefits. These teas are ingested with little expectation of anything other than a slight sense of short-lasting benefit. However, many Mexicans self-treat themselves with herbal preparations with much greater expectations, particularly if an elder family member is the authority who recommends that the specific treatment be used.

At present, there is little evidence that Mexican herbs offer exceptional health benefits. The popularity of certain herbs for diabetes, however, has encouraged researchers to investigate the potential value of the commonly used nopal (prickly pear cactus leaf), and clinical studies are justified for other herbs, such as aceitilla, aloes, bricklebush, chia, cholla, hawthorn, horehound, matarique, topozan, and trumpet bush. Other studies may be justified for herbs popularly used to treat skin problems (e.g., aloe, ragwort, comfrey, and jojoba) and perhaps some other disorders. The potential value of popular herbs to become drugs is seen in the success of one Mexican (or South American) herb: chile pepper, which is the source of the well-known pharmaceutical, capsaicin.

Selected Mexican Herbs*

Mexican Name**	Latin Name	English Name(s)	Alleged Value/Common Uses
Abedul	*Betula alba*	birch	astringent, diuretic, melanoma
Acacia	*Acacia greggii*	uña del gato, catclaw	pain, urinary problems, gastritis, infection
Aceitilla (Picao preto)	*Bridens pilosa (Odorato bidens)*	burr marigold	diabetes, diuretic, digestive
Achiote	*Bixa orellana*	annatto	skin diseases, anti-inflammatory, colorant
Ajo	*Allium sativum*	garlic	hypertension, hypercholes-terolemia,cough
Albahaca	*Ocimum basilicum*	basil	inflammation, infection, colic, earache
Aloe vera	*Aloe barbadensis*	aloe vera	skin irritation, constipation
Ambrosia	*Ambrosia acanthicarpa*	ragweed	parturition aid, cough
Anis de Estrella	*Illicum verum*	star anise	colic, digestive disorders, gas
Arnica	*Tithonia diversifolia*	Mexican sunflower	skin infections, aches, bruises, varicosities
Atlinan	*Rumex pulcher*	sorrel	colds, sore throats, cuts, diarrhea
Avena	Avena sativum	red oat	tonic, energizer
Azar de Naranjo	*Citrus aurantium*	bitter orange blossom	insomnia, tonic, colds
Balsamo	*Myroxylon balsamium*	tolu balsam	diuretic, colds, skin sores
Boldo	*Pneumus boldus*	boldo	liver/gallbladder disorders, colds, nervousness
Borraja	*Borago officinalis*	borage	antipyretic, tonic, anti-inflammatory
Bougainvillea	*Bougainvillea glabra*	bougainvillea	expectorant
Canela	*Cinnamomum zeylanicum*	cinnamon	flatulence, cough, fever, antimicrobial
Cebola	*Allium cepa*	onion	analgesic, antibiotic, diuretic, expectorant
Chayote	*Sechium edule*	vegetable pear	diuretic
Chía (Pinole)	*Salvia columbariae*	chia sage	nerve tonic, hair loss, colds, diabetes
Chicalote	*Argemone mexicana*	prickly poppy	sedative, analgesic, laxative, eyedrops
Chili (Aji)	*Capsicum annuum*	chile	analgesic, cardiac tonic
Cholla	*Opuntia acanthocarpa*	cholla	diabetes, wounds

(Table continued on next page.)

Mexican Name**	Latin Name	English Name(s)	Alleged Value/Common Uses
Cilantro	*Coriandrum sativum*	coriander	sedative, diuretic
Cola de Caballo	*Equisetum arvense*	shavegrass	urinary infection, kidney stone, varicosities
Copal	*Bursera confusa*	elephant tree	cough, analgesic, insect bites, toothache
Cuachalalate (Chalalate)	*Amphipterygium adstringens*		gastritis, ulcers, hypercholesterolemia, blood purifier, anti-inflammatory
Damiana	*Turnera diffusa*	damiana	aphrodisiac, infertility, diabetes, insomnia
Encino	*Quercus* species	oak	astringent, tonic
Epazote	*Chenopodium ambrosioides*	wormseed	flatulence, worms, depression, amenorrhea
Escutelaria	*Scutellaria laterifolia*	skullcap	nervous tension, epilepsy
Estafiate (Ajenjo)	*Artemesia mexicana*	wormwood	gastro-intestinal discomfort, gaseousness, gynecologic disorders, asthma
Eucalipto	*Eucaliptus globulus*	eucalyptus	asthma, bronchitis
Gobernadora	*Larrea tridentata*	chaparral, creosote bush	fever, herpes, indigestion, arthritis, infection
Gordolobo	*Verbascum thapsus*	mullein	cold sores, bronchitis, colic, hemorrhoids, pain
Guayaba	*Psidium guajava*	guava	diuretic, gastritis, diarrhea, skin irritation, cholesterol
Guayacan	*Guaiacum officinale*	lignum vitae	expectorant, diuretic, antiseptic
Hoja de Laurel	*Laurus nobilis*	bay leaf	gas, cramps, tonic
Jamaica	*Hibiscus sabdariffa*	hibiscus, Jamaican sorrel	diuretic, nervousness, tonic, hypertension
Jojoba	*Simmondsia californica*	jojoba	shampoo, sore throat, vaginitis, asthma
Llantén	*Plantago major*	plantain	constipation, diarrhea, anti-inflammatory
Maguey (Agave)	*Agave americana*	century plant, false aloe	diuretic, purgative, toothache, syphilis
Malabar (Berenja)	*Solanum verbascifolum*	malabar mix	antiseptic, diuretic, inflammation, digestive, diabetes
Manita	*Chiranthodendron pentadactylon*	flower of manita	antispasmodic, heart disease
Manzanilla	*Matricaria chamomilla*	chamomile	digestive, sedative, menstrual pain

(Table continued on next page.)

Selected Mexican Herbs* *(Continued)*

Mexican Name**	Latin Name	English Name(s)	Alleged Value/Common Uses
Manzanilla del Rio	*Gnaphthalium species*	cudweed	colds, cough, diabetes, anti-inflammatory
Manzanita (Pinguica)	*Arctostaphylos uva-ursi*	uva ursi, bearberry	urinary and prostate problems, gall-bladder disease
Marrubio	*Marrubium vulgare*	horehound	expectorant, tonic, carminative, diabetes
Matarique	*Psacalium decompositum*	Indian plantain	diabetes, purgative
Mercadela	*Calendula officinalis*	marigold	pharyngitis, anti-inflammatory
Mesquite	*Prosopis julifera*	mesquite	antibacterial, astringent, eye irritation
Milenrama (Plumajillo)	*Achillea millefolium*	yarrow	wounds, antipyretic, colds, antiseptic
Mostaza negra	*Brassica nigra*	mustard	digestive, aches, fever, colds
Nopal	*Opuntia species*	prickly pear	diabetes, abscess, toothache, diuretic, cholesterol
Orégano	*Origanum vulgare*	marjoram	cough, digestive, worms, rheumatism
Orozús (Regaliz)	*Glycyrrhiza glabra*	licorice	expectorant, tonic, gastric ulcers, antiseptic
Ortiga verde	*Urtica dioica*	nettle	diuretic, tonic, anti-allergy, astringent
Osha (Chuchupate)	*Ligusticum porten*	lovage	wounds, colds, anti-inflammatory, infections
Pasiflora (Pasionaria)	*Passiflora incarnata*	passion flower	insomnia, relaxant, headaches, convulsions
Pinon	*Pinus species*	pine	antiseptic, diuretic, stimulant, cough
Popotillo	*Ephedra viridis*	Mormon tea	diuretic, astringent, tonic, venereal diseases
Prodigiosa (Rodigiosa)	*Brickellia grandiflora*	bricklebush	diabetes, digestive, diarrhea, biliousness
Raiz del Manzo	*Liriosma ovata*	muira puama	astringent, sore throat, aphrodisiac, tonic
Romero	*Rosmarinus officinalis*	rosemary	gynecologic problems, digestive
Rosa de Castilla	*Rosa woodsii*	rose petals	child's laxative, eye problems, relaxant
Ruda	*Ruta graveolens*	rue	gastrointestinal upset, menstrual problems, nervousness, diabetes
Sabila	Agave socotrina	aloes	burns, wounds, toothache, indigestion, diabetes

(Table continued on next page.)

Mexican Name**	Latin Name	English Name(s)	Alleged Value/Common Uses
Sabino (Enebro)	*Juniperus* species	juniper	diuretic, antiseptic, carminative
Salvia	*Salvia officinalis*	sage	digestive, antiseptic, tonic, sedative
Sauco	*Sambucus nigra*	elder flower	fevers, colds, colic, inflammation
Santa maria	*Tanacetum parthenium*	feverfew	migraine, arthritis, menstrual pain
Sauce blanco	*Salix alba*	white willow	pain, fever, rheumatism
Sueldo	*Symphytum officinale*	comfrey	anti-inflammatory, skin diseases, astringent
Te limon	*Cymbopogon citratus*	lemongrass	fever, stomachache, stress
Tejocote	*Crataegus mexicanus*	hawthorn	diuretic, tonic, colds, cough, diabetes
Tila	*Tilia mexicana*	tilden (linden)	sedative, insomnia, antipyretic, colds, colic
Toloache	*Datura* species	jimson weed	pain, sores, bruises, chest problems
Tomillo	*Thymus vulgaris*	garden thyme	expectorant, anti-inflammatory, pain, toothache
Topozan	*Buddleia americana*	butterfly bush	diabetes, tonic, menstrual pain, gastritis
Toronjil	*Agastache mexicana*	giant hyssop	antispasmodic, circulation, gastritis, nerves
Trebol morado	*Trifolium repens*	red clover	cough, colds, sedative
Tronadora	*Tecoma stans*	trumpet bush	diabetes, gastritis, antibiotic, air purifer
Tusilago	*Tussilago farfara*	coltsfoot	cough, expectorant, sedative
Uña de gato	*Uncaria tomentosa*	cat's claw	anti-inflammatory, antimicrobial, ulcers
Uvalama	*Vitex agnus-castus*	chaste tree	menstrual problems, expectorant
Valeriana	*Valeriana officinalis*	valerian	sedative, soporific, antispasmodic
Verbasco	*Senecio longilobus*	gordolobo yerba	substitute for gordolobo
Verbena	*Verbena officinalis*	vervain	colds, influenza, stomach problems
Yerba buena	*Mentha* species	mints	digestive, colic, antiseptic, anti-inflammatory
Yerba del Buey	*Grindelia aphanactis*	gum weed	expectorant, tonic, antispasmodic

(Table continued on next page.)

Selected Mexican Herbs* *(Continued)*

Mexican Name**	Latin Name	English Name(s)	Alleged Value/Common Uses
Yerba del Golpe	*Oenothera kunthiana*	evening primrose	anti-inflammatory, anti-spasmodic, expectorant
Yerba del Indio	*Aristolochia pentandra*	birthwort, Indian root	snakebite, antimicrobial, stomach ache
Yerba del Manzo	*Anemopsis california*	lizard tail	arthritis, pain, infections
Yerba maté	*Ilex paraguayensis*	mate	appetite suppressant, hangovers, stimulant
Yuca	*Yucca schidicera*	Joshua tree	arthritis, cholesterol, anti-inflammatory
Zábila	*Aloe vera*	aloe vera	cuts, burns, purgative
Zapote blanco	*Casimiroa edulis*	sapodilla	insomnia, hypertension, malaria
Zarsasparilla	*Smilax officinalis*	sarsaparilla	astringent, diarrhea, diabetes, diuretic

* This table has been compiled from many sources. It is not an evidence-based list, and information on alleged value and common uses is not definitive nor complete. It is intended primarily as a selected guide to familiarize health professionals with the array of traditional Mexican herbal medicines that are used by patients.

** The names of plants are not always clear from accounts, or from purchases made from herbal outlets. The list of alleged benefits is usually quite long; a few of the more popular ones have been selected for this table. For references, see general chapter references. Additional research provided by Yda Ziment.

Hundreds of Mexican herbal products (see table) are available, sold by retailers in the Southwestern U.S. and in supermarkets and drug stores catering to the Hispanic community. The accurate identification of a specific herb is often impossible because of the lack of consistency in different published accounts. The English and Spanish names can vary considerably, and many names may be given to an individual herb. The properties of and the indications for each herb are usually quite extensive. Note that there is little evidence—other than custom and practice—to support these claims, and many experts disagree about them. It can be concluded that despite the popularity and widespread usage of many of these herbs, it is probable that most of them only result in the particular effect that the individual prescriber or the specific user devoutly expects the herb to deliver.

references

Websites (Accessed March 2001)
www.acusd.edu/~alperson (Mexican herb usage)
www.clnet.ucr.edu/library/rescoll.html
www.conabio.gob.mx/biodiversitas/diverset.htm (The Herbolaria)

www.egregore.com/misc/herbindx2

www.herbsofmexico.com (This site provides extensive information, but contains numerous errors.)

www.herbweb.com/herbage

www.nos.net/yerbamex/herbs1.htm

www.williecolon.com/health/latinofolkremedies.htm

www.rice.edu/projects/HispanicHealth/Courses/mod7.html (Neff N: Folk Medicines in Hispanics in the Southwestern United States)

Journals

Heinrich M, Ankli A, Frei B, et al. Medicinal plants in Mexico: Healer's consensus and cultural importance. Soc Sci Med 47:1859–1871, 1998.

Yarnell E. Southwestern and Asian botanical agents for diabetes mellitus. Altern Complement Ther 6:7–11, 2000.

Books

Davidow J. Infusions of Healing. New York, Simon and Schuster, 1999.

Kay MA. Healing with Plants in the American and Mexican West. Tucson, University of Arizona Press, 1996.

IV: Essays & Commentaries

Aromatherapy

Pleasant and pungent smells have always been of importance to human societies.[1] The ancient Egyptians made perfumery an art, and numerous fragrant plants were used in cosmetics and medicines; such plants were also of great importance in religious ceremonies that employed aromatic incenses.[2,3] The close relationship between perfumes and incenses is expressed in the meaning of the word perfume (per = through, fume = smoke). In the Old Testament, a holy anointing oil was described in detail for use in the official appointment of the high priest, or messiah (from the word for "the anointed one"), and the mixture for holy incense to be used in temple ceremonies was also stipulated.[4]

Incenses and strong aromas have continued to have a powerfully evocative effect, which varies from the spiritual to the satanic, and from the sensually romantic to the utilitarian and antiseptic. Thus, perfumes are also related to fumigation, and have a long association with disease treatment.[2]

History

In biblical times, exotic and precious aromatic herbs were imported over incredible distances to satisfy priests and aristocrats.[4] In the Middle East and in the Roman Empire, extraordinary attention was given to the use of exotic tastes and smells, and this refined appreciation persists in many Arab countries to this day. In Western society, the art of the fragrance creator transcends far beyond basic appreciation of the delight of exotic essences.

Increasingly, aromas are being used in imaginative and flamboyant fashions, which couple sensory refinement with extravagance.

Educated people willingly suspend rationality when they purchase expensive soaps, skin creams, and perfumes based on wildly exaggerated claims about valuable combinations of minute amounts of essential oils in a simple, inexpensive base. This phenomenon attests to the powerful influence of creative advertising and olfactory stimulation, both of which have subtle but potent effects on mood, impulse, and behavior. Thus, the psychic benefits of aromatherapy—particularly when accompanied by other pleasing sensory input, such as massage—may create healing feelings that can modify disease processes or improve physiologic or functional deficits.

Imagination and sensitivity guided the ancient perfumers and incense-makers, who employed a number of well-recognized herbs such as cinnamon, frankincense, and myrrh along with more obscure odiferous plants such as cassia, calamus, stacte, galbanum, onycha, and spikenard.[3] A host of newer aromatic essences became popular over the millennia, and most are now obtained by extracting them from biologic sources via a process of distillation not too different from that which was first developed about a thousand years ago. The essential oils that are marketed to the public are generally named after their source (such as eucalyptus oil) and rarely by their major chemical components (such as cineole).

Current Aromatherapy

Currently, an increasing number of herbalists concentrate their skills on the practice of aromatherapy, using floral essences and other odiferous components to help the partaker "feel good" rather than "feel better." These therapists are more concerned with relieving the "dis-ease" of psychologic stress and physical fatigue, than with treating diseases that are based on organic pathologic damage. Aromatherapy can be simplified to the point of using pleasant-smelling incenses, bath soaps or oils, cosmetics, shampoos, and fragrances, or it can be used more imaginatively in douches, body wraps, massages, and inhalations from various diffusers, sprayers, vaporizers, and nebulizers.

The benefits of aromatherapy include relaxation, relief of tension, increased energy, refreshment, purification, and sensual stimulation.[5] The health-related value of aromatherapy has been reported in a variety of settings including hospices, nursing homes, and hospitals.[6] In Europe, health spas cooperate with healthcare providers to use aromatherapy in a sophisticated fashion to meet the individual patient's health or illness requirements. In the U.S., health spas are generally separated from conventional medical practice, and are therefore perceived as providing unorthodox or alternative therapy.

Home aromatherapy, which is catered to commercially by a huge variety of incenses, perfumed candles, creams, and lotions, can be obtained more simply, and can have a spiritual quality. Certain groups use incense and candle aromas with herbal drugs in an "aromantic" mixture with dance, religious, spiritual, shamanistic, astrologic, sexual, or healing practices.[7] The availability of commercial aromatherapy products demonstrates the range of the appeal of olfactory stimulants: they are found in markets, pharmacies, music outlets, and sex shops, and are sold by cosmetic purveyors, tarot-card readers, and health food providers.

Many recommendations on the use of the healing properties of herbs and proprietary aromatherapy products are available in books, magazines, and brochures. An incredible wealth of information is available on the internet,[8–11] and many foreign suppliers of herbs and exotic products make themselves available to the curious inquirer or the seeker of new experiences in alternative medicine. However, the range of misinformation and imaginative, unscientific dogma is impressive. Nevertheless, the growth and popularity of this alternative medical practice clearly indicate that it is deserving of scientific evaluation, and studies are gradually being undertaken.[20,21]

Flower Therapy. One of the most successful of the commercial aromatherapy products is Bach's flower remedies.[12] Dr. Bach prepared 38 healing flower essences targeted at alleviating psychological distress. Thus, crab apple is used to treat self-hatred; rockrose to relieve terror and panic; honeysuckle to counteract excessive nostalgia; and so on. These remedies are often presented as a form of alternative, but nevertheless scientific, treatment, although there is no clinical evidence that demonstrates the validity of the claims that are made.

The wide availability and popularity of these curious remedies provide potent testimony to the influence of olfactory stimulation and to the value of these substances in addressing individual perceptions of psychic distress. For example, Bach offers a "Rescue

Remedy"—a creative combination of cherry plum, clematis, impatiens, rockrose, and star of Bethlehem—for use in emergencies, such as to counter the stress of taking an exam. These and similar healing modalities appeal to people who may feel dissatisfied with the offerings of modern science and are more accepting of simple, natural remedies or are fascinated by the poetic claims of the marketers.

Aromas powerfully resonate at an emotional and psycho-spiritual level to evoke a sensation of relief from disease, arising out of a deep feeling that responds to forces more basic than the logic of modern medical science. Thus, the physicochemical response to aromatherapy is bound up in emotional alchemy rather than in the mechanics of organic chemistry.

Essential Oils. Manufacturers make many claims for their aromatherapy agents (see table). It is evident that the claims are based on imagination and differ according to the individual author's whims; thus many of the alleged benefits for a specific aroma are directly contradictory. Nevertheless, these arbitrary indications are selectively accepted by professional aromatherapists and people who seek their advice and services. Most of the available aromas are supposed to exert their alleged effect by means of inhalation of the vapor of the essential oil, or by application of the oil to the skin. Some aromas are claimed to be beneficial for the skin or hair,[22] and even are touted as having a healthy effect on both the state of mind and the symptoms of specific illnesses such as cancer.[23] A number of these agents may serve as mild expectorants, or may help soothe a cough,[4] but there is no good evidence that they have any substantial therapeutic benefit on organic disease, even though some may be absorbed when used topically or given by inhalation.

Several aromatherapy agents have *in vitro* antimicrobial properties when used alone or in combination,[13] but there is little reliable evidence that they can treat clinical infections of the skin or internal organs. Overall, a number of studies are credited with having shown evidence of antibacterial or antifungal effectiveness for such aromatherapy agents as cinnamon, chamomile, sandalwood, lavender, ylang ylang, peppermint, neroli, lemon grass, basil, rose, and various mixtures,[14] but most of these reports are in nonscientific journals and lack adequate substantiation. However, herbal remedies for skin disease care are attracting the attention of orthodox medicine,[15] and further studies are justified.[19]

Partial Listing of Aromatherapy Agents: Manufacturer Claims*

Herb	Key Properties†	Alleged Benefits	Special Properties
Angelica	balancing	revitalizing, strengthening, stimulating, anchoring	improves immunity
Anise	cheering	euphoriant, relaxing, toning, sense-enhancing	deodorant
Basil	strengthening	clearing, stimulating, refreshing, soothing, uplifting	clears the mind
Bay	illuminating	soothing, relaxing, warming	migraine, colds, pain
Benzoin	soothing	warming, uplifting, decongesting, comforting	tired muscles, skin therapy
Bergamot‡	uplifting	refreshing, stabilizing, sedating, normalizing	skin therapy
Black pepper	penetrating	stimulating, warming, relaxing, vitalizing, aphrodisiac	muscle aches
Camphor	balancing	stimulating, decongesting, toning, cooling, clarifying	skin conditioner
Cardamon	toning	stimulating, sensual, warming	skin conditioner
Carrot seed	revitalizing	nourishing, cleansing, restoring	skin therapy
Cedarwood‡	soothing	calming, composing, stabilizing, decongesting	skin therapy
Chamomile‡	soothing	calming, relaxing, sedating, comforting, nourishing	skin therapy
Cinnamon‡	energizing	relaxing, balancing, stimulating, warming, vitalizing	anti-inflammatory
Citronella‡	pungent	uplifting, refreshing, stimulating, purifying	repels insects, deodorant
Citrus oils‡	revitalizing	uplifting, refreshing, cleansing, stimulating	skin therapy, anxiety
Clary sage	relaxing, euphoriant	warming, sensual, soothing, centering, euphoriant	fatigue, PMS
Clove	energizing	stimulating, numbing, warming, sense-enhancing	relaxant
Cypress	improves circulation	astringent, toning, soothing, purifying	fatigue, oily skin, deodorant
Eucalyptus‡	clearing, energizing	invigorating, refreshing, soothing, decongesting	fatigue, colds
Fennel	female tonic	toning, detoxifying, stimulating, cleansing, warming	cellulite, PMS, mouthwash
Frankincense‡	meditative, uplifting	rejuvenating, relaxing, harmonizing, clarifying	rejuvenative for skin
Gardenia	perfumey	uplifting, sensual	aphrodisiac

(Table continued on next page.)

Partial Listing of Aromatherapy Agents:
Manufacturer Claims* *(Continued)*

Herb	Key Properties[†]	Alleged Benefits	Special Properties
Geranium	balancing	stabilizing, sedating, stimulating, uplifting	PMS, mood swings, skin
Ginger	spicy, stimulating	fortifying, toning, warming, anchoring	tonic, tired muscles, colds
Hops	soporific	calming, sedating	for sleep pillows
Hyssop	stability	warming, relaxing, healing, refreshing, cleansing	bruises, rheumatism
Jasmine	aphrodisiac	relaxing, sensual, euphoriant, stimulating, asserting	skin tonic, perfume
Juniper	purifying	stimulating, cleansing, strengthening, fortifying	acne, cellulite, fatigue
Lavender[‡]	immunity, relaxing	soothing, rejuvenating, sedating, balancing	first aid for skin, aching
Lemongrass[‡]	astringent, refreshing	tonifying, stimulating, sedative, vitalizing	oily skin, deodorant, aching
Linden	rejuvenating, luxurious	relaxing, harmonizing	perfume
Marjoram[‡]	sedating	soothing, warming, comforting	tired muscles, sleep
Melissa	soothing	cheering, uplifting, relaxing, sedative	headaches, skin, depression
Mints	cooling	refreshing, clearing, soothing, reviving	fatigue, headache
Myrrh[‡]	resinous	rejuvenating, astringent, preserving, centering	skin therapy, spiritual
Neroli	renewal	rejuvenating, relaxing, soothing, sedative, centering	skin therapy, fatigue, anxiety
Niaouli[‡]	protective	anti-inflammatory, inhalant	upper respiratory infections
Patchouli[‡]	pervasive, sensual	soothing, relaxing, rejuvenating	skin therapy, hair
Pine[‡]	invigorating	refreshing, clearing, stimulating	deodorant, air freshener
Rose	sensual	uplifting, soothing, rejuvenating, balancing	aphrodisiac, skin therapy
Rosemary	stimulant, reviving	invigorating, clearing, clarifying, warming	skin therapy, mental fatigue
Rosewood	calming	relaxing, clearing, strengthening	PMS, skin therapy
Sage[‡]	energizing	stimulating, cheering, warming	soothing

(Table continued on next page.)

Herb	Key Properties†	Alleged Benefits	Special Properties
Sandalwood	expression, balancing	relaxing, sensual, stimulating, soothing, centering	tonic, skin therapy
Tea tree‡	revitalizing	cleansing, soothing, diaphoretic, purifying	insect bites, sores, first-aid
Thyme‡	strengthening	warming, soothing, stimulating, balancing, purifying	increases strength
Yarrow	tonic	balancing, soothing, rejuvenating	skin therapy, hair, perfume
Ylang-ylang	enticing, sensual	soothing, relaxing, stimulating, uplifting, euphoriant	stress, insomnia, anger, skin

* This list is summarized from a variety of information sources, each of which gives somewhat different indications, properties, and benefits. It is not an evidence-based list. There are many other herbs used in aromatherapy.

† Information based on claims of proponents; for example:
  Tisserand Aromatherapy, Petaluma, CA (Brochure)
  Nelson & Russell Aromatherapy (www.nelsonbach.com)
  Aura Cacia Aromatherapy, Weaverville, CA (Brochure)
  www.quinessence.com/essentialoils
  www.fragrant.demon.co.uk/aroma

‡ Has alleged or purported antiseptic properties

Many scented compounds that are found in plants have measurable chemical and medical effects, and some do merit further clinical evaluation. Some essential oils cause allergic or phototoxic reactions in sensitive people, and many can be poisonous if ingested orally (e.g., wormwood oil, pennyroyal oil).[5] Several volatile oils have been shown to have relaxant effects on airway muscles in laboratory animals,[16] but adequate clinical studies are lacking.

Nevertheless, aromatherapy may help relieve stress and induce relaxation in various conditions, which accounts for the interest in using essential oils in palliative care, as well as in nursing homes and hospitals.[23] Much of the current medical literature on aromatherapy is in nursing journals, and this attests to the value of pleasant olfactory stimuli in improving the well being of chronically ill patients.

Aromatherapy and Homeopathy

Aromatherapy uses minute doses of natural agents to liberate the inner self-healing response, and thus has a striking resemblance to homeopathy, which relies on many botanical remedies—a few of which are popular in aromatherapy (e.g., cinnamon, rockrose, bitter orange, jasmine, wintergreen) but for different in-dications.[17] Indeed, homeopathy is closely allied to Bach's flower remedies; each treats people according to their personality rather than in accordance with the pathology of the disease. However, in the case of homeopathy, there is some clinical trial evidence of ef-ficacy in disorders such as asthma and hayfever that has been accepted by orthodox peer-reviewers who practice allopathic medicine.[18] Interestingly, Samuel Hahnemann, who introduced the alternative medical practice of homeopathy, came to believe that enormously diluted drugs (such as camphor and strychnine) could be effective when experienced by "smelling" the medica-tions rather than by swallowing them.[19]

Conclusion

Aromatherapy is the most ancient form of sophisticated herbal-ism. It combines sense with sensibility, pleasure with faith, and practicality with magic. By so doing, aromatherapy achieves the therapeutic goal of making the partaker feel better. Thus, like the placebo effect, aromatherapy must be given serious attention, since it provides us with an excellent example for understanding the healing effects of all varieties of herbal medications. Scientific rationalism and evidence-based medicine can be used to evalu-ate the benefits of individual essences, but do not offer the opti-mal tools for examining the success of aromatherapy. As with other traditions that combine pleasant sensory stimuli with belief and hope as part of the individual's psychological experience of the healing response, the effectiveness of aromatherapy is inde-pendent of the practical outcome of pharmacologic intervention in the pathophysiology of disease.

Aromatherapy arises from history and tradition, yet relies heav-ily on modern methods of advertising, which tend to overstate benefits as well as encourage a perception of need for luxuries in everyday life. Aromatherapy unites humans with nature and beauty, and thus appeals to the inherent spiritual qualities that dif-ferentiate them from animals. More importantly, it constitutes an evolutionary bridge between the material response of the individ-ual patient's concepts of health and illness, and the metaphysical response resulting from the individual's faith, hope, and imagina-tion. Without these latter three components, healing in many dis-orders could not occur. Certainly personal experience and faith are extremely relevant in the course of most illnesses, and these aspects of healing may prove to justify greater use of some of the treatments encompassed by aromatherapy.

references

1. Morris ET. Fragrance: The Story of Perfume from Cleopatra to Chanel. New York, Charles Scribner & Sons, 1984.
2. Majno G. The Healing Hand: Man and Wound in the Ancient World. Cambridge, MA, Harvard University Press, 1975.
3. Manniche L. Sacred Luxuries. Fragrance, Aromatherapy, and Cosmetics in Ancient Egypt. Ithaca, NY, Cornell University Press, 1999.
4. Ziment I. The messianic relationship between inspiration and expectoration. In Baum G, Priel Z, Roth Y, et al (eds): Cilia, Mucus, and Mucociliary Interactions. New York, Marcel Dekker, 1998, pp 383–389.
5. Lawless J. The Illustrated Encyclopedia of Essential Oils. Rockport, MA, Element Books, 1995.
6. Vickers A, Zollman C. ABC of complementary medicine. Massage therapies. BMJ 319:1254–1257, 1999.
7. Worwood VA. Aromantics. London, Pan Books, 1987.
8. Aromatherapy Global Online Research Archives: www.nature-helps.com/agora
9. The Guide to Aromatherapy: www.fragrant.demon.co.uk/aroma2.html
10. www.quinessence.com/essential-oils (Accessed March 15, 2001)
11. www.aromaweb.com/essential_oilsaf (Accessed March 15, 2001)
12. Dr. Edward Bach Center. Accessed March 15, 2001 at www.bachcenter.com
13. Lis-Balchin M, Deans S, Hart S. A study of the changes in the bioactivity of essential oils used singly and as mixtures in aromatherapy. J Altern Comp Med 3:249–256, 1997.
14. Buckle J. Aromatherapy. In Novey DW (ed): Clinician's Complete Reference to Complementary and Alternative Medicine. St. Louis, Mosby, 2000, pp 651–666.
15. Brown DN, Dattner AM. Phytotherapeutic approaches to common dermatologic conditions. Arch Dermatol 134:1401–1404, 1998.
16. Reiter M, Brandt W. Relaxant effects on tracheal and ileal smooth muscles of the guinea pig. Arzneimittelforschung 35:408–414, 1985.
17. Ullman D. First aid with homeopathic medicines. Accessed March 15, 2001 at www.homeopathic.com/ailments
18. Ziment I, Tashkin DP. Alternative medicine for allergy and asthma. J Allergy Clin Immunol 106:603–614, 2000.
19. Hael R. Samuel Hahnemann. His Life and Work. Delhi, B. Jain Publishers, 1995.
20. Cooke B, Ernst E. Aromatherapy: A systematic review. Br J Gen Pract 50(455):493–496, 2000.
21. Lis-Balchin M. Essential oils and aromatherapy: Their modern role in healing. J R Soc Health 117:324–329, 1997.
22. Hay K, Jamieson M, Omerod AD. Randomized trial of aromatherapy. Succesful treatment of alopecia areata. Arch Dermatol 134:602–603, 1998.
23. Kite SM, Maher EJ, Anderson K, et al. Development of an aromatherapy service at a cancer centre. Palliat Med 12:171–180, 1998.

The Placebo Effect and Herbs

Many of the criticisms having to do with efficacy that are leveled against herbs can be charged equally against many orthodox medicines. Pharmaceutically designed and tested drugs that are approved by the FDA are not always effective, despite their popularity with physicians and patients. Although this applies in particular to over-the-counter drugs, the value of many prescription drugs can also be questioned. Some of the questionable products disappear spontaneously by attrition, and others are removed by the FDA, but many continue to be available for decades despite the continuing concern that they lack effectiveness. A major example of the latter is the class of drugs known as mucokinetics or expectorants: any effect on secretion clearance from the respiratory tract is difficult to determine for virtually all drugs in this class. Nevertheless, clinicians and patients tend to favor using them for conditions such as bronchitis.[1]

Orthodox drugs usually have potent pharmacologic effects; thus, they also have potent side effects. In contrast to the vast majority of herbs, numerous orthodox drugs are extremely dangerous. The National Institute of Medicine has shown that hundreds of thousands of patients are harmed and many thousands are inadvertently killed each year by such medications. These disturbing outcomes can result from inappropriate use of drugs and—all too often—from medical personnel error.[2]

In contrast, appropriately used herbs are relatively safe. Mistakes in herbal medicine, while a rare cause of worrisome toxicity, are unlikely to result in severe morbidity or in mortality. Thus we have an interesting dichotomy: while health-giving drugs can dispense danger and death, the majority of the known herbal medicines, though not convincingly effective, cannot. Herbal remedies rarely cause significant or serious effects, and therefore are often considered to be harmless placebos.

The Placebo as a Token

All experienced healers try to treat mild illnesses with nontoxic, harmless modalities; if such remedies help patients, then both the healer and the patient have reasons to be equally pleased.[3] The art of the healer is to understand which patients can gain maximum healing from minimal therapy. The conscientious healer who uses drugs will strive in all cases to provide the least toxic choice that will relieve the patient's symptoms or cure the illness. The empathetic healer realizes that, in many cases, the prescribed medication serves as a token, enabling the patient to feel reassured that helpful support is provided while Nature fosters the healing process.

For some patients, it is appropriate to prescribe a harmless token medicine such as an expectorant, a vitamin, or a well-known herb. The prescriber may be fully aware that the medication has no healing properties, but the patient believes the opposite. This is the basis of the term *placebo*, which implies that the physician knowingly provides an inert medicine, with the expectation that by so doing he or she will please (literally, "I will please") the patient. In such cases, the prescriber hopes for an "intentional placebo" response to a deliberately given, inert medication.[4] This does not constitute fraud, unless the prescriber or provider is cynical and exploitative, or frankly unethical, and knowingly provides useless therapies that could even lead to worsening of the illness, at inflated costs.

Placebos are also used by clinicians, patients, and families like lottery tickets, since it is felt that patients with horrible diseases have little to lose (apart from a variable expense) by taking a chance with a "cure" that has a remote chance of being effective. The patient who knowingly elects to try a recommended placebo invests hopeful expectation in the outcome. Evidence shows that a beneficial outcome can result from a sympathetic relationship with a healer who endorses a placebo as a means of fostering a hopeful attitude.[5,6] It is possible that one- to two-thirds of people who receive placebos feel better, and are likely to believe that the "medicine" caused the improvement.[6]

Similarly, placebos are used in double-blind, randomized trials because it is recognized that the placebo effect in any group of study-patients may be considerable.[7] Physicians know that placebos have been the mainstay of therapeutics throughout history, and many believe that most herbs and other forms of alternative medicine that are in use today serve as placebos, just as they did in the past (see table).

Reasons For Regarding Many Herbal Medicines as Placebos

- There is a lack of high-quality clinical evidence to convincingly demonstrate the benefits of most herbal medicines.
- Historically, most of the safe herbal medicines were placebos.
- Currently, many herbs are promoted because they are very safe, even in large dosages; this implies lack of any major effect.
- The great variety of dosages for specific herbs suggests that they are both harmless and useless, or of very low potency.
- The numerous indications, with lack of proof of value, suggests that the value of many "panacea" herbs is non-pharmacologic.
- Herbs are often recommended for nonspecific, milder illnesses that will spontaneously improve by regression to the mean.
- Some herbs are recommended even though proof of effectiveness is difficult or impossible to obtain, e.g., for prevention of feared diseases or of aging.
- Many patients who use herbs selectively accept anecdotal recommendations and ignore scientific refutations.
- Many orthodox medicines are popular, even though they have no active effect; thus, both drugs and herbs can be used as placebos.
- Many of today's herbs are the modern equivalent of favored placebos of the past, such as mustard plasters and leeches.

Placebos and Nocebos

Patients can either improve or worsen significantly after taking a placebo (as compared to no treatment), and the response usually reflects the individual patient's expectations.[8] A positive placebo response has clearly occurred in as many as 62% of patients in some controlled drug studies, and may have been higher in others.[6,9] The placebo effect is likely to be even greater in uncontrolled clinical studies (which is the situation with the majority of older reports on herbs), particularly when the investigator is convinced of the value of the treatment. Anxious patients who seek out herbal therapy are more likely to benefit, since it has been shown that the positive placebo effect is greater in subjects with high anxiety scores.[10]

Most clinicians learn of the importance of the negative (or *nocebo*)[8,10] effect as well as the positive placebo effect, since some anxious or untrusting patients are convinced that taking a harmless remedy caused unpleasant consequences. Physicians and other health providers usually recognize that their interaction with the patient can strongly influence the direction of this effect. The keenly aware clinician strives to influence the outcome positively, and carefully assesses the response as would an experimentalist. Improvement can occur in physiologic processes with placebo therapy, and in some cases the symptomatic benefit may be experienced without any measurable change in physical parameters; this has been clearly shown in functional dyspepsia.[9]

If a trusted clinician does not believe that a remedy will work, and tries to dissuade the patient from taking a probable placebo, the patient is less likely to gain benefit from taking that medication. However, even this outcome varies, since other influences—family, friends, religious belief, advertising claims—may reinforce the effect of a placebo and thereby counteract the clinician's negativism. Some patients take great satisfaction in telling their doctors that a treatment worked in spite of the physician's doubts, and this is often the situation when the patient chooses to supplement orthodox therapy with one or more alternative remedies. On the other hand, some patients claim that a simple or harmless therapy had an inexplicable harmful effect, even though this was unlikely to have been a direct outcome of the treatment. The wise clinician carefully evaluates the outcome to try and decide whether his or her own expectations were founded on incorrect assumptions.

Repeated experiences with multiple patients help each clinician draw conclusions as to which are "useful" placebos and which are "useless," or which are "harmful" nocebos as opposed to being "harmless." The thoughtful therapist can determine which option should be offered to a particular patient. Since experienced clinicians cannot rely solely on evidence-based data, they will naturally rely on empirical information to influence their clinical decision-making. Thus, they are likely to have differing opinions about the effectiveness of various herbal treatments.

Does the Placebo Effect Exist?

It has been repeatedly pointed out that the value of the placebo may have been overstated.[11] There are many means by which illnesses improve while patients are taking either active or placebo therapy, and the change may be independent of the treatment given. All symptoms in a spectrum of patients with similar manifestations merge closer to the average when subjected to repeated evaluation. This phenomenon of "regression to the mean" suggests that—irrespective of whether active treatment or placebo treatment is given to any group of patients with disorders such as dyspepsia, asthma, depression, or pain—there will be a tendency for the group to show improvement over time.[12,13]

Many herbalists and herbal authorities recommend that phytomedicinals be used for several weeks to months before judging their effectiveness. Although a slow onset of action is often attributed to the herb's "gentle" nature, or its abilities to "naturally and slowly" stimulate the body's own healing process, the phenomenon of the regression to the mean is a more likely explanation for the delayed onset of action of many of these therapies. Other explanations for apparent improvement include observer bias, patient bias, misinterpretation of meaningless responses, the simultaneous use of other unrecognized treatment, and several less-obvious variables.[13]

Recently, an analysis of clinical trials suggested that the taking of a placebo leads to responses that are not significantly more effective than those attained by giving no treatment at all.[14] However, an editorial commentator criticized this interpretation as being too wide, particularly since there is evidence that placebos do produce better pain relief than no treatment.[15] Furthermore, the situation in clinical trials is very different from real life, since study patients are extensively screened and monitored, and they give informed consent when participating in studies that use an experimental protocol. This cannot be compared to a personal advisor simply prescribing a placebo for an individual patient, using it as a deliberate choice for a specific condition.

The Placebit Effect

It may be assumed that the most successful placebos are those believed by clinicians to be effective—even if they are remedies proven to have no effect or are inadequately evaluated.[5] The belief of the prescriber can synergize with that of the patient to maximize the benefit of a placebo. This response to a noneffective treatment, or one of uncertain effectiveness, with both prescriber and taker believing in its value, can be called a *"placebit"* effect, from the Latin, "It will please," (i.e., the treatment will please both the prescriber and the patient). The outcome of placebit therapy is likely to be more satisfactory for both prescriber and user, than the outcome of a placebo therapy in which the clinician considers the agent ineffective.

This discussion of the placebo and the placebit effect may be of the highest significance in complementary and alternative therapies and may be particularly relevant to a course of herbal medicine. The beneficial effect of an ineffective herb prescribed by a convinced herbalist or integrative clinician to a patient who specifically seeks out this therapy can be considered a placebit effect. Any improvement in health, however, can be considered a true benefit. Moreover, the prescriber is correct to deny the scientifically proved ineffectiveness of the herb, since in its ability to foster a beneficial outcome, it is, in practice, effective.

It is more difficult to explain how an inactive herbal preparation can be effective when taken as self-therapy by a patient without the input of an herbal prescriber. In this instance, the placebit effect can still exist, because the patient's belief is synergized by the collective belief of the manufacturers, marketers, writers, and other individuals who may have influenced the patient to select the herbal remedy. Moreover, a prolonged course of any therapy is usually accompanied by improvement in most illnesses, thus convincing a patient that the phytomedicine worked and thereby encouraging further self-experimentation with other herbal therapies for subsequent health problems.

Mechanisms of the Placebo Effect

Physiologic explanations of the placebo response have been sought, although studies on placebos in humans are more often carried out by psychologists and behaviorists than by physiologists, anatomists, and biochemists. Cerebral mechanisms involving endogenous opioid or endorphin release have been postulated to explain the analgesic response to placebos given for pain.[16] However, the overall placebo response has not been adequately elucidated as a physiologic phenomenon, and suitable animal models do not exist to aid in the investigations of the neuropsychologic or neuroimmunochemical mechanisms.

Ancient physicians, and those who succeeded them prior to modern times, were very certain that there was a need for the intervention of a divine force in the healing process. Current medical terminology relies on more prosaic explanations: the time course and the variabilities of natural repair and healing are understood, and there is awareness that the improvement of a chronic or prolonged illness may occur as a consequence of regression of the illness to the mean. Nevertheless, the old concept of the positive influence of spiritual forces such as hope, faith, and prayer is still accepted.

Physicians in the 18th century invoked the *vis medicatrix natura* or the *vis vitalis;* this is the natural healing spirit that was described by Hippocrates and emphasized by Paracelsus.[17] This powerful force undoubtedly can be used as an explanation (particularly for responses to homeopathic medications), although it is not physically identifiable or quantifiable. It has been pointed out that the romantic plays a role in medicine as much as the rational[6]; thus healing can occur as a response to the warm "poetic resonance" created by a sympathetic healer as well as to the cold "scientific prose" that is the more usual tool of the practicing physician.

The sensitive healer can recognize, assess, and harness the individual patient's ability to self-heal, and can facilitate the process with sympathetic intervention based on knowledge, inherent skills, experience, and authority—with, or even without, drug therapy of any type.

Should the Placebo Effect Be Used Therapeutically?

The placebo/placebit effect is potent, and it is legitimate. It can be used as effectively as a well-known song or verse of poetry to capture the mind and the soul of the patient in a resonant relationship whereby healer and patient interact in a psychospiritual harmony. Thus, "poetic healing" can evoke physical responses that the prose of conventional medicine is unlikely to stimulate. The placebo effect works as an effective psychic tool, and it may be used consciously or unconsciously when the patient feels a special rapport with either the healer or the tools of healing—be they herbs or other therapeutic modalities.

Undoubtedly, the appropriate use of a placebo can help bring about more rapid or complete healing in disorders that can spontaneously resolve. It can also be used as an adjunct to routine treatment or to enhance well being in chronic diseases for which there is no cure. The response can be very effectively employed in treating irreversible and fatal diseases for which orthodox therapy may have been tried and found to be useless, insufficient, harmful, or merely of temporary benefit.

In many situations, an herbal medicine, whose value may be unclear but whose danger appears to be minimal, can offer significant benefits to the majority of patients who believe in natural or herbal healing. This can be particularly effective when the herbal remedy is prescribed by an understanding practitioner in an integrative regimen along with orthodox medical treatment. The value of many herbal therapies lie somewhere between that of a known placebo and a clinically proven medication. However, with most herbs, the quality of the evidence fails to provide adequate proof of the claimed benefits. Thus, it is often unknown which herbal medicines act purely as placebos and which offer pharmacologic properties that may serve to complicate the "placebo effect" of the herb.

In addition, dangers can accompany the overuse or exaggerated use of herbs (e.g., in serious diseases, when herbal medicines are heavily relied on despite the availability of more effective options). Costs must also be considered, as well as the lack of quality control and regulatory oversight of herbal therapies, and the possibility that presumed placebo herbs may be truly harmful. Thus, placebo herbs and potent herbs all merit knowledgeable and thoughtful analysis when considered as components of the patient's therapy, so as to ensure maximal benefit with minimal harm.

Conclusion

Much of the discussion in this book emphasizes evidence-based analysis in an effort to separate the pharmacologic effects from the placebo effects of herbal medicines. However, not only is it often difficult to make this distinction, it is understood that a sympathetic and effective clinician does not always base therapeutic decisions on a foundation of evidence-based medicine. There are additional avenues of healing, and many herbal therapies can be employed not only as medicines with potential pharmacologic benefits, but as harmless placebos, resulting in a good therapeutic response for the patient.

Both placebo and pharmacologic effects can have health-improving value, and their use must be individualized to the patient's needs. The goal of any treatment is to ensure that both the prescriber and the user "will be pleased," whether the tool is a potent pharmacologic therapy, a valued herbal token, or perhaps a sensitive ear, a kindly touch, or a few sympathetic and encouraging words. The recent phenomenal increase in popularity of herbal

remedies is in large measure a reaction to the relatively imper-
sonal nature of healthcare provider services, which are increasingly replacing the traditional caring physician. Herbs do not
provide an overworked practitioner with an ideal tool, but they do
offer opportunities for communication with the patient and for an
enhanced therapeutic relationship.

references

1. Ziment I. Respiratory Pharmacology and Therapeutics. Philadelphia, WB
   Saunders Company, 1978.
2. Richardson WC, Berwick DM, Bisgard JC. The Institute of Medicine report on
   medical errors. N Engl J Med 2000; 343:663–665. (Letter and response)
3. Brown WA. The placebo effect. Sci Am 1998; 278:90–95.
4. Champion DG. Unproven remedies, alternative and complementary medicine. In Klippel JH, Dieppe PA (eds): Rheumatology, 2nd ed. London, Mosby,
   1998.
5. Benson H, Friedman R. Harnessing the power of the placebo effect and re-
   naming it "remembered wellness." Ann Rev Med 1996; 67:193–199.
6. Spiro H. The Power of Hope. A Doctor's Perspective. New Haven, Yale
   University Press, 1998.
7. Quitkin FM. Placebos, drug effects, and study design: A clinician's guide. Am
   J Psychiatry 1999; 156:829–836.
8. Weil A. Health and Healing. Boston, Houghton Mifflin Company, 1988.
9. Mearin F, Balboa A, Zarate N, et al. Placebo in functional dyspepsia:
   Symptomatic, gastrointestinal, motor and gastric sensorial responses. Am J
   Gastroenterol 1999; 94:116–125.
10. Hahn RA. The nocebo phenomenon: Scope and foundations. In Harrington E
    (ed): The Placebo Effect. An Interdisciplinary Exploration. Cambridge, MA,
    Harvard University Press, 1997, pp 56–76.
11. Shapiro AK, Shapiro E. The placebo: Is it much ado about nothing? In
    Harrington E (ed): The Placebo Effect. An Interdisciplinary Exploration.
    Cambridge, MA, Harvard University Press, 1997, pp 12–36.
12. Bland JM, Altman DG. Some examples of regression towards the mean. Br
    Med J 1994; 309:780.
13. Kienle GS, Kiene H. The powerful placebo effect: Fact or fiction? J Clin
    Epidemiol 1997; 50:1311–1318.
14. Hróbjartsson A, Gøtzsche PC. Is the placebo powerless? An analysis of clini-
    cal trials comparing placebo treatment with no treatment. N Engl J Med 2001;
    344:1594–1602.
15. Bailar JC III. The powerful placebo and the Wizard of Oz. N Engl J Med 2001;
    344:1630–1632.
16. Fields HL, Price DD. Toward a neurobiology of placebo analysis. In Harrington
    E (ed): The Placebo Effect. An Interdisciplinary Exploration. Cambridge, MA,
    Harvard University Press, 1997 pp 93–116.
17. Osler W. The Evolution of Modern Medicine. New Haven, Yale University
    Press, 1921.

What We Have Learned

The editors of this text and most of the contributing authors pursue orthodox medical careers in academic teaching centers. We are accustomed to questioning the logic and apparent effectiveness of most forms of therapy. We recognize that many patients seek medical help for health disorders that will either remit without specific treatment or become a relatively acceptable, chronic component of the patient's life. There are doubts as to the effectiveness and safety of many of our orthodox therapies, but there is little doubt that popular over-the-counter remedies as well as a healthy diet and exercise can be as beneficial as some corresponding prescription drugs. Undoubtedly, the placebo effect is a potential component in the majority of therapies, as there is a psychological or emotional component to any disorder that is affected by the therapeutic alliance between clinician and patient, whatever form of therapy is used.

The modern promotion of herbs relies largely on the powerful influences of popular magazines, the internet, persuasive advertisements, celebrity recommendations, and other media reports. These sources tend to appeal to the increasing public belief that orthodox medicine is at fault for being too scientific, too authoritarian, too cautious, too elitist, too expensive, too dangerous, too much the captive of the pharmaceutical industry—having all the faults that herbal medicine lacks. Herbs are often praised for being providential, natural, sanctified by tradition, proved by long experience, and studied in depth by enthusiasts whose minds remain fresh and open. In addition, there is a huge scientific and pseudo-scientific literature on the pharmacologic and clinical effects of herbs, which is now entering mainstream medicine and the public consciousness. The implication is that herbal medicine is a resurrected, rapidly evolving, popular science that is amassing increasing proof in favor of old claims, while unearthing newly discovered benefits for treating illness, improving health, and preventing severe disease.

Questions To Ask About Herbs

We have read many of the major books on herbs, and have evaluated hundreds of articles including translations of many studies not originally available in English. We have visited innumerable websites, delved into historical texts, reviewed herbal magazines and journals, and held discussions with herb providers and users. We have evaluated European and Native American herbal medicines, Ayurvedic and Chinese traditional medicinal therapies, homeopathy, Bach's flower essence therapy, aromatherapy, nutraceuticals, and food supplements of many classes. Throughout this study, the following questions have been asked about each of the herbal remedies under consideration:

- Why are therapeutic claims made for specific herbal medicines?
- What is the scientific and clinical evidence underlying or supporting these claims?
- What is the relationship between the differing indications for a single herb?
- What uniformity is there in the recommendations made for specific herbal medications by various authorities?
- Is there a potential biochemical or pharmacologic explanation for a claimed benefit?
- What information is published in respected (or, preferably, peer-reviewed) journals in support of claims?
- Have large-scale clinical studies using modern, double-blinded, randomized trials with placebo controls been published?
- What subsequent verification is there for any individual study's findings?
- Does the therapeutic claim make sense? Does it fit in with our own experience of the way drugs, or chemicals in general, function as therapeutic agents?

Objectivity in Herbal Medicine

This deep, objective enquiry has led to the conclusion that most herbal studies have so far failed to meet strict scientific requirements when evaluating the various clinical claims that are made for these healing agents. The typical lists of recommended indications for herbs generally lack acceptable validation. Fortunately, modern scientific investigation techniques are beginning to be applied to help evaluate increasing numbers of herbs.

Overall, too many unrealistic claims have been made for herbal medicines, and sophisticated patients recognize that exaggerated recommendations undermine the credibility of herbs in general. Many newer controlled clinical trials show that herbs are less effective in severe diseases than their proponents have long claimed; indeed, most of the effective herbs are only of limited benefit for milder disorders. It is also obvious that herbs should not be used as the basic treatment for severe diseases that can be treated effectively by orthodox medications administered under the careful guidance of qualified physicians.

The recent recognition that some herbs can be harmful or even dangerous has certainly reduced the enthusiasm of patients who had favored herbs because of their apparent benefits accompanied by an apparent lack of toxicity. Objective assessments of herbal therapy have started to "weed out" many of the less effective agents and are limiting the potentially harmful preparations. The public has become aware of the exaggerated claims for herbs and the equally incorrect assurances about their totally benign nature, and as a result herbal sales have recently declined. However, some individuals will continue to collect and dose themselves with numerous herbs, vitamins, and other supplements in an effort to alleviate minor ills, prevent major health problems, and prolong their life.

There are solid reasons why orthodox medicine is concerned about the flourishing herbal market (see table). The major problems with many studies on herbs are the lack of high-quality, controlled clinical trials; the use of studies without clear clinical outcomes; and the over-reliance on *in vitro* or other nonclinical data to make exaggerated claims. The most balanced and reliable herbal experts emphasize that the majority of herbs cannot be endorsed until more work is done to define indications. Additionally, these experts call for established, scientific study techniques and objective, randomized, controlled trials. Although it is not unusual for authors to state that studies have confirmed certain effects, referral to the original sources often reveals only dogmatic opinions by writers who cite preliminary or inappropriate scientific investigations. In cases where there are controlled clinical trials that can be evaluated, all too often they are unacceptable as indicators of clinical responses in humans. The following table documents the major faults with such studies, which sometimes merge science

Problems With Herbal Therapies

- Anecdotal information rather than scientific evidence predominates, and is often perpetuated.
- Inadequate or unreliable studies, and the resulting claims of benefit, are confusing.
- Publications in nonscientific medical journals, usually without peer review, create doubts as to the validity of the findings.
- Failure to replicate important clinical findings is common.
- Frequent failures of herbs to perform well in scientific studies is a concern.
- Results that are too good to believe are frequently used in marketing.
- Mixture of science with art and imagination is characteristic in advertising.
- Bizarre combinations of herbs reduce the credibility of the whole discipline.
- Recommendations on treatment are often made by unqualified salespersons.
- Multiple contrasting claims for specific herbs are confusing.
- Use for "untreatable" conditions (e.g., cancer or aging) is worrisome.
- Rapid introduction of new exotic herbs suggests opportunism.
- Herbs can be readily marketed to exploitable hypochondriacs.
- There is little or no regulatory oversight or quality assurance of herbal products.
- Contamination and adulteration of herbs is well documented.
- Use of herbs as flavors, novelties, and tonics reduces their status as medicines.
- Many herbal products are simply expensive sources of food constituents.
- Lack of agreement of herbal indications in different sources reduces credibility.
- Many herbs lack any proof of effectiveness, and are marketed as expensive placebos.
- Evidence-based medicine suggests that even effective herbs offer only minor benefits.
- There are no herbal "generic equivalents"; each product is unique.
- Ineffective herbal therapies used in place of more effective orthodox drugs can be detrimental to patient care.

with the self-deception that once characterized alchemy (see table below).

Typical Problems in Studies of Herb Effects

In Vitro Studies
- Studies carried out on the behavior of blood cells, micro-organisms, and malignant cells when exposed to herbal extracts cannot readily be extrapolated to human disease.
- Many non-Western scientists use *in vitro* tests that are not standard studies in Western medical research.
- Certain study models show significant effects that may have no clear relevance to clinical conditions or to disease. For example, numerous herbs are antioxidants, but their value in disease treatment or prevention is unclear.

Animal Studies
- Responses of small laboratory animals may be irrelevant, and are too often inappropriately extrapolated to human illnesses.
- Studies in large animals are not carried out for herbs, mainly because of the expense.
- Herbal doses used in animal studies are often very large compared to human dosing levels.

Human Studies
- Many herbal studies do not adequately stipulate selection criteria, end points, or objective outcome measures, thus resulting in nonevaluable results.
- Double-blind, placebo-controlled, randomized studies with high methodologic quality are rarely performed on herbal remedies in standardized, repeatable fashion. (This is changing, as many newer clinical trials are of better quality.)
- Herb studies often involve small numbers of subjects; the results lack the statistical power for any decisive interpretation.
- Many older studies that report excellent responses have not been repeated and have not been independently verified, and thus their significance is dubious.
- Clinical trials from Asia and Eastern Europe in particular have many methodologic limitations.
- Many European and other foreign studies are not only sponsored by, but appear to be conducted by, the manufacturer of the herbal product.
- There are no generic equivalents among herbal products; thus, results of a given study often cannot be extrapolated to other products containing the same herb.

Herb Versus Drug

Another problem in the study and application of herbal therapeutics is that of clearly defining an herbal medicine. When is a plant-derived medicinal product considered an herbal medicine, and when is it considered a drug? Much of this controversy and debate depends on the context of the word *drug*. One popular definition of a drug is any substance that has pharmacologic effects and is used therapeutically. After reviewing the literature on the chemistry, toxicology, and clinical science of herbal products, there is no doubt that many plants and plant-derived chemicals have pharmacologic activity in humans, which can be therapeutic or toxic, depending on the dose.

However, using a less scientific but accepted legal definition, a drug is also considered to be any substance that is licensed and marketed as such. Thus, herbal products and other dietary supplements (as legally classified by the U.S. Dietary Supplemental Health and Education Act of 1994) cannot be called drugs by government authorities, despite any pharmacologic properties that may have been demonstrated. This same law has restricted the labeling of herbal and other dietary supplements to that of simple "structure and function" claims, which are vague and poorly understood. This semantic discrepancy that separates legal definitions from common usage of drug and herbal products has created confusion and controversy among orthodox healthcare providers, public health authorities, and consumers.

Nevertheless, many well-known traditional herbal therapies have become the source or basis of valued pharmaceutical drugs in modern therapeutics. Several appear to also have beneficial clinical effects. While their clinical effects may be minor or less effective than established pharmaceutical drugs, some of these agents are coming to be accepted in allopathic medical practice. These herbs, however, are a relatively small proportion of the large number in popular use, and the vast majority of herbal medicines will not achieve this evidence-based status of effectiveness.

Although few herbal medicines have been proven to be clinically effective, there is no doubt that many have benefits that are not yet elucidated. As discussed in several chapters of this book (see especially "The Placebo Effect and Herbs"), there are many reasons why patients or clinicians favor and use herbal therapy (see table).

- Historical value and acceptance suggest effectiveness.
- Many current medicines are derived from herbs.
- Increasing popularity with the public indicates that herbs offer useful benefits.
- Herbs are readily available without a physician's prescription, and can be inexpensive.
- Patients can experiment with harmless herbs for minor or chronic diseases.
- Information published by knowledgeable experts is now more readily available for consumers.
- Failure of an herb to have a therapeutic effect may be an indictment of the manufacturer/provider (who may market inferior products) rather than the herb.
- Herbs are natural and appeal to people "in touch" with Nature.
- Many criticisms against herbs apply equally to orthodox drugs, but drugs are more toxic.
- Many drugs cause harm to, or even kill, patients; herbs are much safer in general.
- Herbs may treat conditions that orthodox medicines cannot help.
- Today's herbs may become tomorrow's drugs.
- New herbs can enter the marketplace much more rapidly than drugs, and may offer new healthcare options.
- Many herbs are useful as placebos, as are many drugs (but herbs are safer).
- Herbs can be used as adjuncts to regular drugs in integrative therapeutic regimens.
- Herbs are being used by physicians to fill gaps in orthodox medicine's pharmacopeia.
- Several herbs have achieved acceptable therapeutic status based on randomized, controlled trials.

Herbal Science Versus Herbal Magic

A more spiritual or psychological view of herbal medical practice suggests that this explosively popular component of modern healing unites the physical and the metaphysical. Many herbal medicines, though not pharmacologically active or even beneficial, remain popular and well utilized. Herbalism bridges scientific thinking to imaginative expectations, and enables sensitive, intuitive healers to combine the intellectualism of pharmacology and physiology with the poetic license of the artist. Herbalism is to allopathy as poetry is to prose, and it is evident that many patients who cannot respond with confidence to medical prosaism will respond to the healing message of "natural" herbal medicines.

Most modern, allopathic medical practice is logical and scientific, whereas complementary medicine is humanistic and focused on spiritual healing. Thus, there are clear reasons why many patients favor herbalism as an alternative to orthodox medicines (see table below). Herbs also offer some real benefits, and they bridge some of the therapeutic gaps left by orthodox medicine.

Recognizing that herbalism can be effective without being scientific, one can empathize with the imaginative claims of nonscientific herbalists who credit herbs with vague properties such as "strengthening the circulation," "stimulating hepatobiliary function," "cleansing and purifying the blood," and "regenerating the immune system." Note, too, that many herbal claims were developed in prescientific eras. Self-conviction impels herbalists to confidently advise, for instance, the treatment of allergies with a mixture of chamomile, ginkgo, stinging nettle, reishi mushroom, sage, goldenseal, yarrow, horseradish, and licorice. Such combinations, based to some extent on acceptable science, convey a healing message of inspiration and "natural" care that can be very persuasive to the suffering consumer. Patients may feel that herbal mixtures are the gifts of a beneficent Mother Nature, and they may choose to believe that these mixtures are more potent than any factory-produced, chemical antihistamine. The magic of the herb can readily outweigh the science of the drug.

Efforts by organized medicine to validate, discredit, or even objectively evaluate botanical therapies have met with multiple difficulties. In the interim, dedicated entrepreneurs have created innovative herbal remedies and marketing programs, so that all segments of the public are now being encouraged to experience the magic of herbal therapy. Additionally, the introduction of Asiatic and other exotic herbs to the U.S. marketplace has led many people to self-diagnose problems by matching symptoms to the unusual curative properties of these herbs.

The Challenge for Orthodox Medicine

The allopathic profession has been overwhelmed by the startling growth of herbal medicine and all its extraordinary manifestations.

Government agencies are not equipped to intervene when manufacturers of herbs or nutritional products, food supplements and additives, nutraceuticals, and dietary support products make extravagant claims. Traditional organized medicine and academic researchers are attempting to respond to the need to evaluate these products and to bring their findings to the attention of the public. More effort is being made to challenge the numerous inappropriate health claims and pseudo-scientific promotions by the parallel health industry of alternative medicinal therapies. It is appreciated that many of the herbs currently in use may become the sources of future orthodox medicines for treating very specific indications—but first the facts must be sifted from the fantastic.

The established medical community of academicians, investigators, and researchers is becoming more willing to contend with the powerful marketing forces that have propelled herbal medicine into a major industry. Currently, there is increasing recognition of the obligation to either corroborate or refute the claims made by herbal promoters. The relative inertia of conventional medicine during the last few decades has led to a failure to condemn faulty thinking, deliberate misrepresentation, and unsophisticated enthusiasm—or sophisticated over-commitment—in the practice of herbalism (see table below).

Reasons For Orthodox Medicine's Inability To Effectively Challenge the Excesses/Exaggerations of Herbal Medicine

Health Professionals

- Herbal medicines are not taught in most professional schools; the resurgence of an old field is relatively foreign to most clinicians.

- Physicians and other orthodox clinical professionals have so much to learn, they cannot afford to spend time critically evaluating herbal medicine.

- The public has confidence in alternative medicine; any criticisms from orthodox medicine could result in further distrust of physicians.

- Since most herbal medicines are harmless, health professionals are willing to tolerate their use.

- Many members of health professionals' families (and significant numbers of physicians, nurses, etc.) take herbal medicines.

(Table continued on next page.)

Health Professionals *(Cont.)*

- Knowledgeable clinicians advocate the use of effective herbs, and tolerate their patients' use of other herbs that may act as harmless placebos.

- Many patients have acquired more knowledge about herbs than their orthodox health advisers have, and therefore clinicians recognize that their advice about herbs will seem to be prejudiced rather than informative.

- Multiethnic patient populations use numerous exotic, alternative remedies that clinicians are unqualified to pass judgment on.

Researchers

- Manufacturers of herbal medicines are unlikely to support research that could reach negative conclusions about their products.

- Orthodox researchers can more readily obtain support from pharmaceutical companies and research funding agencies to conduct orthodox drug studies than to investigate herbs.

- It is a daunting challenge to conduct thorough studies on an herb that is made available by numerous manufacturers in a great variety of product formulations.

Organized Medicine

- Many organizations representing orthodox medical professionals are reluctant to criticize any other health-providing sector of the community.

- Organized medical societies rarely sponsor research, and are cautious about sponsoring critical subject reviews that may result in a reaction from other organizations whose interests may be offended.

- The National Institute of Health's National Center for Complementary and Alternative Medicine (NCCAM) has allocated a relatively small budget for research into alternative therapies, and only a small number of herbs are being studied.

- The Dietary Supplement, Health and Education Act (DSHEA) of 1994 opened up a burgeoning market for herbal supplements; marketers can act much more quickly than clinical researchers or organized medicine can respond.

One reason that organized medicine has had trouble condemning the apparent excesses of herbalism is because so many proponents of herbal therapy are idealistic, dedicated, knowledgeable, and experienced in a field of study that is foreign to conventional physicians. Under these circumstances, it is more comfortable to respect the fence between orthodox and unorthodox, and to accept the existence of the alternative practices rather than upset patients by criticizing herbalism in general or specific herbs in particular. Moreover, the patients who are convinced that herbs help are not going to be swayed by simple arguments, and it may be necessary and even helpful to guide them in their forays into alternative medicine.

It must be emphasized that many herbal products exhibit enough potential to justify cautious support for their use, and to call for society to make a much greater commitment in supporting scientific investigation into the more promising agents. But equally in need of emphasis is the importance of condemning the many obviously useless herbs and inappropriate proprietary mixtures that are being promoted to susceptible consumers. Since many different herbs are used for the same minor purposes (such as treating bowel, respiratory, and rheumatic discomforts), it is advisable to focus on the more promising herbs in each class, and to encourage the less-needed herbs to enter obsolescence. Expensive herbs that are used for minor purposes cannot be justified if there is no evidence to support their use.

Orthodox medicine is now doubly challenged: to help the public avoid the false hopes of inappropriate alternative therapies, and, importantly, to help identify effective herbal phytochemicals that offer sufficient advantages to justify their being incorporated into conventional medical practice. However, the ease with which knowledgeable marketers can bring a new herbal product into retail outlets will always exceed the speed of reaction of orthodox medicine to adequately respond to their claims.

The unsatisfactory performance of an herb in a standard randomized, double-blind, placebo-controlled (RDBPC) trial does not necessarily mean that the herb lacks useful effects. However, the RDBPC trial is the standard method for evaluating orthodox drugs, and health professionals, scientists, statisticians, and pharmaceutical companies commit enormous effort to subjecting such drugs to rigorous clinical testing. Thus, the herbal industry must acknowledge the value of the RDBPC trial, and if an herb does not demonstrate value in such testing, serious consideration must be given to the question of why the herb failed. Empiric herbalists (who rely on personal clinical experience) and scientific health practitioners (who more often require objective proof in addition to clinical experience) often have different answers to the same questions about herbal remedies. These differences must be resolved by both groups working together to ask the most appropriate questions and to design the most meaningful studies.

Finally, we recognize that there are herb promoters and herb users who clearly see the controversial issues, and who strongly believe in the value of herbal therapies. We have evaluated these issues and prepared responses to some of the major claims (see table).

Our Evaluation of Herbal Medicine Claims

Issue	Herbal Claims	Evaluation
Herbs are natural and are less harmful to the body than drugs	Herbs contain mixtures of chemicals that make them safer than single drugs	Herbs can be as harmful as drugs; many well-known poisons are herbs
Herbs can cure diseases that drugs cannot	Herbs are anti-cancer, anti-AIDS, anti-aging, anti-hepatitis, etc.	Such uses are difficult to prove; claims are often inaccurate or exaggerated
Herbal medicines are rarely dangerous, even in large dosages	Side-effects are uncommon and are usually not serious; their complications are very rarely fatal	This is generally true, although there are "toxic" exceptions
Multiple dosage forms and recommendations allow for careful selection to treat any condition	Expert herbalists provide product guidance and dosage selection for individual diseases	Uncertain quality and dosages make it difficult for consumers or clinicians to use herbs with confidence
Expert practitioners use herbs empirically to treat clinical diseases	Clinical trials are far less useful than clinical experience	Experience alone is inadequate; proper trials are essential
Herbs offer unique values that are not provided by orthodox drugs	Adaptogens, anorectics, immunostimulants, aphrodisiacs, etc. help improve life	There is little objective clinical evidence in support of these important herbal claims

(Table continued on next page.)

Issue	Herbal Claims	Evaluation
Asian herbs are valuable therapies that need to be introduced in the West	Ginsengs, astragalus, cordyceps, ashwagandha, etc. offer new approaches to health care	Most of these herbs have no clinical proof of value, and are used as exotic, seductive "panaceas"
Multiple herb formulations offer special advantages	Proprietary mixtures result in valuable synergistic effects	Mixtures rarely have demonstrated clinical advantages; they are usually concocted as marketing strategies
Antioxidants are of special value; orthodox medicine is slowly appreciating this	We live in a toxic world; antioxidants offer specific help against cancers, aging, etc.	Their value has been exaggerated; positive results from high-quality trials are lacking
MDs criticize herbs because they do not control their use nor understand their value	Doctors are not trained to use herbs and do not appreciate how effective they are in numerous conditions	MDs criticize herbs because of a lack of quality evidence
Many herbs have been scientifically validated in objective clinical trials	Placebo-controlled studies have showed some herbs to be effective	True, but high-quality studies are uncommon, and the effect is usually small
Whatever one says against herbs, those who use them find them helpful	Whatever the mechanism may be, herbalists know herbs can be beneficial	We agree; however, we are more cautious and selective in our recommendations

Conclusions

While herbal medicines clearly have a great potential for beneficial effects, very few are backed-up by convincing, high-quality clinical evidence. Moreover, many exaggerated and nonsensical claims are being advertised to the public by overly creative marketers, and the more reasonable and appropriate benefits and indications of potentially effective herbal remedies are being diluted.

The authors of this text are practicing clinicians who understand the role of both humanism and marketing in medical practice. We can accept the appeal of herbal healing, but we strongly oppose the pseudo-scientific claims and opportunism that is currently rampant in the herbal and supplement industry. We recognize that a host of ingredients may be added to herbal medicines, just as they are to expensive cosmetics, to create an individual marketing niche. It is often difficult to challenge the exaggerated claims that are made for these products.

Failure to take herbal medicine seriously may deprive many patients of significant benefits. Conversely, a lack of serious examination may condemn herbalism to increasing obscurity once its fashionable counter-culture status has waned. Herbs may be regarded as useful placebos, or as an example of fraudulent marketing, or as potentially valuable adjuncts that merit a place in integrative medical practice. Those of all shades of opinion who are challenged by the unresolved status of herbal medicines should seize the opportunity to work toward integration and to bring rationality and honesty into this debate. Perhaps our evidence-based approach to phytomedicines will help health professionals gain a more thorough understanding of herbal remedies and develop a deeper appreciation of their patients' interest in them.

V: Appendices

Resources for Herbal Medicine Information

A large number of books, monographs, pharmacopeias, newsletters, and web sites that summarize the herbal medicine literature are now accessible. Many strive to be objective, critical, and well referenced, and each has their strengths and weaknesses. The better resources are those that base efficacy or adverse effects claims on the primary clinical literature or high-quality systematic reviews. Accounts that cite other secondary (or indirect) sources of herbal information are generally not as reliable—all too often they are based on "expert" or "authoritative" statements or opinions that may be unsubstantiated. While some authors carefully analyze and describe the available data (or lack thereof), others inappropriately extrapolate claims from animal or *in vitro* experiments; misinterpret or exaggerate pharmacologic studies or case reports; or structure their advice on the basis of information obtained from sources that lack a scientific basis. Much of the published herbal information comes from a historical background of old data that are difficult to interpret, and, as a result, inaccurate, unclear, or questionable information is perpetuated.

The following list of herbal information resources is not comprehensive. There are many other sources with a wide variety of formats, and new resources are rapidly becoming available. Comprehensive lists of information sources have been published.[1,2] However, the following includes a selection of the more popular, important, evidence-based, or useful resources that may serve the needs of health professionals in clinical practice. We have tried to indicate which resources are especially useful for the clinical practitioner in a busy clinic, office, or hospital practice (who needs quick, practical information), and which are appropriate for the health professional or researcher who is interested in more details of herbal pharmacotherapy. Of course, all prices are subject to change, so check with the publishers.

Books & Monographs

American Herbal Pharmacopoeia and Therapeutic Compendia: These are scientific, 20- to 30-page, evidence-based monographs. Only a handful has been completed to date, with more monographs scheduled to be published each year. Comprehensive and well referenced, they review the herbal and scientific literature and focus on botanical descriptions, chemical constituents, and analytical techniques. The clinical extrapolations are not always appropriate. The individual monographs are comprehensive and informative, but are too detailed for use in an office/clinic setting. (Available for $20 per monograph from the American Herbal Pharmacopoeia, Santa Cruz, CA; tel. 831-461-6335; www.herbal-ahp.org)

American Pharmaceutical Association's Practical Guide to Natural Medicines (Peirce, 1999): This publication reviews popular herbal and other natural supplements for consumers. Although using mostly secondary sources of information, it is well written and competently researched. It balances information from the German Commission E with other sources, and is one of the most commonsensible, balanced books written for consumers. (Available for $35; published by Stonesong Press, New York, NY)

Herbal Medicines: A Guide for Health-Care Professionals (Newall et al, 1996): Includes 141 detailed herbal monographs commissioned by the Royal Pharmaceutical Society of Great Britain. It is a comprehensive source of scientific data, and also summarizes key information from European pharmacopeias. The book contains numerous tables of herbal contents, pharmacologic effects, adverse effects, and interactions. Although concise enough for the clinic/office setting, it is now somewhat outdated, and is more suitable as a reference text. (Available for $60; published by the Pharmaceutical Press, London)

Herbal Medicine: Expanded Commission E Monographs (Blumenthal et al, 2000): This book is an update of a 1998 English translation of the German Commission E monographs, which first introduced U.S. readers to the sophistication of German herbal medicine. Many herbal sources cite these monographs as authoritative standards. The Commission E was an authoritative body appointed by the German equivalent of the U.S. Food and Drug Administration; the Commission published official monographs for over 300 herbal medicines from 1978 until 1994. The original evaluations suffer from the inappropriate extrapolation of pharmacologic data to make clinical claims and from a lack of details, critical analyses, and references, and and many of them have become outdated. The new Expanded Commission E Monographs, written in English, provides 107 selected monographs with revised, updated, and referenced information. It offers detailed discussions on each herb and corrects many of the deficiencies of the original Commission E Monographs. This new book contains concise, well-referenced summaries of the important clinical studies in the worldwide literature, and it collates useful information in appendices. It is useful for more detailed reading, but is less well formatted for clinic/office use. (Available for $50 from the American Botanical Council, Austin, TX; see below)

Mosby's Handbook of Herbs & Natural Supplements (Skidmore-Roth, 2001): This handbook is written by nurses, and provides a well-formatted guide of over 270 natural products. It offers patient-oriented information, but lacks appropriate criticism. It over-relies on secondary sources of information, makes too many inappropriate extrapolations, lacks important references, and is insufficiently discriminating as to the value of each herb. (Available for $33; published by Mosby, a division of Harcourt)

Natural Medicines Comprehensive Database: A clinical resource written primarily by pharmacists, it was first published in 1999 and is available in both book and web site versions. It is well formatted to enable the reader to find clinical information; evaluations of over 1000 herbs and other natural substances concisely summarize the known clinical and scientific data. The contents are not always reliable, however, as much of the original data was extracted from secondary sources of herbal information that were not critically reviewed. The extensive use of equivocating terminology such as "possibly . . . ," "probably . . . ," and "likely . . . ," while often accurate, can be confusing. Daily literature updates and references are added to the web version. It is a practical comprehensive resource for clinic/office use. (Available in book or web version for $92/year from the Editors of the Pharmacist's Letter/Prescriber's Letter; tel. 209-472-2244; www.NaturalDatabase.com)

PDR for Herbal Medicines, 2nd ed. (2000): Unlike other Physician Desk References, this book does not contain package insert information because there are no "official" package inserts for herbs or other dietary supplements. Thus, the information is not necessarily in agreement with manufacturer's claims. It is closely based on the German Commission E Monograph information. The book contains more than 600 herbal evaluations, including many rarely used herbs; the reliability of the information on unusual herbs is questionable. Although the 2nd edition has better-referenced clinical information than the 1st edition, this book is not as well written or as helpful as other resources. It is somewhat useful for the clinic/office. (Available for $60; published by Medical Economics Co., Montvale, NJ, tel. 888-859-8053)

Principles and Practice of Phytotherapy: Modern Herbal Medicine (Mills & Bone, 2000): A 643-page, hardcover textbook that can be considered the herbal equivalent of a combination "Goodman & Gilman" for pharmacology and a "Harrison's" for internal medicine. It is written by two respected scientific herbalists, and synthesizes the best of the scientific herbal literature with the best of the traditional herbal philosophies. The textbook contains detailed scientific evaluations of only 45 specific herbal medicines, but provides comprehensive information on herbal pharmacology, principles of herbal therapy, and dosing, as well as discussions of cultural herbal systems, and much more. It addresses both Asiatic and Western herbs. Although critical and evidence-based, there is a "pro-herb" bias by the authors. This textbook's strengths are the careful explanation of both the art and science of herbal medicine, and the extensive lists of comprehensive references. This text is written for the clinician or researcher who desires to learn about the details of herbal pharmacotherapy; it is not as useful in a busy office/clinic practice. (Available for $72; published by Churchill Livingstone, Edinburgh, Scotland)

Professional's Handbook of Complementary & Alternative Medicines, 2nd ed. (Fetrow and Avila, 2001): Written by clinical pharmacists, this handbook contains summaries of over 300 herbal and other natural products. Monographs are well organized and clinically relevant, and provide reasoned evaluations. The authors note the lack of sufficient clinical evidence for most herbal products. One drawback is the adverse reaction sections, which are not always evidence-based; many of the listed side effects are inappropriately extrapolated from nonclinical data, and may not be clinically applicable. The handbook is useful for office or hospital-based clinicians. (Available for $46; published by Springhouse Corporation, Fort Washington, Pennsylvania)

Rational Phytotherapy: A Physicians' Guide to Herbal Medicine, 4th ed. (Schulz et al, 2001): This is a translation of a well-written German text. It critically reviews and summarizes European scientific and clinical literature, much of which is not available in other sources, for clinicians. The authors are often critical of traditional herbs, and they tend to emphasize herbs and teas that are popular in Germany. It is useful for additional reading and research, but not for clinic/office practice. (Available for $49; published by Springer, Berlin, Germany).

Trease and Evans' Pharmacognosy (Evans, 1996): This textbook of pharmacognosy (the study of natural substances, principally medicinal plants) is an excellent resource for the chemistry and pharmacology of plant-based orthodox and herbal medicines. Suitable for interested researchers, it does not, however, contain clinical information. (Published by WB Saunders, Philadelphia, Pennsylvania)

Several other books deserve mention because they are appropriate for a clinic or office library: Boon & Smith's *The Botanical Pharmacy: The Pharmacology of 47 Common Herbs; Tyler's Honest Herbal;* LaValle's *Natural Therapeutics Pocket Guide; Healthnotes Clinical Essentials; Micromedex-AltMedDex Monographs.* Similarly, for additional research of the scientific literature, here are a gew good resources: *ESCOP Monographs on the Medicinal Uses of Plant Drugs; WHO Monographs on Selected Medicinal Plants;* Leung and Foster's *Encyclopedia of Common Natural Ingredients Used in Foods, Drugs, and Cosmetics.*

Newsletters

Alternative Medicine Alert and *Alternative Therapies in Women's Health:* Monthly newsletters that frequently feature herbal medicines and other dietary supplements, providing practical, evidence-based reviews for health professionals. (Available for $219 and $199 per year respectively, from American Health Consultants; discounts for students/residents; tel. 800-688-2421).

The Review of Natural Products: A loose-leaf binder of monographs on hundreds of herbal and other natural products. A large amount of scientific information is presented, which is well referenced although usually not critically reviewed. Updated monographs are mailed to subscribers monthly. This recently was published as a book. (Subscription is available for $195 from Facts and Comparisons; tel. 800-223-0554)

Web Sites

• *HerbMed (www.herbmed.org):* The Alternative Medicine Foundation's extremely well-organized database provides useful links to Medline articles and other primarily evidence-based sources. Provides a wealth of references on over 100 herbs. Useful for searching the primary medical literature.

• *The Longwood Herbal Task Force (www.mcp.edu/herbal):* Provides comprehensive evidence-based herbal monographs on a limited number of herbs. Each lengthy monograph is extensively referenced with primary literature citations.

• *The Natural Pharmacist (www.tnp.com):* Provides well-written, evidence-based herbal monographs that appropriately review the clinical trials for both consumers and clinicians. Much of the information is adapted from *Clinical Evaluation of Medicinal Herbs and Other Therapeutic Natural Products*, by Bratman and Kroll, published by Prima Health Publishing; it is updated quarterly. The web site is user-friendly, and the information is referenced and concise.

• *ConsumerLab.com (www.Consumerlab.com):* An independent quality-control lab that tests different brands of herbs and supplements. A few brand names that meet their quality criteria are posted on the web site, but details on all the brand names are available for a yearly subscription fee (about 20–30 different brands for each herb or supplement).

Organizations & Associations

The American Botanical Council (ABC): A nonprofit herbal research and educational organization. Although it has a "pro-herb" bias (its mission is to promote herbs), it is a very useful and responsible source of information. Its quarterly journal, HerbalGram, contains relevant news items, scientific herbal reviews, conference reports, business analyses, and literature updates. The ABC also has an extensive book catalog, and is one of the best sources for purchasing herbal reference texts. (Subscriptions to HerbalGram are $29/year; tel. 512-926-4900; www.herbalgram.org)

The Herb Research Foundation (HRF): A nonprofit research and education center similar to the ABC. It offers bibliographic researching services, information on web sites, and other useful links. ($35/year; tel. 303-449-2265; www.herbs.org)

National Center for Complementary and Alternative Medicine (NCCAM): Established in 1998 (previously the Office of Alternative Medicine), this NIH Center sponsors and supports research, education, and dissemination of information about validated complementary and alternative therapies. Does not provide information on individual herbs or supplements, but has useful web-links. (http://nccam.nih.gov)

NIH Office of Dietary Supplements (ODS): Established in 1995, the ODS internet site has a bibliographic database on dietary supplements, consumer fact sheets, and links to other herbal and dietary supplement news and web sites. The ODS also supports academic research on herbs and other dietary supplements. Of limited value for obtaining information on individual herbs, but has useful web-links. (http://dietary-supplements.info.nih.gov)

references

1. Jackson EA, Kanmaz T. An overview of information resources for herbal medicinals and dietary supplements. J Herbal Pharmacotherapy 2001;1:35–61.
2. Miller LG, Hume A, Harris IM, et al. White paper on herbal products. Pharmacotherapy 2000;20:877–891.

Selection of Additional Herbal Medicines[1]

Common Name (Latin name)	Typical Uses or Indications[2]	Special Properties[2]					Approximate Oral Dosing Range of Crude or Dried Herb (g/day)[3]
		Anti-inflammatory	Anti-microbial	Anti-oxidant	Immuno-stimulant		
Agar (*Gelidium amansii*)	laxative						4–32
Agrimony (*Agrimonia eupatoria*)	astringent, stomatitis, diarrhea, diuretic, diabetes	√					3–12 (T)
Alfalfa (*Medicago sativa*)	hypercholesterol, tonic, diuretic, diabetes, phytoestrogen	√			√		1–30
Andrographis (*Andrographis panniculus*)	tonic, colds, urinary infections, dyspepsia	√	√	√	√		2–6
Arnica* (*Arnica montana*)	skin and muscle bruising, stomatitis, varicose veins, colds, bronchitis, pain	√	√				— (T)
Artichoke (*Cynara scolymus*)	choleretic, liver protection, hyper-cholesterol, dyspepsia, diuretic						3–12
Asparagus (*Asparagus officinalis*)	diuretic, bladder disorders, rheumatism						40–60 (T)
Barberry (*Berberis vulgaris*)	diarrhea, fever, cough, biliary disorders, urinary infection, dyspepsia	√	√				1.5–3 (T)
Benzoin (*Styrax benzoin*)	skin and oral lesions, skin protectant, expectorant						— (T)
Bitter melon (*Momordica charantia*)	diabetes, antiviral, cancer		√				—
Blackberry (*Rubus fructicosus*)	diarrhea, stomatitis, sore throat, astringent, diabetes	√					4–20

Herb	Uses			Dose
Bloodroot* (*Sanguinaria canadensis*)	expectorant, antiplaque (dental), skin lesions	✓		— (T)
Blue cohosh (*Caulophyllum thalictroides*)	uterine stimulant, antispasmodic, rheumatism	✓		1–3
Boldo (*Peumus boldus*)	diuretic, choleretic, liver disorders, digestion, sedative		✓	2.5–4.5
Boneset (*Eupatorium perfoliatum*)	fever, diaphoretic	✓	✓	2–6
Bromelain (pineapple enzyme extract) (*Ananas comosus*)	wounds, post-traumatic edema, digestion	✓		0.16–1.5 (T)
Buchu (*Agathosma betulina*)	urinary disinfectant, diuretic	✓		3–6 (T)
Bupleurum (*Bupleurum falcatum*)	post-traumatic edema, colds, liver disease, sedative	✓		1.5–12
Burdock (*Arctium lappa*)	gout, rheumatism, diabetes, skin infections, antipyretic, diuretic	✓		3–18 (T)
Butcher's broom (*Ruscus aculeatus*)	diabetes, diuretic, venous insufficiency, arthritis			—
Butterbur* (*Petasites hybridus*)	spasm, cough, dyspepsia, analgesic	✓	✓	1–7
Calendula (Marigold) (*Calendula officinalis*)	wounds, dermatitis, immune stimulant, dyspepsia, spasmolyyic	✓	✓	2–15 (T)
Cascara sagrada (*Rhamnus purshiana*)	cathartic	✓		0.09–0.36
Celery (*Apium graveolens*)	diuretic, urinary antiseptic, rheumatism, sedative, hypertension, diabetes	✓		0.4–6

(Table continued on next page.)

Selection of Additional Herbal Medicines[1]

Common Name (Latin name)	Typical Uses or Indications[2]	Special Properties[2]				Approximate Oral Dosing Range of Crude or Dried Herb (g/day)[3]
		Anti-inflammatory	Anti-microbial	Anti-oxidant	Immuno-stimulant	
Chaparral (Creosote bush)* (Larrea tridentata)	bronchitis, arthritis, cancer, HIV, cutaneous disorders, snakebite	✓		✓		— (T)
Chicory (Chichorium intybus)	dyspepsia, diuretic, laxative, tonic, sedative					1–5
Chinese cucumber (Tricosanthes kirilowii)	AIDS, cancers, abortant, cough, diabetes		✓		✓	9–20
Cinnamon (Cinnamomum verum)	diarrhea, colds, rheumatism, colic, dyspepsia, dysmenorrhea	✓	✓	✓		0.5–4
Clove (Syzygium aromaticum)	toothache, analgesic, diarrhea, dyspepsia, colic, antiseptic	✓	✓			0.12–0.3 (T)
Codonopsis (Codonopsis pilosula)	adaptogen, fatigue, dyspepsia, HIV, cancer				✓	1–15
Colchicum* (Colchicum autumnale)	gout, arthritis, brucellosis	✓				—
Coleus (Coleus forskolin)	asthma, glaucoma, eczema, hypertension, heart failure	✓				0.25–0.75
Cordyceps (Cordyceps sinensis)	adaptogen, anti-aging, stimulant tonic	✓		✓	✓	3–9
Cowslip (Primula veris)	expectorant, bronchitis, sedative					3–7.5
Damiana (Tumera diffusa)	aphrodisiac, headaches, anxiolytic, depression, hallucinogen					1.2–12

Herb	Uses					Dose
Dandelion (*Taraxacum officinale*)	diuretic, choleretic, dyspepsia, digestion					6–30
Dill (*Anethum graveolens*)	carminative, colic, dyspepsia					3–12
Elecampane (*Inula helenium*)	expectorant, dyspepsia, worms, sedative	✓				4.5–12
Eucalyptus (*Eucalyptus globulus*)	respiratory disorders, congestion and cough, fever	✓				4–12 (T)
Eyebright* (*Euphrasia officinalis*)	conjunctivitis, catarrh, astringent			✓		3–12 (T)
Fennel (*Foeniculum vulgare*)	carminative, spasmolytic, dyspepsia			✓		5–20
Flax (Linseed) (*Linum usitatissimum*)	constipation, irritable bowel, hypercholesterol, hypertension			✓		10–50 (T)
Frankincense (*Boswellia carteri*)	anti-inflammatory, arthritis, colic			✓		—
Garcinia (*Garcinia cambogia*)	anorexiant, diabetes, hypercholesterol			✓		0.25–3 (extract)
Gentian (*Gentiana lutea*)	anorexia, digestion, dyspepsia, sinusitis, tonic					2–6
Glucomannan (extract of *Amorphophallus konjac*)	laxative, hypercholesterol, diabetes, weight loss					3–7 (extract)
Goldenrod (*Solidago spexies*)	diuretic, spasmolytic, wounds			✓		3–20
Grape seed (*Vitis vinifera*)	vascular disorders, cancer prevention, heart disease prevention		✓	✓		0.04–0.3 (extract)
Green tea (*Camellia sinensis*)	digestive, heart disease prevention, hypercholesterol, cancer prevention		✓	✓	✓	— (1–10 cups)

(Table continued on next page.)

selection of additional herbal medicines   453

Selection of Additional Herbal Medicines[1]

Common Name (Latin name)	Typical Uses or Indications[2]	Special Properties[2]					Approximate Oral Dosing Range of Crude or Dried Herb (g/day)[3]
		Anti-inflammatory	Anti-microbial	Anti-oxidant	Immuno-stimulant		
Guar gum (Cyamopsis tetragonoloba)	laxative, diabetes, hypercholesterol, weight loss						3–15
Guarana (Paullinia cupana)	stimulant, anorexiant, diuretic			√			3–6
Guggul (Commiphora mukul)	hypercholesterol, arthritis, weight loss, gingivitis	√	√				3–16
Gymnema (Gurmar) (Gymnema sylvestre)	diabetes, hypercholesterol, acne	√		√			2–4
Hibiscus (Hibiscus sabdariffa)	diuretic, laxative, cardiac disease, skin and mucosal inflammation, colds						— (T)
Hops (Humulus lupulus)	hypnotic, sedative, phytoestrogen	√	√				0.5–2
Horseradish (Shavegrass) (Armoracia rusticana)	arthritis, pharyngitis, bronchitis, urinary disorders, diuretic	√	√				2–20
Horsetail (Equisetum arvense)	diuretic, urinary disorders, bone strengthening, wounds						6–10 (T)
Huperzine A (extract from Chinese club moss)	dementia, memory, myasthenia gravis, arthritis	√		√			50–400 mcg (extract)
Hyssop (Hyssopus officinalis)	expectorant, cough, sedative, antispasmodic, dyspepsia			√			3 (T)
Jimson weed* (Datura stramonium)	asthma, cough, spasmolytic, anticholinergic						0.075–0.225 (T)

Herb	Uses				Dosage (g)
Juniper (*Juniperus communis*)	diuretic, cystitis, dyspepsia, antiseptic, anorexia, rheumatism	√			2–20 (T)
Kelp (*Laminaria* species, others)	goiter, weight loss, respiratory disorders, arthritis, dyspepsia				—
Kudzu (*Pueraria lobata*)	alcoholism, allergy, gastritis			√	9–27
Lavender (*Lavandula angustifolia*)	hypnotic, sedative, neuralgia, astringent, dyspepsia, cancer	√	√		0.8–1.6 (T)
Lily-of-the-Valley* (*Convallaria majalis*)	sedative, cardiac disease, urinary disorders, wounds				0.2–0.6 (T)
Linden (*Tilia* species)	colds, antipyretic, sedative				2–4
Lovage (*Levisticum officinalis*)	urinary infections, stones, diuretic dyspepsia	√			4–8
Marshmallow (*Althaea officinalis*)	cough, expectorant, demulcent, gastritis	√			5–15 (T)
Mastic (*Pistacia lentiscus*)	peptic ulcer, dentistry	√		√	1–2 (T)
Mayapple* (*Podophyllum peltatum*)	liver tonic, warts, cathartic, cancer			√	1.5–3 (T)
Meadowsweet (*Spiraea ulmaria*)	astringent, fevers, rheumatism, colds, bronchitis, dyspepsia	√		√	2.5–25
Mistletoe (*Viscum album*)	hypertension, sedative, cancer	√		√	6–18
Motherwort (*Leonurus cardiaca*)	cardiac disorders, anxiety, neurosis, cramps			√	2–12
Mugwort (*Artemisia vulgaris*)	GI problems, menorrhagia, analgesic, (used in moxibustion)				1–15
Muira puama (*Ptychopetalum* species)	aphrodisiac, rheumatism, performance enhancer				0.25–2

(Table continued on next page.)

selection of additional herbal medicines 455

Selection of Additional Herbal Medicines[1]

Common Name (Latin name)	Typical Uses or Indications[2]	Anti-inflammatory	Anti-microbial	Anti-oxidant	Immuno-stimulant	Approximate Oral Dosing Range of Crude or Dried Herb (g/day)[3]
		Special Properties[2]				
Myrrh (*Commiphora myrrha*)	skin and mucosal inflammation, mouthwash, colds	√	√			0.5–1.3 (T)
Neem (*Azadiracta indica*)	antimicrobial, psoriasis, gastric ulcer, spermicide	√	√			0.5–1.5 (T)
Noni (*Morinda citrifolia*)	heart disease, arthritis, GI upset, diabetes, tonic				√	—
Oats (*Avena sativa*)	anxiety, eczema, hypercholesterol, GI disorders, varicose veins, gargle		√			— (T)
Olive leaf (*Olea europaea*)	viral infections, diabetes, allergies, tonic, hypertension		√		√	4–8
Oregon grape (*Mahonia aquifolium*)	colds, astringent, diarrhea, rheumatism, skin problems	√	√	√		1.5–3 (T)
Pau d'arco (*Tabebuia impetiginosa*)	dysentery, cancer, colds, fungus infections, psoriasis, aphrodisiac		√		√	1.5–3.5
Prickly pear (Nopal) (*Opuntia* species)	diabetes, hypercholesterol, diuretic, prostatic hypertrophy					100–500
Psyllium (*Plantago* species)	laxative, hypercholesterol, diabetes, furuncles					2–30 (T)
Pumpkin seed (*Cucurbita pepo*)	bladder problems, prostatic hypertrophy, antihelminthic, diuretic					10–60
Pycnogenol (extract from *Pinus pinaster* and others)	microcirculation, cancer, anti-aging	√	√	√		0.025–03 (extract)

Herbal medicine	Uses				Dosage (g)
Red rice yeast (*Monascus purpureus*)	hypercholesterol		✓		1.2–2.4
Rosemary (*Rosmarinus officinalis*)	dyspepsia, rheumatism, cancer prevention, circulation	✓	✓		4–10 (T)
Reishi (*Ganoderma lucidum*)	adaptogen, hepatitis, cancer, infections, hypercholesterol, hypertension, fatigue	✓	✓	✓	0.45–15
Rue (*Ruta graveolens*)	spasmolytic, menstrual disorders, uterine stimulant, pain, worms	✓	✓		0.5–1 (T)
Sage (*Salvia officinalis*)	pharyngitis, mucosal inflammation, mouthwash, dyspepsia, sedative	✓	✓		3–12 (T)
Sarsaparilla (*Smilax* species)	psoriasis, rheumatism, diuretic	✓			3–12 (T)
Sassafras* (*Sassafras albidum*)	diuretic, rheumatism, sedative	✓			3–12
Schisandra (*Schisandra chinensis*)	adaptogen, liver prevention, heart protection, HIV		✓	✓	1.5–15
Scotch broom* (*Cytisus scoparius*)	diuretic, hypotension, emetic, anti-arrhythmic, cardioactive				3–8
Scullcap (*Scutellaria* species)	sedative, depression, spasm, seizures, tonic, cancer	✓	✓		2–9
Senega (Snakeroot) (*Polygala senega*)	bronchitis, cough, diabetes			✓	1.5–3
Senna (*Senna alexandria*)	cathartic, skin diseases, liver disorders				0.5–30
Snowdrop* (*Galanthus nivalis*)	dementia, myasthenia, myopathy				—
Sorrel* (*Rumex acetosa*)	GI problems, diuretic, sinusitis	✓			—

(Table continued on next page.)

selection of additional herbal medicines   457

Selection of Additional Herbal Medicines[1]

Common Name (Latin name)	Typical Uses or Indications[2]	Special Properties[2]				Approximate Oral Dosing Range of Crude or Dried Herb (g/day)[3]
		Anti-inflammatory	Anti-microbial	Anti-oxidant	Immuno-stimulant	
Soy (*Glycine max*)	hypercholesterol, liver disease, phytoestrogen, menopause, cancer					20–60 (soy protein)
Squill (*Urginea maritima*)	diuretic, hypertension, cardiac effects, expectorant					0.1–0.75
Stevia (*Stevia rebaudiana*)	sweetener, diabetes, hypertension, weight loss		✓			1–20
Sweet clover (*Melilotus officinalis*)	colic, diarrhea, lymph and venous disorders, bruises	✓			✓	3–30 (T)
Thuja (Cedar) (*Thuja occidentalis*)	diuretic, expectorant, rheumatism, cancer	✓	✓		✓	—
Thyme (*Thymus vulgaris*)	expectorant, spasmolytic, dyspepsia, disinfectant	✓	✓	✓		3–12 (T)
Vervain (*Verbena officinalis*)	purgative, anxiolytic, sedative, colds, analgesic, depression			✓		6–12 (T)
Wild yam (*Dioscorea villosa*)	female vitality, dysmenorrhea, spasmolytic	✓				— (T)
Wintergreen (*Gaultheria procumbens*)	muscle pain, neuralgia, rheumatism	✓				0.2–3 (T)
Witch hazel (*Hamamelis virginiana*)	astringent, bruises, varicosities, hemorrhoids	✓				3–9 (T)
Yellow Dock (*Rumex crispus*)	skin diseases, cathartic, cough, colds, fever	✓	✓			2.5–15

Yerba maté (*Ilex paraguariensis*)	fatigue, headache, stimulant, diuretic	3–12 (T)
Yerba santa (*Eriodictyon californicum*)	expectorant, coughs, bruises, rheumatism, diuretic √	3–15 (T)

Notes

(1) This table is not evidence-based; it is intended primarily as a selected guide to familiarize health professionals with the array of herbal medicines that are used by patients. Herbs listed do not appear in the evaluation section; they include predominantly Western herbs or those used in Western countries. For additional Chinese, Indian, and Mexican herbal medicines, see appropriate chapters.

(2) The typical uses, indications, and properties tabulated here vary considerably in the literature and are not necessarily evidence-based. They are compiled from a variety of herbal publications and textbooks (see references below). Many traditional uses lack scientific or clinical validation.

(3) Doses are in g/day of crude or dried herb, unless otherwise noted. The recommended oral dosages are taken from several sources, and may range widely; specific doses depend on the plant part used (root, leaf, whole herb) and the method of preparation or administration (solid form, tea, etc.). The more variation there is in dosage, the less reliable the herbal benefits are likely to be. Note that many commercial extracts are also available; because each individual product is unique, doses may vary considerably among different formulations and extracts.

— indicates insufficient information or wide variable; (T) indicates that a major use is as a topical skin or mucosal agent

* Oral dosing may cause marked adverse effects or dangerous toxicity, especially in excessive doses.

References

Blumenthal M, Goldberg A, Brinckmann J (eds). Herbal Medicine: Expanded Commission E Monographs. Newton, MA, Integrative Medicine Communications, 2000.
Boon H, Smith M. The Botanical Pharmacy: The Pharmacology of 47 Common Herbs. Kingston, Ontario, Quarry Press, 1999.
DerMarderosian A (ed). The Review of Natural Products. St. Louis, MO, Facts and Comparisons, 2001.
Drug Topics Red Book. Montvale, NJ, MEdical Economics Company, 2000.
Fetrow CW, Avila JR. Professional's Handbook of Complementary & Alternative Medicines. Springhouse, PA, Springhouse Corporation, 1999.
Foster S, Tyler VE. Tyler's Honest Herbal, 4th ed. New York, Haworth Herbal Press, 1999.
Jellin JM (ed). Natural Medicines Comprehensive Database. Stockton, CA, Therapeutics Research Facility, 2001, www.NaturalDatabase.com.
LaValle JB, Krinsky DL, Hawkins EB, et al. Natural Therapeutics Pocket Guide. Hudson, OH, Lexi-Comp Inc, 2000.
Mills S, Bone K. Principles and Practice of Phytotherapy: Modern Herbal Medicine. Edinburgh, UK, Churchill Livingstone, 2000.
Newall CA, Anderson LA, Phillipson JD. Herbal Medicines: A Guide for Health-Care Professionals. London, The Pharmaceutical Press, 1996.
Peirce A. The American Pharmaceutical Association Practical Guide to Natural Medicines. New York, William Morrow and Company Inc, 1999.
www.holisticonline.com

selection of additional herbal medicines   459

Index